The Secret Worlds of Stephen Ward

Sex, Scandal, and Deadly Secrets in the Profumo Affair

Anthony Summers
and Stephen Dorril

headline

This edition first published in 2013 by
HEADLINE PUBLISHING GROUP

1

Cataloguing in Publication Data is available from the British Library

Paperback ISBN 978 1 4722 1664 9

Typeset in Goudy Old Style by Avon DataSet Ltd,
Bidford-on-Avon, Warwickshire

Printed and bound in Great Britain by Clays Ltd, St Ives plc

Headline's policy is to use papers that are natural, renewable and recyclable
products and made from wood grown in sustainable forests. The logging and
manufacturing processes are expected to conform to the environmental
regulations of the country of origin.

HEADLINE PUBLISHING GROUP
An Hachette UK Company
338 Euston Road
London NW1 3BH

www.headline.co.uk
www.hachette.co.uk

Anthony Summers is the award-winning author of eight bestselling non-fiction books. As a BBC journalist, he covered events in the United States and wars in Vietnam and the Middle East for *Panorama*. His most recent book *The Eleventh Day*, co-authored with Robbyn Swan, was a finalist for the 2012 Pulitzer Prize for History. It also won the Crime Writers' Association's Gold Dagger award for best non-fiction. Summers is the only author to have won two Gold Dagger awards for non-fiction.

Stephen Dorril is an acknowledged authority on the activities of the British Security and Intelligence services (MI5 & MI6). He is the author of an acclaimed history of MI6 and has been a consultant and researcher for many television and radio programmes on post-war covert operations. He lectures on investigative journalism at the University of Huddersfield.

Also by Anthony Summers

The Eleventh Day: The Full Story of 9/11 and Osama bin Laden
(with Robbyn Swan)

Sinatra: The Life
(with Robbyn Swan)

The Arrogance of Power: The Secret World of Richard Nixon
(with Robbyn Swan)

Official and Confidential: The Secret Life of J. Edgar Hoover

Goddess: The Secret Lives of Marilyn Monroe

Not in Your Lifetime: The Assassination of JFK

The File on the Tsar
(with Tom Mangold)

Also by Stephen Dorril

Blackshirt: Sir Oswald Mosley and British Fascism

MI6: Fifty Years of Special Operations

The Silent Conspiracy: Inside the Intelligence Services in the 1990s

Smear!: Wilson and the Secret State
(with Robin Ramsay)

'The System's just a story we tell to the people that aren't running it, and they're supposed to just mind their own business and believe it . . .'

George V. Higgins

For Robbyn
      – A.S.

For Guy Debord
      – S.D.

Contents

A Convenient Death

Midnight on Tuesday, 30 July 1963. A man in a white Jaguar, driving through the streets of central London. Fifty-one-years-old and tired, though younger-looking, lean, his hair slicked back behind his ears. He had recently become world-famous – more correctly infamous – but passed unnoticed that night. At about 1 a.m., he turned into a quiet road in fashionable Chelsea.

There, in Mallord Street, the man let himself into an unpretentious flat where a friend had given him refuge. There was coffee and a cigarette – he smoked a lot – and it seems he stretched out on the sofa. That is where the friend found him in the morning, his face purple, hardly breathing, deep in a coma from which he would never recover. Beside him, near the coffee cup and the cigarette stub, lay several letters and an empty bottle of Nembutal sleeping pills.

The man was Dr Stephen Ward. Six months earlier, he had been a man about town, an osteopath by profession who also had a flair for portraiture, virtually unknown to the public. Now he was dying in a firestorm of notoriety. For Ward had become the focus of a crisis that effectively destroyed a British Conservative government and rocked an Establishment already off balance: the sex and espionage scandal remembered as the Profumo Affair.

To the avid millions it entertained at the time, the Affair came over as a series of titillating sideshows around a seamy centrepiece – but one redolent of something darker. The Secretary of State for War, John Profumo, aged forty-six, had had an affair with a nineteen-year-old named Christine Keeler. The very weekend of their meeting, Keeler had also taken up with thirty-seven-year-old Captain Yevgeny Ivanov, nominally a Soviet assistant naval attaché in London but also an officer in Soviet military intelligence, the GRU.

It was as a result of her friendship with Stephen Ward that Christine Keeler became acquainted with British Minister Profumo and the Soviet agent. Ward had befriended her when she was just seventeen and working as a showgirl at a London nightclub. It was he who introduced her to Profumo on 8 July 1961, at the country mansion of a wealthy aristocrat, Lord Astor. The couple met at the mansion's swimming pool, which Ward – who was renting a house on the Astor estate – was allowed to use.

The alarming fact that Keeler had had simultaneous involvements with the British Minister for War and a Soviet spy remained hidden for two years. It emerged only when she began blabbing about it – to the police, to Members of Parliament, to the press and others. Captain Ivanov left London as soon as she did so – presumably for Moscow.

Publicly, the scandal began in earnest in March 1963, when Labour Party Member of Parliament George Wigg, a close confidant of Opposition leader Harold Wilson, asked a question in the House of Commons. Next day, following a dawn conference with high-ranking Conservatives, including the Attorney General and the Solicitor General, Profumo claimed in Parliament, flanked by Prime Minister Macmillan and other Cabinet members, that there had been 'no impropriety' in his relationship with Christine Keeler.

Within a week, Wilson – who headed the Labour Party – wrote to the Prime Minister expressing concern about national security. His memorandum, based on information supplied by Dr Ward, supported Profumo's denial of impropriety while declaring that the Security Service, MI5 – the domestic arm of British intelligence – had been briefed from the start on the fact that Keeler was seeing both Profumo and the Russian. Ward's own friendship with the Soviet spy, he said, had been 'used in the interests of the country'.

The Prime Minister, under pressure, ordered the Lord Chancellor, Britain's senior judge, Lord Dilhorne, to look into the matter. Then, on 4 June, Profumo admitted that he had lied to Parliament about his relations with Christine Keeler and resigned. He was found guilty of contempt of the House of Commons and removed from his post on the Privy Council.

The Minister's personal disgrace aside, the government now took a severe beating in a 'no-confidence' debate on national security. The Prime Minister came under pressure to resign – and would do so four months later, though on the grounds of ill health. Lord Denning, who headed the Court of Appeal, was asked to investigate whether the Profumo episode had endangered national security, and to examine the performance of British intelligence. In autumn 1963, following an inquiry held in secret, Denning reported that there had been no security breach and that British intelligence had been competent. So ended a year-long crisis, the most public shaming endured by a British government in the twentieth century.

Though Stephen Ward had testified to Lord Denning, he did not survive to read the Report, which vilified him in death while being hugely polite to the minister whose sexual folly had triggered the scandal.

* * *

In the spring of the year, as Ward had begun supplying information to the Labour leadership, the police had embarked on an extraordinary probe into his activities. Ostensibly, this was prompted by letters sent to the police, claiming that Dr Ward had been living on the proceeds of prostitution. The letters – said to have been anonymous – have never been produced. It is likely significant that the police pursuit of Ward began within days of a meeting between the Home Secretary, the Commissioner of Police and the head of MI5.

In the weeks that followed, the police conducted interviews with 140 people, all to look for evidence that one man had acted as a pimp. Then, just as the crisis for the government was becoming more serious, Ward was arrested, charged with living on the immoral earnings of three women, of procuring abortions – abortion was still illegal at that time – and of conspiring to keep a brothel.

In mid-July 1963, while the Denning inquiry was under way, Ward went on trial at the Old Bailey on the charges of living on immoral earnings. The trial, which held the attention of the world for ten days, was a mockery of justice. Of two prostitutes called to give evidence, one admitted in court that her initial testimony had been false, and a second later said as much to a reporter. Both claimed the police had persuaded them to give false evidence.

Christine Keeler admitted that she had given money she had received from men to Ward. She said, though, that she gave Ward the cash because she owed him money, and that she usually owed him more than she ever made. Mandy Rice-Davies, an eighteen-year-old who had also been Ward's protégée, said that she had taken money from a wealthy financier with whom she had sex on several occasions, Dr Emil Savundra – he used to leave cash on the dressing table. Rice-Davies also said that, though she occasionally gave Ward money to pay for food, she – like Keeler – had been getting funds from Ward.

Ward was indeed perhaps unusually fascinated by sex, did delight in young women, and ingratiated himself socially by introducing them to affluent male friends with similar tastes. It was nonsense, though, to suggest that this well-paid osteopath and artist had lived on prostitution. Nevertheless, following an aggressive lecture from the judge on the precise letter of the law, the Old Bailey jury found Ward guilty on the charges involving Keeler and Rice-Davies.

Stephen Ward never heard the verdict. By the time it was handed down, he was in hospital on life support, following the barbiturate overdose that was to kill him. A distinguished observer wrote at the time that, 'There were many people in Britain who, on hearing the news, felt a little ashamed, a little diminished . . .'

The writer Henry Fairlie defined the British Establishment as 'A small group of men who use their contacts and influence to put a stop to the things they disapprove of, to promote the reliable, and to preserve the *status quo*.' Though it has been described as being time-hallowed, the Establishment had the odour as much of corruption as of sanctity – as it still does all these years later. It provided the principal villains in the Profumo Affair.

Talking with a friend in his last conscious hours, Ward had said, 'Someone had to be sacrificed, and it was me. One or two people can still vindicate me, but when the Establishment want blood, they get it.'

In the summer of 1963, there was a growing threat that more top names would be tarnished. Allegations considered in these pages suggest that a Cabinet minister offered to resign at the height of the affair, out of concern that the investigation would reveal his relationship with the Duchess of Argyll, the subject of a recent sensational divorce. And then there was the Royal Family.

Ward, as a fine artist, had sketched no fewer than eight members of the Royal Family in 1961. Prince Philip he knew already – they had been acquainted since the late 1940s – and Philip had attended a party given by Ward. Philip's cousin and close friend, David, Marquess of Milford Haven, had cause for fear. Information to be examined in this book indicates that Ward provided women for sex parties given by the Marquess.

During Ward's trial, a London art gallery held an exhibition of his sketches, including those of several members of the Royal Family. No sooner had the exhibition opened than a mysterious emissary arrived and bought up all the royal portraits.

A feature of the Profumo furore, meanwhile, was a story about an orgiastic dinner at which one male guest waited on the others dressed only in a waitress' apron and a black mask. There followed years of speculation as to his identity. The authors report who he was to a virtual certainty – a member, now dead, of a famous aristocratic and political family.

In 1963, then, there was a cause for panic in the ranks of the Establishment. That, though, hardly explains the decision to try Ward on trumped-up charges. There was, after all, a real risk that prosecuting Ward would goad him into exposing those he had imagined to be his friends. Why did those who made the decision take that risk?

Putting the osteopath on trial had the effect of making many matters sub judice, strictly limiting how the scandal could be discussed in the press and even in Parliament. As significantly, publicity about Ward's sexual peccadilloes – dressed up as crimes – created a diversion. Lurid headlines and bedroom revelations titillated as many people as they outraged. It made Ward and his girls, and the sexual capers, rather than John Profumo and the government, the focus of public attention. That was a diversion from the far more important issue – national security.

Harold Wilson was right when he told Parliament, just before Ward's trial: 'What concerns us . . . is whether a man of high trust, privy to the most secret information available to a Government . . . imperilled our national security or created conditions in which a continued risk to our security was allowed to remain . . .' Wilson understood something the authorities preferred the public not to think about – that Minister for War Profumo had laid himself open to blackmail.

It mattered not that he had supposedly terminated his affair with Christine Keeler well before the scandal became public. The very fact of the affair left him vulnerable. Some tried to calm such fears by suggesting that Profumo did not, in any case, have access to much really sensitive material. As we shall show, he did.

Lord Denning's report made light of one specific allegation: that Ward, prompted by Ivanov, had asked Christine Keeler to get information from Profumo on 'when the Americans were going to supply the atomic bomb to Germany'. Put like that, it was a nonsense. There never was any question of giving West Germany 'the bomb'. In 1961, though, there was real Soviet concern as to whether American Sergeant and Crockett weapons systems in West Germany were to be armed with nuclear warheads and, if so, when.

Nevertheless, the possibility of espionage in the Profumo case was not considered in any depth in the Denning Report. Nor were a string of questions concerning the role of British intelligence. According to the Denning Report, MI5 did not learn until early 1963 that Profumo and Keeler had been lovers. In fact, as we shall show, MI5 officers learned of the affair much earlier. What were the security services up to? The answer lies in the title of the first, 1987, edition of this book – *Honeytrap*.

A 'honeytrap', in intelligence parlance, refers to the entrapment of an espionage target through sexual compromise. If there was a honeytrap involved in the Profumo episode, who was hunting whom? The Denning Report considered whether the Soviets had lured the Minister for War into his folly as part of a Soviet plan to sow disunity between Britain and the United States. The British would appear to be unreliable at a very senior level and trust between Washington and London would be eroded. If that was the plan, it succeeded to some extent.

What, though, was Ward's true role? He spent a good deal of time with the Soviet attaché and sometimes aired sympathy for the Soviet Union. During the crisis following the erection of the Berlin Wall, and later during the Cuban Missile Crisis, he acted as an intermediary for Soviet diplomatic initiatives. Was he simply a naïve dupe, the Soviets' messenger boy? Was he a witting traitor? Or did he act on behalf of British intelligence?

The Denning Report did not pursue this last possibility, that this was a British game, and Soviet attaché Ivanov the eventual target. We piece together the way Ward was effectively recruited by MI5, two years before the Profumo scandal, in hopes of softening up Ivanov as a potential defector. For MI5, Profumo's affair with Keeler may have been only an unforeseen hitch in an operation that continued after the affair was over. If so, and not least once the scandal broke, that would have been something British intelligence would have been determined to keep secret. There is also evidence on Ward's Soviet connection that did not surface at the time. We discovered that a second Soviet, a diplomat, was in touch with Ward. His calling card was found in Ward's pocket after his death.

Our research, moreover, located another prostitute, not

identified in 1963, who admitted that Ward sent her British Members of Parliament – and Americans – as clients. This all raised new questions about Ward's true allegiance, and led us into an area that escaped notice in 1963: the American connection.

What was known at the time was that three American airmen based at the US Third Air Force headquarters in Britain were found to have associated with Christine Keeler. They were flown back to the United States, questioned, then returned to duty in England when it was decided there had been no security leak. Much later, with access to US Air Force and FBI files – the Bureau's dossier was code-named 'Bowtie' – it emerged that a fourth airman had had sex with another prostitute Ward knew, at his flat. At Ward's trial, the prostitute first gave false evidence, then admitted she had done so following police pressure, and subsequently fled to the United States.

Another, perhaps the most extraordinary, piece of the puzzle lifts the story into the stratosphere of scandal. According to a combination of official documents and human sources, the Profumo Affair touched the President of the United States, John F. Kennedy.

At least one woman linked to Ward may have met and had sex with Kennedy during the transition between his election in 1960 and inauguration in early 1961. So alleged Mariella Novotny, who, though only eighteen at the time, had travelled to New York to work as a prostitute. We established that she spoke at the time of having dallied with the President-elect – as distinct from merely cooking up a juicy story long afterwards – and we obtained an unpublished memoir in which she described the experience in detail.

We also obtained a mass of US official documents on a young actress called Suzy Chang who attracted intense federal interest at the time of the Profumo scandal. A major American newspaper linked her with 'one of the biggest names in American politics' – on the day in 1963 that the President was in England visiting

Prime Minister Macmillan. Kennedy promptly assigned his brother, Attorney General Robert Kennedy, to mount a ruthless damage-control operation.

As for Mariella Novotny, she had met with Stephen Ward the day before she began the trip to the United States during which she allegedly had sex with John F. Kennedy. Later, she would say that she believed she had been a pawn in a plot designed to compromise him. Her alleged encounter with Kennedy took place – as did all the central events in the Profumo case – at the very height of the Cold War. Just as the British Minister of War was compromised by his mistress' link to a Soviet spy, so too were there efforts to link Novotny, the daughter of a Czech father, with the communist bloc.

At the height of the Profumo furore, Labour Party leader Harold Wilson referred darkly to 'evidence of a sordid underworld network, the extent of which cannot yet be measured'. His chief adviser on the Affair, George Wigg, claimed flatly in Parliament: 'There are three gentlemen actively connected with blackmail on an international scale who got out of London as quickly as they could when they knew that Dr Ward had been arrested.'

Were there really such 'blackmailers'? What really triggered the Profumo scandal? We shall analyse the strange circumstances in which the story broke surface, and the odd way Profumo's lover, Christine Keeler, suddenly began pouring out her tale to anyone who would listen. She did so partly because of one man's personal vendetta against Dr Ward. But was there in 1963 a plot within a plot, one that could have had the effect of harming even the President of the United States?

What is not in doubt is that this was a graver international drama than was understood publicly at the time. A former Deputy Director of the FBI told us: 'This was a time when there was a feeling that we had been deceiving ourselves, that we had felt more secure than we should have done, not least because we depended a great deal on the security capability of the British. And then to find that the President was perhaps involved with somebody involved in the British security scandal. Nobody was grinning . . .'

The involvement of President Kennedy aside, some accounts have claimed the extent of the American ramifications of the scandal was largely inflated by the press, that no national security issues were involved. Documents released to the authors, however, show that the scandal led to a crisis in the security relationship between the United States and Britain. American fears that secret information was making its way to Moscow led to a suspension of cooperation with MI5.

The truth behind the Profumo Affair was very obviously obscured at the time – and has remained so to this day. The authorities deliberately misled the public in many ways. In spite of the passage of time, it is certain that some British intelligence documentation remains closed, or was long ago destroyed. In the United States, the Freedom of Information Act is a fine-sounding law that has been thwarted by obfuscation, censorship and – again – destruction of records.

A measure of the resistance to full disclosure was a 1987 attack on the BBC – made by a group of peers in the House of Lords – for plans it had made, then dropped, to produce a documentary about Stephen Ward. Lord Grimond, former leader of the Liberal Party, said it had been 'extremely irresponsible' for the BBC even to have considered making such a programme. Lord Denning, for his part, deplored the way the BBC had been re-examining past court cases. 'Does not this conduct,' he asked, 'tend to shake people's confidence in the courts and in the police, and is it not therefore to be condemned?'

We live in a time when probing journalism is discouraged in

many ways and for multiple reasons, when newspapers and broadcasters are intimidated as never before. Curbing irresponsible reporting and abuse of press freedoms cannot justify Orwellian strictures. The best reporting, non-fiction books and broadcast programmes have exposed serious government misdemeanours, professional malpractice and miscarriages of justice. Long after all other appeals have been exhausted, living men have walked free and dead men have received posthumous pardons. False history has been corrected. Sometimes, journalism and literature can be the court of last appeal.

Lord Denning declared of the Profumo Affair that he had heard all the evidence and 'was quite satisfied that there was no miscarriage of justice at all'. Yet, in a report of more than a hundred pages, Denning devoted only two paragraphs to the Ward trial. Our investigation suggests that the public never learned the true facts about the Profumo case, and remained woefully uninformed about the role of the British security and intelligence services.

We reached these conclusions by compiling our own dossier, based on many dozens of fresh interviews. Apart from the new American documents, we were permitted – for the first time – to see official transcripts of the Ward trial, a record that had always been denied to researchers. Finally, we obtained a typewritten outline for a memoir Ward himself assembled shortly before he died. Part of it was written by hand in Brixton Prison and taken out in sections by a visiting friend, part was apparently dictated into a tape recorder.

Some of what he claimed may have been self-serving, less than the truth, but it is evident that he was used, then made a scapegoat – while sordid truths about the 'great and the good' were covered up in both Britain and the United States. This book is an effort to open a window on an episode the Establishment preferred kept tightly shut.

CHAPTER I

Learning the Game

'The story must start with Stephen Ward,' Lord Denning was to write at the beginning of his report on the Profumo Affair. There was no reason why his report should start thus. The focus should have been on Minister for War John Profumo. Nevertheless, like Denning, we open our story with Dr Ward.

He was born Stephen Thomas Ward on 19 October 1912, the year the *Titanic* went down. One of those who perished in the shipwreck was millionaire Jacob Astor. His relative, young Bill Astor, one day to become Lord Astor and Ward's patron, was about to start school. John Profumo, the son of a line of Italian aristocrats, would be born three years later. Harold Macmillan, future prime minister, was about to go to Eton, the launch pad for political stardom and marriage to the daughter of a duke. Beside these lucky inheritors of privilege, Stephen Ward's silver spoon seemed somewhat dull.

Stephen was born to Arthur, a Hertfordshire vicar, and his wife Eileen. Reverend Ward, described by his bishop as 'a forthright preacher of fiery sermons and modern ideas', was scholarly and somewhat austere. Eileen Ward enhanced the social clout of the family. She came from the Vigors family of County Carlow in Ireland, landed gentry who had produced a steady stream of clerics, magistrates, High Sheriffs and officers for the British Army.

Later, Stephen Ward would make a point of telling people he was from a 'good' family. He had social aspirations, and his mother supplied excellent credentials. She doted on her boy and thought he was 'brilliant'. There were prayers at Stephen's christening for 'a happy and holy life', and Eileen told a close friend: 'One day my boy will be famous.'

As vicars must, Ward's father moved his family from parish to parish, eventually settling amidst the genteel seaside folk of Torquay. The Reverend Ward's church was St Matthias, still flourishing today. Young Ward had two brothers and twin sisters. He was educated first by a private tutor, then at a private 'prep' school, and finally sent to the empire-building academy of the old British class system, a public school.

Just as Ward was born into a middling-upper-class drawer rather than the one reserved for the crème de la crème, so his public school was – as a luckier acquaintance later sniffed – 'second-rate'. Canford, in Dorset, was for those whose parents wanted their sons in a privileged school, but had to settle for less than the best. Stephen wanted to impress his father. 'I wanted to be good at everything,' he was one day to tell his close friend the journalist Warwick Charlton, 'I wanted to pass exams brilliantly, to be noticed for my fine mind. I also wanted to be good at games.'

It did not happen. In a world of achievers, Ward was not especially good at anything. He was lazy, a bit of a dreamer, but he could not dream his way out of what public-school enthusiasts like to call their 'code'. Forty years later, at the height of the Profumo Affair, Ward told Charlton about an incident in the dormitory at Canford. Someone, not Ward, had hit a boy who was snoring during the night. In the morning, the boy was found unconscious with a fractured skull.

'Someone,' Ward said, 'had to be punished. If no one confessed, then the entire dormitory had to be punished. I knew who it was,

2

but one was not supposed to tell. There would have been great fury if I'd said anything and in any case I was completely indoctrinated. I had a horror of being a sneak. The upshot was I was taken away and thrashed in front of the whole school and I jolly well nearly got the sack, too. Of course, all the other boys thought I was a famous fellow. I'd done the right thing. I hadn't split . . .'

Long afterwards, Ward asked one of his former masters whether he and his colleagues had really believed he was the culprit. 'No,' came the reply, 'but someone had to be whacked. It just happened to be you.' During the Profumo Affair that ancient episode evidently still rankled. 'I suppose they expect me to go along with this stupid public-school convention that good chaps don't tell. Well, I didn't tell once. But not this time. If I'm going down then they're going with me. I promise you that.'

When it came to it, Ward died without splitting on his friends. At one stage he even lied in public to protect John Profumo. Like so many of its victims, he was bound to the public-school code to the end. Good chaps don't tell.

At the age of seventeen, after the dormitory incident, Stephen Ward told his father he wanted to leave school and get a job. 'He was puzzled,' Ward recalled. 'In my father's world young boys simply did not chuck up their schooling and get jobs for which they had no apparent training. Gentlemen's sons didn't behave like that.' In the twenties, gentlemen's sons certainly did not take jobs at the Houndsditch Carpet Warehouse. That is where Ward first worked, and it is here that he takes up his own story – in the memoir he drafted before he died.

'I was paid twenty-seven shillings a week and no overtime,' Ward said of the spell at the warehouse. 'It was rather amusing . . . I spent the day turning over carpets and taking wholesale buyers to various departments. I wasn't there very long, I think the Christmas rush finished me.' Within months, he was off to Germany and a return to something a little closer to a gentleman's existence. Though his German was poor, an uncle found Ward a job as a translator for Shell Oil. He played football for a Hamburg team, joined the local British tennis club, took long weekend trips on the river – and went out with Lieselotte Peters, the Swedish consul's daughter.

Ward's sex life began in Hamburg. He recorded, without elaboration, how he 'explored the extensive night life of the famous Reeperbahn'. The Reeperbahn was then as now Hamburg's brothel district. The job in Germany, he wrote, ended the day 'I imprisoned my very fat boss behind a door and made him yell for mercy. Paris was next on the list.' Ward joined a young friend, Paul Boggis-Rolfe, who was studying in France. Boggis-Rolfe remembered Ward as 'a delightful person, awfully nice', and let him use a bed in his room at a Left Bank pension.

Ward registered for a course on 'Civilisation' at the Sorbonne, but did little studying. He supplemented his allowance by giving English lessons, guiding tourists and working in a nightclub called Chez Florence. The writer John Doxat, 'Britain's foremost thinking drinker', who met Ward in Paris, remembered him as 'an ebullient character, a bit of a laugh. He was doing a stupendous amount of drinking. I was just beginning, he was a past master.'

In later years, Ward drank only moderately. Living in the Latin Quarter, though, he formed some traits that would last. There, he cultivated the easy charm that would later make him popular in London. Ward perfected the insouciant pose, the white shirt, sleeves rolled up to the elbow, the Gauloise cigarette at the lip, the black coffee in hand. He had a gift for portraiture, especially in chalks, and practised a lot in Paris – drawing girls.

Ward took parties of tourists to Le Sphinx, a famous brothel where 'the girls were all naked and danced with the customers'. As he put it later, 'It didn't take me long to find out that people were more interested in real live girls than in the *Mona Lisa*.' As Boggis-Rolfe remembers it, Ward himself showed little interest in actual sex with girls. That was how it would be in the 1950s and early 1960s. He would gather girls around him, draw them, and introduce them to wealthy friends. Many noticed, though, that he had little sexual appetite for them himself.

His friend Boggis-Rolfe would go on to become a soldier, then a member of MI6 during World War II. Ward returned to England in 1932, aged twenty, and breezed into county society and a whirl of hunt balls and parties. His mother at first proved generous with funds, and Ward acquired a red two-seater MG sports car. Then, when he had an affair with a married actress, a former Ziegfeld Follies girl, Ward's mother cut off his allowance. He left home for a while and, for the first and perhaps the only time, fell in love.

The girl was Mary Glover, the beauteous daughter of a local insurance man. She would recall: 'At first I thought Stephen rather arrogant, vain and snobbish, but as time went on I found myself in love with him.' Ward said, 'Mary gave me the confidence that I could accomplish anything I set my heart on.' There was talk of marriage, but Ward had no job and no money. In London, his uncle Edward Vigors, an Examiner of Standing Orders to both Houses of Parliament, decided to intervene. He introduced Ward to Jocelyn Proby, an aristocratic friend then playing a leading role in introducing the British to osteopathy. Proby, who had returned from the United States, where osteopathy originated, suggested Ward go to America to learn the profession. Ward saw that he had to 'make good' for Mary Glover, and agreed.

In the autumn of 1934, Ward found himself aboard the SS *Mauretania*, in third class, watching the towers of Manhattan appear on the horizon. By Greyhound bus, he travelled on to Kirksville College in Missouri, the home of osteopathy, and began medical studies that were to last four years.

Far in the future, during the Profumo Affair, the press would suggest that Ward was a quack doctor who had performed poorly at college. In fact, Ward worked hard and passed his examinations with credits. In the United States, an osteopath had to qualify fully in conventional medicine, and Ward devoured pathology, gynaecology and surgery. Jocelyn Proby said Ward 'could memorise whole paragraphs of *Gray's Anatomy* at one sitting'. In America, the young doctor discovered, there was an ample supply of bodies available for dissection – the corpses of poor black people, purchased from bereaved families for fifty dollars apiece. 'When we did obstetrics,' he recalled, 'we were often taken to remote farms, sometimes in winter over deep snow and on snowshoes. We did surgery on kitchen tables, and deliveries of the most abstruse type, without help.'

Soon came a blow, a letter from home telling Ward that his sweetheart Mary Glover had decided to marry someone else. Ward hurried home to try to stop the marriage, but failed. 'This was my first brush with pain,' he wrote, 'I wondered how anyone could possibly reject me like that . . . I decided that I would never again become so seriously involved with anyone.' He never did have a stable, long-term affair with a woman.

Back in America, Ward threw himself into his studies – and into exploring the continent. He travelled to every state in the Union and to Mexico. He hitchhiked to Florida and survived a bear attack in Wyoming. He went to Hollywood to meet the film star Madeleine Carroll, who was a relative by marriage – the beginning of his fascination with show business. In Chicago, he met the gangster Ralph Capone, Al's brother, and – following a pattern he would keep to in every great city – he made for the red-light district.

Ward like sexual game-playing. He told his friend Warwick Charlton that he had vastly enjoyed the 'petting' ritual then much practised in America: 'You touch the girl's hand. She must make a sign of withdrawal. Never take this seriously. From the hand you move to the lips. You kiss. The lips, of course, are closed. Once you have kissed, then you caress. More expertly, more lingeringly. You may touch the body. But petting must be staggered over a period. There's an art in this sort of stimulation. I found it an exciting emotional experience.'

'Stephen,' Charlton thought, 'refined the art of petting until it became almost a perversion. Consummation was never supremely important to him. A sort of body closeness, a hint of dangerous pleasures to come, a smoothly placed hand, a dextrous slip of silk against skin. These were the delights of Stephen Ward. Pleasure was always to be round the corner. Never to be taken now.'

In 1938, still only twenty-six, Ward brought his medical experience home to England. Dr Stephen Ward, the gifted osteopath, set up a practice in Torquay, close to the clock tower on the Strand. He became sought after for his medical skill, and his social charm soon made him a favourite in the county set. In January 1940, the South Devon Debating Society's records show, he spoke at a debate on 'Modern Sex Problems'. A female acquaintance remembered first hearing about him because 'he had young girls staying in his tent' during a Dartmoor camping holiday. Ward might have remained obscure enough, in the West Country, had World War II not intervened.

As soon as war broke out, Ward volunteered for the Royal Army Medical Corps. He was rejected, for the army did not recognise osteopathy. Conscripted instead into the Armoured Corps, Ward was sent for training at Bovington Camp. Once installed, he got his own way in any case. The colonel in charge of the regiment discovered his talents, and Ward was soon running an unofficial clinic from his very own Nissen hut. This lasted only until the medical officer – whose name was also Ward – objected.

Ward was commissioned and transferred to the Medical Corps. He was banned from practising medicine, however, because he had obtained his qualifications abroad. Ward began a campaign to get the Army to recognise osteopathy.

However naïvely, he believed that an individual could beat the system, that justice would be obtained if he took his case to the very top. It was a notion that would remain with him until scandal burst around him in 1963, when he fired off letters to the Home Secretary and other public figures. As it would fail Ward then, it failed him during the war.

In March 1945, Ward was aboard ship beginning a posting to India. There were compensations – 3,000 young women on a vessel carrying only 300 men. 'The longer it took,' said Ward, 'the happier we were.' In India, and with the war winding down, Ward was in his element. His osteopathic prowess won him friends from exclusive clubs to maharajahs' palaces. When Ward treated Gandhi for a stiff neck, the Indian leader greeted him with: 'It is strange to have a visit from a British officer who has not come to arrest me.' Years later, when Winston Churchill in turn became a patient and was regaled with the Gandhi story, he grunted: 'Pity you didn't twist it [the neck] right off.'

Meanwhile, Ward's tussle with the military bureaucracy had not ceased. With the Army continuing to ignore his qualifications, using him merely to draw anatomical specimens for other medics, he fought to have osteopathy recognised. By the time his military service ended, he had appealed in vain to Churchill, even to the King. Eventually Ward suffered some sort of nervous collapse. According to Dr Ellis Stungo, a psychiatrist who knew him in India and later became a friend in London, he was shipped home in 'an anxiety state'. He returned to England aboard a hospital ship in October 1945. Once home, he recalled, he was permitted off base to go to art classes in Oxford – accompanied by a military policeman. Ward was discharged soon after, the record shows, 'on account of disability'.

Dr Jocelyn Proby, the osteopath who had first encouraged Ward to become a doctor, thought his protégé became seriously disturbed during this period and 'may have attempted suicide'. Psychiatrist Stungo knew of no suicide attempt at that time, but knew from first-hand experience of one a few years later. Ward's was a fragile ego, and his reaction to rejection was always extreme. Dr Proby, who liked Ward and continued to help him, was one of the first to understand the instability behind the smiling charmer that was Ward's front to the world. He remained, he thought, 'utterly irresponsible and emotionally immature, someone who could not settle down and was largely ruled by the impulse of the perverse.'

In 1946, with Proby's help, Ward began to practise as an osteopath in London. He was employed, at first, to practise at the Osteopathic Association's clinic in Dorset Square, tending to clients not wealthy enough to go to a private consultant. The starting salary was ten pounds a week.

Not just because of the humble salary, Ward was not satisfied with his post for long. 'I believe that in medicine, as in all things,' he was to say, 'you finish up as you start. If you want to finish up at the top, you've got to start at the top. Get one or two good patients and, if you're any good, you'll soon be treating nobody but top people.'

The man with the impulse of the perverse was on his way.

CHAPTER 2

The Doctor Goes
to Town

One morning in 1946, a few months after Ward began working in London, the telephone rang at the Dorset Square clinic. Ward, who happened to take the call, found himself talking with an official at the US embassy who was in search of an American-trained osteopath, 'the best in town,' to treat an eminent dignitary.

Ward grabbed the opportunity. 'Our best man is Dr Stephen Ward,' he told the caller. 'I'll get him to phone back.' Soon afterwards, after a pause during which he arranged to borrow a consulting room at a smart Park Lane address, he rang back to fix an appointment. The important patient turned out to be none other than the ambassador himself, Averell Harriman. 'He told me he always visited an osteopath every week,' Ward was to recall. 'It was the only thing that kept him going . . . I decided to let him in on my prank. He thought it was a terrific joke.'

Years later, at the height of the Profumo Affair, Harriman would say he could 'not recall' having been treated by Ward. That, though, was at a time when all Ward's famous acquaintances were running for cover. The man who was serving as ambassador in 1963, David Bruce, accepted – as one of his diary entries shows – that Ward had indeed treated Harriman. Ward always spoke of

Harriman with gratitude. He 'dropped my name in high places,' he said, 'and soon I began to get private patients.'

'He was very clever, very knowledgeable, and he was considered a good and talented osteopath, rightly much sought after,' fellow osteopath William McClurg told the authors – and several other medical colleagues concurred. Soon after treating the ambassador, Ward took over a practice just around the corner from Harley Street, in Cavendish Square. 'Pretty soon,' he later said proudly, 'my patients included King Peter of Yugoslavia, several maharajahs, six members of the Churchill family, Elizabeth Taylor, Ava Gardner, Danny Kaye, Frank Sinatra, Mary Martin, Mel Ferrer and dozens more. My appointment books read like the invitation lists to film premieres.'

Ward treated Winston Churchill – at home – a dozen times. 'He hopped out of bed to get on to my portable treatment table,' he remembered, 'forgetting that he was wearing only the top half of his pyjamas.' Ward and the former prime minister seem to have got on well: they discussed their mutual interest in painting, and Churchill showed Ward some of his canvases. Ward had been recommended, he said, by his daughter Diana.

Ward lived in a large first-floor flat above his consulting rooms. It became open house for his friends, who included a bevy of young women. One was Eunice Bailey, a redhead from Bexleyheath who became Ward's second real love. She broke it off, though, and went on to marry the son of Sir Harry Oakes, the millionaire victim in a famous Caribbean murder case. The rejection was a shattering blow and, probably for the second time, he attempted suicide.

Ward took a barbiturate overdose, to be rescued by the psychiatrist Dr Ellis Stungo, the friend he by now called 'Pops'. Stungo administered a lifesaving injection, and Ward woke up in the Middlesex Hospital. The psychiatrist thought the overdose had been more a cry for help than a serious attempt to kill himself.

In the summer of 1949, when he was thirty-six, Ward did get married – to a twenty-one-year-old model and former beauty queen named Patricia Baines. This was a calculated decision. 'I decided at the very first meeting that I wanted her,' Ward later reminisced. 'I worked it out quite calmly. She would grace the practice. She would be useful. She was also desirable.' The new wife, according to a friend, bore an astonishing physical resemblance to Ward himself.

There were rows even on the honeymoon in Paris, and it was an unhappy couple who headed back for England on the boat train. The marriage was over, bar the legalities, within six weeks. 'I was desperately unhappy with him,' the former Mrs Ward recalled years later. 'He was virtually a stranger to me, and he was a very unhappy man. But he did have a lot of charm. I think basically he was in conflict with himself most of the time . . . I was left at home while Stephen was out socialising.' Ward, for his part, maintained that, 'She was always wanting things, and pretty soon I couldn't stand the sight of her. Soon she had divorced me on the grounds of adultery, which wasn't difficult.'

Michael Eddowes, a wealthy former solicitor who met Ward at this time and will later play a role in this story, offered a hilarious and revealing anecdote on the marriage episode. 'Ward,' said Eddowes, 'always had a penchant for streetwalkers. He was always disappearing from the flat where they lived, for a couple of hours at a time, and Pat didn't know what he was up to. One evening she decided to find out and hid in the back of the car – the boot opened into a sort of jump seat. When the car stopped she jumped out, to find Ward chatting up a prostitute!'

The sad end of the tale came from the actor Jon Pertwee, who later starred as Dr Who in the famous television series, and was a loyal friend from the 1940s until Ward's death in 1963. Ward's enraged wife, he related, 'came out over the back of the car like an avenging angel, and practically gave Stephen a heart attack. The poor prostitute fled in a state of terror, and fire and brimstone was poured on his head.'

Ward had always patronised prostitutes. Now, in London, whores served as a regular diversion. Michael Eddowes recalled visiting Ward at his flat one evening when several men were drinking there. 'Ward disappeared out,' he said, 'and returned thirty minutes later with a couple of real tarts. He put one in the consulting room and one in the bedroom, then disappeared into the consulting room and came out a few minutes later, laughing and doing up his flies. He then went into the bedroom and, presumably, had the other one too.'

The prosecuting counsel at Ward's trial in 1963 was to call him 'a thoroughly immoral man'. Tens of thousands of men, then as now, in fact regularly seek sex for hire. Prominent amongst them, not least because they could afford it, were the well-heeled upper-class customers seen ducking out of red-lit doorways from Mayfair to Soho every day. It was the exposure of the carnal antics of some of those customers that would lead to Ward's eventual ruin. What set him apart from the rest was his dedication to the sport of sex, his resourcefulness in always having a girl on hand – whether pretty protégée or professional whore. It was a facility that made him the toast of hundreds of well-placed London males.

'I suppose I have been one of the most successful men in London with girls since the war,' Ward wrote with relish in his draft memoir. 'I am the proof that you don't have to be handsome or rich to get the best girls. My technique has been never to force them. Just be gentle, interested, and they come . . .' That was his boast, but – friends noticed increasingly, especially after his second rejection in love – actual intercourse was not a priority. 'I don't think he was interested in sex per se,' said Jon Pertwee.

'He was fascinated by women, fascinated by sex, but not particularly by the act. One of his girlfriends complained rather bitterly that he treated her like a piece of wood . . .'

From now on, though he shared affection with some women, most became commodities. Many were prostitutes, or close to it. 'He was what we call passively aggressive,' said Dr Stungo, 'like a spoilt child who gets his way, in Ward's case thanks to his charm . . . without regard to convention, propriety or suitability.' Dr Stungo, who was well versed on the sex habits of the famous – one of his patients was Errol Flynn, another Judy Garland – thought Ward something of a voyeur, a penchant he did not try to hide. He had a fixation, especially, about legs, loved to have a girl pose in underwear, stockings and suspenders, and high-heeled shoes – showing them off.

Ward, himself a keen photographer, accumulated a large collection of photographs, some just 'girlie' pictures, some blatantly pornographic. While the pornographic ones generally showed straightforward intercourse, Stungo remembered a set of pictures depicting a girl grinding a stiletto-shod heel into a young man's penis. Those pictures excited Ward. Another friend, antiques dealer Hod Dibben, recalled that – at parties – Ward 'liked to have a high-heeled shoe tied around his nose'. The psychiatrists' interpretation is that an individual evincing such behaviour gradually becomes more attached to the idea of sex – as expressed in the pictures – than to the reality of his or her partner. The longer Ward indulged, the less he was interested in real live women, the more intense his liking for the bizarre.

The easiest way to satisfy such a need is by using prostitutes, which is not to say that Ward treated them badly. He enjoyed the company of whores and befriended many. Should he see a loitering street prostitute being hustled by the police, Stungo recalled, he would rush up with an 'I'm sorry I'm late, dear' to get the woman out of trouble. He became, too, something of a connoisseur. 'Stephen had a fascination for prostitutes,' said Pertwee. 'He used to pick them up and talk to them. He used to drive around the park in his car, pick up a girl and sit her in his car, smoke a cigarette and talk to her . . . find out why she did it and all that sort of thing. He was fascinated by the subject.'

Warwick Charlton, a journalist and former army major who served under General Montgomery and Lord Mountbatten – and much later authored an insightful book on the Profumo Affair – was a major source for this book. His role was probably especially significant because – as these pages will reveal – he probably worked with MI6. Ward trusted Charlton as a friend, and shared intimate thoughts with him about sex.

The osteopath, who dabbled in psychiatry himself, said he respected prostitutes who provided top service. 'They knew, more than any psychologist, what was needed by certain types of men,' he told Charlton. 'These girls accepted sex as sex. To them it was a job. Whippings, beatings, the lot – what did it matter to them? I really believe they felt they were performing just as good and necessary a service as a doctor. Perhaps, indeed, they were.'

The Cavendish Square apartment, with its spacious old-world rooms, became the venue for much partying, often impromptu. The osteopath Jocelyn Proby was one night woken at 3 a.m. by Ward erupting into the flat with a bevy of girls from the Windmill Theatre – in those days still the nude revue that boasted 'We Never Closed', or, as the wits had it, 'We Never Clothed'.

Though Ward's income was now far better, he was usually broke. Guests at his parties brought their own bottles. He – who never used hard liquor – supplied the glasses and perhaps tonic for the gin. Dr Stungo remembered the moment the bill came one night when he and Ward were dining at the RAC Club with two female companions – Joan Collins, future star of the soap opera

Dynasty, and her sister Jackie, later to become a best-selling author of sexually charged novels. Stungo had to pay, as Ward had left his wallet at home.

Dr Stungo hastened to say that Ward was not a sponger – just not well off enough to 'stand his whack' in the wealthy milieu he cultivated. A journalist friend, Frederic Mullally, put it down to the young osteopath's 'heavy overheads, and a chronic reluctance to have the thrill of the chase constrained by excessive hours working over obese matrons' vertebrae'. For all his tailored suits and fast cars, Ward quickly became known as one of the tightest men in town.

'Ward's objective was esteem,' said Stungo. 'He wanted to impress his acquaintances and be accepted in society.' Thanks to the combination of osteopathic and artistic skills, Ward soon had both distinguished and raffish friends. One of the latter was the portrait artist Vasco Lazzolo, who had met Ward at the end of the war in Oxford, when Lazzolo was attending the Slade School of Art. 'Latin' Lazzolo became a society artist, following years spent working as a commercial artist in Soho, when one of his mistresses married into the aristocracy. He shared many of Ward's characteristics – not least the predilection for young women and prostitutes, and for the world of show business.

Ward was often called to the Hippodrome Theatre, off Leicester Square, to look after the dancers' pulled muscles. Michael Bentine of *The Goon Show* fame, who had heard of Ward's reputation as 'the best physio in town' and met him at the Hippodrome, remembered him as 'a very handsome man, with his black hair combed back very tightly, and smelling eternally of aftershave. He was a charming person, a very good conversationalist and witty.'

Lazzolo aside, Ward's two other closest friends were top-flight portrait photographers. There was Anthony Beauchamp (born

Entwhistle), who married Sir Winston Churchill's actress daughter Sarah. 'Like me,' Ward said of him, 'he knew no barriers of class in his relationships with men and women. He took his friends from all walks of life.' Beauchamp's wife Sarah remembered, rather, his 'wild, insubstantial infidelities'.

The other photographer in Ward's life, the one with by far the greatest influence, was Sterling Henry Nahum, born in England into an Italian-Jewish family, and known to all by his professional name, 'Baron'. After the war, Baron, who used a studio above Lazzolo's in Belgravia and concentrated on photographing 'society', rose, with the support of Lord Louis Mountbatten, to become photographer to the Royal Family. For a photographer, there was nowhere higher to fly in the social galaxy.

Stephen Ward went out of his way to cultivate Baron and became a regular visitor to his unpretentious flat in Brick Street, off Piccadilly. 'I knew he was on the way up,' Ward would recall. 'Everyone seemed to know him, and I felt I had a certain rapport with him.' One reason Ward knew Baron was on the way up was the identity of two of the photographer's close friends – Battenberg cousins David, Marquess of Milford Haven, and Prince Philip of Greece, as of 1947 Duke of Edinburgh and husband to the future Queen Elizabeth.

Twenty-five-year-old Prince Philip, in London after the war and staying at the Belgravia home of his uncle and mentor Louis Mountbatten, had renewed a childhood friendship with the Marquess of Milford Haven. Cruising around town in Philip's red MG sports car, the two young men were sowing their wild oats. It was while they were doing so, in 1946, that Baron and *Tatler* editor Sean Fielding dreamed up the Thursday Club, named for the day of the week on which – for years afterwards – select members would convene for lunch in a private upstairs room at Wheeler's Oyster Bar in Soho's Old Compton Street.

The idea was 'to lighten the gloom that surrounded us all', an aspiration expressed by the weekly treat the men gave themselves. Their weekly meal usually featured oysters and lobster claws washed down with copious quantities of champagne and Guinness. The membership reportedly included Prince Philip, the Marquess of Milford Haven, and Iain Macleod, a future Conservative Member of Parliament who by the time of the Profumo Affair would be Leader of the House of Commons. Other members were artists Vasco Lazzolo and Felix Topolski, Baron's barrister brother Jack, *Tatler* illustrator Pip Youngman Carter, *Daily Express* editor Arthur Christiansen – he drank champagne out of one of his shoes at one Thursday gathering – *New York Post* correspondent Sam Boal, and actors Peter Ustinov, James Robertson Justice and Michael Trubshawe, broadcaster Gilbert Harding, and Larry Adler, the harmonica player. Knightsbridge solicitor Michael Eddowes, who was also a member, would play an interesting role during the Profumo scandal.

Stephen Ward, though not a full-time member of the Thursday Club, was a frequent guest and associate of most of those who were. Felix Topolski remembered airily that Ward was 'always around. I had a drawing of Ward having intercourse with a woman.'

The club was a strictly male affair, its 'lunches' – more accurately described as booze-ups that often lasted into the evening – were occasions for holding forth with stories that tended to be long, funny and, more often than not, bawdy. Baron was a celebrated raconteur, but a club rule dictated that he never be allowed to finish a story. Members honoured the man who had made the biggest fool of himself in recent weeks with the title 'Cunt of the Month'.

Ward's friend Anthony Beauchamp was initially keeper of the club records, a set of visitors' books filled with the bon mots, yarns and caricatures that kept the membership in belly laughs. According to Fleet Street artist member Tony Wyzard, the books were 'very near the knuckle. Whatever the main topic of conversation, the scandals of the day and so on, people would write relevant verse and I would provide the illustrations. Not for publication, as you can imagine!'

Stories about Prince Philip did the rounds. 'We all heard about them, of course,' said club member Larry Adler, 'but we never discussed them. We didn't want to embarrass Philip.' According to Adler, the Thursday Club gatherings continued in the 1950s – and the Prince, accompanied sometimes by his private secretary and old Royal Navy chum Mike Parker, would on occasion attend. This, of course, was long after his marriage to the future Queen.

The gossip columns regularly mentioned the parties held by Baron at his Piccadilly flat, but other bacchanalia went unreported. Vasco Lazzolo was to recall wild affairs, some attended by 'girls dressed only in Masonic aprons'. Ward was a regular at the Baron parties.

Prince Philip was on the organising committee of the Thursday Club and a regular dinner guest at Baron's flat. In 1948, backstage at the Hippodrome Theatre, he was introduced by Baron to Pat Kirkwood, then a leading singer and actress. Kirkwood had emerged from a failed marriage to a theatrical manager and – reportedly – affairs with actor and comedian Danny Kaye and with the actor Peter Lawford, later the brother-in-law of John F. Kennedy. Kennedy's name, as other chapters will show, is also entangled in the Profumo Affair.

Michael Bentine described the actress to the authors as 'a gorgeous, uninhibited Northern lass'. Baron was in love with her, but his love was unrequited. It was with Prince Philip that she danced the night away the night they met – and with whom she breakfasted at dawn. This made the newspapers and – married

19

as Philip was to his daughter – King George VI is said to have been 'incandescent with fury'. The rumours about Pat Kirkwood persisted until her death in 2007.

After the Queen's Coronation in 1953, there would be whispers about the wild goings-on of Philip's Thursday Club pals. Stephen Ward had met Philip in the 1940s, and the Prince attended one, possibly two, of the parties thrown by Ward at the flat in Cavendish Square. In his memoir, Ward drily mentions Philip's appearance at one of the parties 'with a very attractive girl called Mitzi Taylor' – a Canadian model whom Baron had photographed. Dr Stungo recalled having met Prince Philip at Ward's place on a couple of occasions. The lawyer Michael Eddowes also remembered Philip having been present – the Prince had danced with Eddowes' wife.

Ward liked to say he knew Prince Philip, but sneered a little while expounding to Warwick Charlton about high society: 'I've always found [Philip's jokes] schoolboyish,' he said, 'I don't see much fun in turning hoses on photographers and that sort of thing. You see, the superior person should never do that. It is part of the rules that only small fry may take liberties, and balancing the degree of liberty and daring is the whole art of the business. Usually the big people know this and play up to the people who do it cleverly. Philip wants to hold the stage himself. He acts like a little person when in fact he should try to be a big person . . .'

CHAPTER 3

The Rakes and the Royals

Philip's cousin David, Marquess of Milford Haven, knew Ward very well. The Marquess cut a lurid path through society in the 1940s and 1950s, and his closeness to Prince Philip caused anxiety at Buckingham Palace. It was the Marquess who once, at an open-air luncheon at Les Ambassadeurs on Park Lane, gave Ward the sort of opportunity he coveted to 'make a breakthrough' in society.

'I knew,' Ward was to say, 'that one could never afford not to be noticed at these events . . . How to be bright and yet not put one's foot in it? That was the problem. David was talking about shaving. I remember he thought shaving a bit of a bore, and to demonstrate the point he fingered a small cut on his chin. He said he had cut it that very morning. Suddenly I said, without thinking, "Well, what are you worrying about – wasn't it blue?" Everyone though it was very funny, and even David smiled. So that was it, I told myself. The moment. The moment when everyone laughs at something you said . . . You will certainly be remembered as the man who dared to say something daring to someone like Milford Haven.'

From the Royal Family's point of view, the Marquess was thoughtless enough in 1950 to become married for a time to an American divorcee named, as the Duchess of Windsor had been, Mrs Simpson. When the marriage ended, he began a liaison with the Hungarian actress Eva Bartok, who later wrote that she did not wish 'to belong to those who misuse sex'. She hoped, now, to marry a man who 'is not guilty of the frightful sin of having lost his birthright, his title – the only title I respect – a human being. Someone who is not an empty shell in a human shape . . .'

In the mid-fifties, ordinary cocktail parties aside, Milford Haven hosted sex parties for carefully chosen male guests at his flat at 35–37 Grosvenor Square in Mayfair. The evening would begin with card playing and then, when the drink had flowed, young women would be brought in. From that point on, the betting would be for the women, in games with names like 'Chase the Bitch' and 'Find the Lady'. For the winners, the prize was sex in one of the luxurious bedrooms. Brian McConnell, a reporter for the *People* newspaper who investigated the stories, learned that some of the women involved were brought to the flat by Stephen Ward.

Ward's confidant Warwick Charlton gave the authors the names of prominent people who, he said, attended other early parties. He claimed that Prince Philip, lawyer William Rees-Davies – who served as a Conservative MP for twenty years – artist Vasco Lazzolo, photographer Baron and – much later – singer Bing Crosby were all in Milford Haven's social set.

The Marquess and Stephen Ward both had a keen interest in pornography, and the Marquess had inherited one of the largest private collections of pornography in the world. He owned a multitude of books as well as seven albums of erotica, some embossed with the Milford Haven family crest. Shortly before the Profumo scandal broke, and on hearing that his name would crop up, the Marquess would order that the family porn be destroyed. His chauffeur, to whom the task was assigned, instead sold some of the material to the antiquarian bookseller Louis Bondy. A good deal of it – including some donated by one of

Stephen Ward's friends – made its way to the Private Case of the British Museum. Two of the Marquess' albums were acquired by the University of Texas.

Album 7, which reached the British Museum, was described by former curator Dr Eric Dingwall as 'Leaflets, booklets . . . advertising dirty books, tickler condoms, dildoes, photographs and so on.'

Police raided the homes of several of Ward's friends at the height of the Profumo Affair. One target was wealthy American expatriate Beecher Moore, who later said he was told his wife might be charged with running a call-girl racket. There was no foundation to such a charge, but Moore himself was known to be a collector of erotica – he owned thousands of paperback books – and commissioned a great deal of pornographic art. One artist, Tom Poulton, supplied hundreds of sketches on sexual themes – lesbian sex between naval personnel, adulterous couples caught in the act, and orgies. The detail in the sketches suggests that many of them were drawn from life, and it may be significant that Poulton knew Ward.

Beecher Moore, fearing arrest, donated his erotica, too, to the British Museum. Some went to the Kinsey Institute in the United States.

The police also descended on the premises of Vasco Lazzolo, whose collection included pornographic photographs of himself and photographer friends, some featuring sadomasochism, some of young men. The detectives did not find them, he explained later, because he was keeping them elsewhere. 'It wouldn't look good,' he remembered the police telling him, 'if the man who was painting Prince Philip had anything to do with a scandal.'

Lazzolo, who had previously painted the Queen, had – at the time the Profumo scandal broke – been commissioned to paint Prince Philip. This despite an earlier occasion when he and the Marquess of Milford Haven had visited the French Riviera. When Lazzolo suggested he and the Marquess come aboard the Royal Yacht, which was anchored offshore, Prince Philip is said to have snorted, 'Not him! I've got enough problems already.'

In 1986, during preparation of the first edition of this book, a complex sequence of telephone conversations led to a meeting at Liverpool Street Station with a 'Mr Melton'. Melton, who satisfied us that the material he had was the genuine article, showed us many photographs from Ward's own pornography collection. Female associates of Ward were clearly identifiable in some of the pictures – a few of the photographs, somewhat altered for publication, feature in the illustration section of this book.

Baron, the man who had given Ward his entrée to high society, died in 1956. His death and the suicide soon afterwards of playboy photographer Anthony Beauchamp shook the osteopath. Ward had himself long been exploring the notion of holding sex parties – and seeking out women who would join in – in effect, laying the foundations for the disasters of 1963. His own introduction to orgies, he said, had been:

. . . a rather amateurish affair in Hampstead. There was abandon all right, and the sight of naked bodies all over the room . . . It was at this gathering that I met for the first time one of the more determined organisers of these parties in London. I was standing rather bemused when he came up to me and said, 'If you are surprised at this, come round to my flat one day and be really amazed.' This was temptation and I went.

The only excuse I can make is that I really was curious in a sort of detached way. I would be a humbug if I did not confess that I looked forward to it too. There was the start of one of the strangest experiences of my life . . . Looking back, one sees how easy it is to be drawn into a situation out of simply weakness, to be horrified to start with and later to accept it all as normal behaviour or nearly so.

These parties nearly all started in the same way, a few drinks, rather formal introductions, and one or other of the girls would start the ball rolling . . . It was always the girls that seemed most eager – usually one would offer to do a striptease or a belly dance. That was enough. Someone would then suggest what was called 'costumation', which was dressing up in a scanty loincloth, a pretence of fancy dress but in reality a 'clearing of the decks for action'.

One could go to a party like this on Saturday, go home and come back to the same scene on Monday with very few of the personnel changed. How was it achieved? I found out at about the third one I went to. I came across the host grinding up pills in a bowl which he put into everything we drank, whether it was gin, whisky, or just coffee. Benzedrine or Methedrine was used . . .

At one Belgravia party, given by the same man Ward had met in Hampstead, the telephone ceased working just when the host wanted to use it to summon more partygoers. Evidently no longer thinking straight, he tossed a message out of the window requesting the passer-by who might pick it up to call the phone engineers. The bizarre message was indeed picked up – by someone who called the police. On arriving at the door, however, the officers were confronted by a naked woman who said their services were not needed. 'It's girls we want,' she snapped, 'not men.'

'The people involved,' Ward wrote of the parties in his draft memoir, 'never forced any situation . . . The married couples were invariably happy and contented. Possibly this open infidelity prevented anything being hidden and consequently removed one of the biggest obstacles to happy marriage normally encountered

. . . I have never known a couple involved to split up or go off with anyone else. Curious but true . . . I have seen well-known psychiatrists at these parties . . . The other thing, of course, was that a lot of the people were not sexually normal, and such parties allowed them to indulge in anything their mood dictated.'

Ward's artist friend Lazzolo often held sex parties. One of those who attended was an Austrian named Clement von Frankenstein – that really was his name – the tenant of the upper floor of Lazzolo's studio. 'The first two hours,' von Frankenstein recalled, 'were very much like any other social gathering, with well-dressed couples meeting, conversing, and getting to know each another. Yet one knew that most of the women were wearing stockings, garter belts and expensive lingerie under their fashionable cocktail dresses – always arousing to an Englishman – and that if you met someone you were attracted to and you played your cards right, within an hour you would be naked and making passionate love along with at least two-thirds of the other guests. It was the metamorphosis that was the greatest aphrodisiac.'

Once a week, Lazzolo's wife Leila permitted him to enjoy a prostitute whose specialty was sadomasochism. He did so while inhaling crushed ampoules of amyl nitrate, the chemical said to heighten the sexual experience. It was a kink he may have picked up from a friend, antiques dealer Horace 'Hod' Dibben. Ward would write, without naming names, of parties devoted to masochism and sadism, including one that Dibben organised:

I remember one dinner party where all round the room were girls and men tied and gagged in various attitudes and they so remained during the entire meal. Suffering was an essential part of their enjoyment. No cruelty was done – I myself never saw any cruelty, though I certainly heard of it being practised.

It is a kind of ritual sadomasochism . . . One of the most noticeable things about these people is the high standard of intelligence among them . . . rather like an intellectual cocktail party. The ceremonies usually started as follows – a large collection of chairs, straps and apparently fierce instruments would be produced and laid out in a formal manner on a low table. A beautiful girl would step forward and remove her clothes. The master, as he was called, would sit on a kind of throne. The girl would kneel before him and kiss his feet . . . she would be dressed in a wide, studded black leather belt, high-heeled black shoes and straps around her wrists, neck and ankles . . . A ritual punishment was administered. Finally, long bars were fastened to hooks in the straps . . . in such a way that the legs were widely separated . . . and a gag was placed in her mouth.

Drinks would now be brought and the secured girl would be left lying or standing while the guests stood around discussing the finer points . . . When this was over everyone looked normal again . . . There we were back at a normal cocktail party again.

Ward also described satanic rituals – he had a fascination with black magic, according to Michael Bentine. 'At one such party in Kensington, there was a huge and obscene priapic emblem in the middle of the room. All the girls, and there were about a dozen, knelt down round it and made obeisance . . . the spontaneous way in which it was done made me realise they had all done it many times before . . .'

According to Ward, the participants at such sessions were 'quite normal' individuals. 'Of necessity, most of them are attractive . . . The men tend to be older than the girls, who are nearly all very beautiful . . . Many of them are rich and many famous – many faces that are seen in public life and on television. If their public could only see them like this!'

'The two lives of Stephen Ward gave him knowledge of many secrets,' said his friend Warwick Charlton. 'For many highly placed men shared his sexual likings . . . He participated in the pleasures of his circle and that circle was suitably wide . . . He gained confidences from his patients in his consulting room . . . If a few patients had their sexual needs attended to . . . by way of a few little parties and introductions, well, that was life, wasn't it?'

CHAPTER 4

Pygmalion and the Popsies

In 1963 Ward would be dubbed a Pygmalion, a label he was assigned because the musical *My Fair Lady*, based on George Bernard Shaw's play *Pygmalion*, had been running in London for several years. In the ancient Greek myth, Pygmalion was a sculptor who carved a statue of a maiden, then fell in love with his own creation. Ward no longer fell in love with his discoveries, and his relationships did not necessarily include sex. He continued to have affectionate friendships with many women. One of them, whom he encountered before she turned twenty, ended up a countess.

This was Maureen Swanson, a young actress fresh from a break as a dancer in the musical *Carousel*. They met through the *Daily Express*' Logan Gourlay, who asked Ward to do a sketch of Swanson to accompany the interview he was doing. Her future husband, the 4th Earl of Dudley, later said, 'I think their friendship lasted about a year . . . but she realised he was bad news.' Ward described their friendship as 'one long battle . . . Our quarrels were spectacular and occurred all over London . . . She could either have been a ballet star, or the chatelaine of a great house, and happy with children.'

When her husband inherited the title, Swanson became Lady Dudley. The couple had seven children. The 4th Earl's late father had been close to the family of Ward's friend and patron Lord Astor. Swanson and Ward continued to see each other following the marriage, as the author John Grigg once observed at lunch with the noble couple. Ward, he wrote, was 'needling Maureen Swanson throughout, saying, "You were nothing. I absolutely created you, you couldn't act at all!" She was fighting back, saying, "Well. You're no artist . . ."'

For all the bickering, they stayed in touch. When Maureen gave birth to a stillborn son, they asked Ward to sketch the dead baby before the funeral.

The young women around Ward were physically of a pattern, ample-bosomed – the Profumo Affair's Mandy Rice-Davies was an exception – and long-legged. They were usually lower-middle or working class. Ward would coach them in how to speak and eat correctly, and how to improve their sexual technique. Proper diction was important, for Ward wanted his young females to be acceptable to London society. Like Professor Higgins, he helped them iron out their working-class accents.

Young woman after young woman came off the Ward production line, painted human statues fashioned in coffee-bar conversations and late-night drives. Ward's journalist friend Frederic Mullally recalled 'a constant self-renewing flow of them, passing through that benevolently bogus *ashram* in Devonshire Street* . . . Most, when they took shelter there, were nonentities. At a personal count – and I was too often away from England to know the true score – three of them went on to titled marriages, in England or on the Continent, five to international fame as actresses or top models, and four found sterling millionaire or dollar millionaire husbands . . .'

---

* Ward moved his practice from Cavendish Square to Devonshire Street.

The prototype, around 1952, had been a woman who used the name Vicki Martin. Ward had picked her up on the street – the easiest place to find a girl in London in those days. 'I met Vicki in a shower of rain at Marble Arch,' he recalled. 'Blonde, with large eyes set wide apart, and with probably the most exquisite smile you have ever seen, revealing perfect teeth. I used to try to keep her laughing just to see it . . .' Ward hailed a taxi, took Martin back to his flat, dried her hair by the fire, and dressed her – in clothes that had belonged to his ex-wife. Years after her departure, he had not got rid of them.

Martin's real name was Valerie Mewes, the product of a broken home in Staines, Middlesex. She had left school at fourteen and tried nursing before being diverted by dreams of becoming a film star. At seventeen, she found work as a hostess at Mayfair's Court Club, in Duke Street. The club was not only a fashionable night-spot but also a brothel. The male clientele was a mix of the English upper class and racketeers, and the owner, dubbed the 'monster with the Mayfair touch', expected his female staff to have sex with the customers. Ruth Ellis, fated to die on the hangman's rope, was a hostess at the Club and she and Martin had become close – they were sharing a flat at the time Ward met Martin.

It is not clear whether Ward also knew Ruth Ellis, but it seems likely. She had modelled nude at the Camera Club and been photographed – clothed – by Ward's friend Anthony Beauchamp. She had a walk-on part in the film *Lady Godiva Rides Again*, which starred the rising glamour girl Diana Dors and the actress Kay Kendall, future wife of stage Pygmalion Rex Harrison. Kendall was a friend of Stephen Ward, and Dors would recall meeting him. 'I did not take to him at all. He looked devious and something of a show-off . . . He insisted that I go for a quick ride in his new sports car, and he drove around the country lanes at such speeds I was terrified . . .'

'Dandy Kim' Waterfield, a boyfriend of Dors' – and reportedly founder of the first Ann Summers sex shop – knew Ruth Ellis and Vicki Martin, and met Ward. He remembered the osteopath's 'quizzical look with his eyebrows and his stance, a shade camp'.

Martin stayed with Ward for more than a year, for he not only told her she could do better but seemed not to want to use her sexually. 'I really do love girls for themselves and not purely for a sexual reason,' he maintained. 'I have always tried to help them along – often with very good results.' For Martin, the result of the grooming was a breakthrough as a model – she had a body, as Frederic Mullally put it, to 'commit crimes for'. She posed for court photographer Baron, and Lazzolo painted her portrait at about the time he took on the commission to paint the Queen. Through Ward's friend Anthony Beauchamp, she landed a role in the film *It Started in Paradise*, which starred Ward's friend Kay Kendall. Soon, coached by Ward, Martin was being invited to high-society dinners and parties. The gossip columns dubbed her the 'Golden Girl'.

When one of the wealthy men who slept with Martin promised to set her up in a Mayfair flat and then reneged on the agreement, Ward came to the rescue. He brought pressure on the man to pay up or face a lawsuit and exposure, and the money came through. It seemed that the Golden Girl really had struck gold, though, when she began a dalliance with the Maharajah of Cooch Behar – another Ward friend. There was jewellery, exotic travel, even talk of marriage, until the Maharajah discovered that marriage to a non-Indian would mean forfeiting his princely allowances.

Vicki Martin loved fast cars, as did Ward, and hobnobbed with Ward's friends at the Steering Wheel Club. The Club, nominally a watering hole for motor-racing aficionados, had a wider clientele. Regulars included the film-star Douglas Fairbanks Jr, whose name would come up at Ward's trial in 1963, and a number of MI5 officers. For Martin, cars proved a fatal attraction. She made headlines when her maharajah, with her in the front seat, crashed at high speed in Hertfordshire. Later, and again a passenger, she was killed in a head-on nighttime collision on the Maidenhead road. The hundreds who attended her funeral included the Marquess of Milford Haven. 'One man well known in London,' Ward was to say, 'was so overcome he had to go into a nursing home.' Ward got in touch with Martin's relatives and visited them for years afterwards.

It was 1956, and Ward was set on a dangerous path. Vicki Martin had been if not a full-fledged whore, something close to one. Other young women, by no means all whores, would follow in short order. He introduced one of them, dancer and minor film actress Vicki Page, to Anthony Beauchamp, Churchill's son-in-law. A child was born of that affair, an event not reported in the newspapers because of the Churchill connection. Her mother, Page's daughter would recall, 'liked Stephen . . . named my younger brother after him.'

The succession of young females went on. Ward appeared to feel no guilt, to see no peril to himself.

'Ward had no necessity for financial gain from girls,' said fellow osteopath William McClurg. 'He earned well, and was busy.' Dr Stungo made the same point. 'He never lived off the girls or ran a call-girl service. He often had three or four girls staying at his place, because he was so generous and wanted to help people.' Ward once offered Stungo himself the sort of introduction that would one day have lawyers arguing over the fine line between putting a pretty woman a friend's way and acting as pimp.

'Shortly after my divorce,' he said, 'Ward phoned me one evening and asked if I was doing anything. I said I wasn't and Ward said that in that case he was sending over a young girl, a "popsy", because he, Ward, had been called out.' Had Stungo accepted the offer of a woman, then 'looked after' her when she left his bed, the law – as it would be interpreted in the 1963 trial – might have judged it prostitution. Had she, in turn, given any of the money to Ward, it could have been said he was living on immoral earnings.

The risk had been there for some time. 'When she was broke,' Warwick Charlton said of 'Golden Girl' Vicki Martin, 'Stephen sometimes lent her money. When she was affluent she would repay him or make some contribution towards their joint living expenses. It did not occur to Stephen that there was anything wrong in this.'

It did not occur to anyone, not until 1963. 'The accusation that he was this sort of monster who lived off the immoral earnings of women, as far as I could see,' said Ward's friend the play-wright Michael Pertwee, brother of Jon, 'was the most abject rubbish . . . though it would be wrong to paint him in any way as an admirable figure . . . He was known as a man who knew a lot of pretty girls. He was a snob and a social climber, and this was a passport into the kind of circle he liked . . . He was, if you like, a social pimp.'

One of Ward's prominent protégées in the 1950s was a taxi man's daughter from Essex named Anita Wimble. She arrived in London, aged fifteen, with an ambition to go on the stage and with a bosom – an asset displayed in photographs – encased in tight angora sweaters, very evidently unharnessed by a brassiere. Somewhere along the line she got a part in a Tommy Trinder revue, changed her name – to Pat Marlowe – and met Stephen Ward. 'I've decided on my career,' she was to say, 'I'm just going to get rich.' Under Ward's tutelage, she did find a sort of success.

The high life beckoned, and Marlowe forgot about becoming an actress. She became a 'jet-setter' at a time the word was only beginning to be used, ricocheting between New York,

Hollywood, Paris and Monte Carlo. She numbered Prince Aly Khan, the producer Jack Warner and Bill Wallace – Princess Margaret's escort of the day – among her friends. She had the use of a Manhattan apartment when producer Mike Todd was in town, made news when she stripped off at one of Warner's parties in Monte Carlo, and held parties in London for prominent homosexuals.

She had flings with friends of Ward – one, she claimed, with Lord Astor, another with the septuagenarian bandleader and impresario Jack Hilton. She had a baby by Max Bygraves, who would later acknowledge having paid her £10,000 to keep quiet about the child's paternity. She named the baby Stephen.

Millionaires used Marlowe for projects with which they did not want to be associated, and the press described her as 'the shrewdest businesswoman in the West End'. She had achieved her ambition to be rich, but happiness eluded her. In August 1962, the year before the Profumo scandal, one of her homosexual friends found Marlowe dead in bed at her Mayfair flat. 'Pat talked to me about Marilyn Monroe,' the friend said. 'She knew her well from Hollywood . . . said she could understand why she did it.'

Monroe had died only days earlier – more noisily – and, like Marlowe, from an overdose of barbiturates. A doctor admitted at the inquest that he 'doled out' the same tablets to Marlowe for her depression. 'There are always these silly girls around,' Ward said, 'who take some pills, have a drink, and then forget they have taken them, and so take some more.' Marlowe left £100,000 – a very large sum in those days – to her son Stephen.

Young women, Frederic Mullally said, loved Ward 'as a girl might love an elder brother or a father . . . Stephen used girls. But he never abused them, which is more than can be said for many of his betters. In Stephen's London – then as today – young girls were pressing their noses to windows screening the merchandise of luxury and fame. Stephen's sin was to show them the way in from the cold. That he enjoyed himself in the process, that he flourished in the sensual hothouse of a home forever strewn with discarded nylons, lip-printed tissues, cosmetic debris, these were the bounties of a prodigious expenditure of enthusiasm and compassion on the female sex.'

In the oddest way, the Vicki Martin episode was a signpost to the quicksand of Ward's future. Three years after her death, when Martin's name came up in conversation, another young protégée was to exclaim, 'I was at school with her sister!' The girl's name was Christine Keeler.

These events took place in the 1950s. Post-war England had only just begun to feel the beginnings of affluence. Those who enjoyed it first were, as always, those already at the top of the social pile. One day, an MI5 officer would write in a report, 'From what I hear of Ward and his dealings with women and his enormous circle of friends, I strongly suspect that he is the provider of popsies for rich people.' This was precisely accurate and, for many years, it suited everyone nicely.

CHAPTER 5

Osteopath by Appointment – Wooing the Astors

'Stephen was a specialist in lost souls, and Bill Astor was a lost soul.' So said David Astor, brother of Lord William Waldorf Astor, the 3rd Viscount – most definitely a rich person, and one who encountered any number of Ward's popsies. For the boy from a minor public school, Ward's entrée to the Astor family was the most significant single step up in a lifetime of social climbing. It would turn out, though, to have been disastrous social alchemy, a mix that would lead to the death of Ward, the ruin of John Profumo's career, and dishonour for the house of Astor.

Lord Astor – Bill to his intimates – inherited his title in 1952, when he became the last of the line to live at Cliveden, the family's massive home in Buckinghamshire. The family's rise to wealth had begun in the eighteenth century, when a Spanish butcher called Astorga emigrated to Germany. He dropped the 'ga' on the end of his name, and sent his sons to seek their fortune further afield. Two went to London to manufacture musical instruments, another to the United States. In New York, the Astors sold flutes imported from London, started the American Fur Company, became property moguls, and wound up almost as rich as the Rothschilds.

One of the Astor heirs came to England in the late nineteenth century, apparently in hope of being raised to the peerage. Wealth works wonders. William Waldorf became the 1st Viscount Astor and bought the mansion at Cliveden from the Duke of Westminster for – at today's value – more than ten million pounds. He also bought Hever Castle in Kent, and built a village nearby to accommodate additional guests.

Born in 1907, the eldest child of the 2nd Viscount and his formidable wife Nancy, Bill Astor grew to adulthood during the family's British heyday. The Cliveden house and estate, on four hundred acres overlooking the River Thames, was the scene of lavish entertainment on a scale that is barely imaginable today. 'Dinners for between fifty and sixty were very frequent,' said a former staff member. 'Two or three balls for anything up to five or six hundred during the season.' There was an army of servants – the garden alone employed fifty men.

The guests at the Astors' table between the wars included kings and queens, ambassadors and political leaders. One of them, in the 1930s, was Harold Macmillan, who by the time of the Profumo Affair would have risen to become Prime Minister. Back then he was in his thirties, a World War I veteran and fledgling MP, recently married to the eldest daughter of the 9th Duke of Devonshire. The Astors' money brought to Cliveden an aristocratic style that had withered since 1918 and almost disappeared.

In the dusk of a summer's evening, though, on the terrace overlooking the river, some felt uneasy even then. Cliveden felt out of place, as though it ought to be in the Mediterranean – only the fireflies and the grasshoppers were missing. 'To live here would be like living on the stage of the Scala theatre in Milan,' wrote the diarist Harold Nicolson. 'Its beauty is purely scenic . . . There is a ghastly unreality about it all.'

Bill Astor's parents' view of the world was dominated by the idea of 'doing good' – a fine idea, but not necessarily good for their brood of six. Waldorf Astor was remote, and his wife Nancy was trapped by the rigid code in which she had imprisoned herself. 'She felt it her bounden duty,' Bill's brother Michael said, 'to chastise, in and out of season, those weaknesses and uncertainties that beset young men and women as they begin to grow up . . . Trying to do "bad" . . . I came to discover in myself forces which did not recognise these absolute distinctions.'

The two family members whose lives would most entwine with Ward's were Bill Astor and Bobbie Shaw, his half-brother by his mother's first marriage, Bobbie Shaw. Lady Astor sensed that Bobbie was headed for disaster. 'Don't bother about the new baby [Bill],' she wrote to a friend, 'look after Bobbie . . .' Bobbie, ignored by his alcoholic father, was the cuckoo in the nest, with no rights of succession to the Astor peerage. As if to compensate, his mother smothered him with love, cold-shouldering the unfortunate Bill. Having at first excessively depended on her, however, Bobbie came to resent her. He served in the trenches in the First World War, then entered manhood psychologically maimed. Handsome as a god he might be, witty and charming – but programmed to fail.

In 1929, aged thirty-one, Bobbie was drummed out of the Royal Horse Guards for being drunk on duty. Two years later, having been caught performing a homosexual act, he was sentenced to four months in jail. Years later, when Lady Astor was planning her autobiography, another of her sons told her the truth would be too horrifying. 'What d'you mean, horrifying?' asked her ladyship. 'Because you are so possessive,' he responded. 'That's why we are all cases of arrested development. Though I admit . . . Bobbie is the only one of us actually to have *been* arrested.' The author Christopher Sykes, a family friend, thought Bobbie 'a cynic and secret debauchee'.

Probably as a result of meeting him at an osteopathic consult-tion, Bobbie had a lengthy association with Stephen Ward. Years later, David Astor recalled, Bobbie adamantly refused to accept attention for an infected arm from any doctor other than Ward. The younger Astor disapproved. Ward, he said, 'liked to have people on strings. There was no reason why he should want to control Bobbie, except for the lust for power and influence.'

Some wondered whether Ward himself was homosexual. MP William Shepherd thought his voice 'rather irritating. It had a phoney, almost homosexual intonation. His whole manner was one to arouse suspicion.'

'There was a precision about him that seemed significant,' the American columnist Dorothy Kilgallen would write during his trial in 1963, 'a soft reluctance in the way he used his fine hands. He did not strike me as a man who would be attractive to a woman except as a friend who would be kind and amusing, and always ahead of the game in knowing which Greek island will be fashionable next year . . . They send flowers and thoughtful notes on birthdays, they can be funny or wicked or nice, but they are not usually interested in women in the conventional way. The evidence at the trial, however, indicated that I was wrong, or that there were two sides to the defendant . . .'

Ward knew what people thought. Once, when he was stripped to the waist shaving, Warwick Charlton commented on his soft, pale skin. 'You mean my ambidextrous look, eh?' Ward grinned, then added quickly, 'Hair on the chest isn't a sign of virility, Warwick.' It is not, but Ronna Riccardo, a prostitute who testified at Ward's trial, said Ward 'couldn't manage normal sex'.

Many of Ward's male friends were 'ambidextrous'. Robin Drury, a publicist who 'managed' Ward's protégée Christine Keeler at the time of the scandal, was openly bisexual. Ward was very close in the early 1960s to John Hamilton-Marshall, who was also bisexual.

He was friendly with Toby Roe, who ran the Rockingham, London's first overtly homosexual club.

The travel writer Robert Harbinson, who wrote under the name Robin Bryans, knew both Ward and Astor step-son Bobbie Shaw. Himself bisexual – and disarmingly open about it – he had no doubt that homosexual society was another of Ward's secret worlds. Harbinson says the osteopath had sat as a model for the prominent artist Frank Slater, who in 1953 painted the first portrait of Queen Elizabeth following her accession. 'Stephen was a very vain person,' Harbinson thought. 'That's why he posed for Frank – he was very proud of it.'

Ward also associated with the Scots painters Robert Colquhoun and Robert Macbryde, familiar kilted figures around Soho. 'It was a very gay group,' Harbinson recalled. 'Not only gay but extremely wild. The sort of orgies that Stephen was supposed to have gone to – these people were there.'

Mandy Rice-Davies, who with Christine Keeler was one of the two most prominent female characters in the Profumo Affair, said Ward often dined with the homosexual columnist Godfrey Winn. Winn, a poseur and hypocrite, was to dump Ward as soon as the scandal broke and excoriate him in print.

Through Bobbie Shaw, Ward had gained entrée to the people around the Astors and to friends among influential homosexuals. One such connection was the Very Reverend Monsignor Hugh Montgomery, a controversial churchman who – Harbinson claimed – was a lover of Albino Luciani, the future Pope John Paul I. Ward met often with another of Monsignor Montgomery's lovers, businessman, former British diplomat and – in the late 1950s – Permanent Under-Secretary of State for Commonwealth Relations, Sir Gilbert Laithwaite. At the Travellers' Club, the hallowed watering hole of diplomats and intelligence officers, Laithwaite, red carnation in buttonhole, would often lunch with Ward. As a supporter of the extreme right, he sometimes found Ward's liberal comments intolerable.

Ward's course through life had brought him into a strange eddy of the social stream, the so-called 'Gay Establishment'. This was a tight little world peopled by upper-class homosexuals of the generation that produced the most infamous British traitors of the twentieth century: Burgess, Maclean and Sir Anthony Blunt. Sir Gilbert Laithwaite was a friend of Blunt, the then highly respected Surveyor of the Queen's Pictures. Monsignor Montgomery's brother Peter was Blunt's longtime homosexual lover. Robert Harbinson cheerfully acknowledged having had sex with Guy Burgess. On the one hand, Ward was at just one remove from the enemy within, while simultaneously – as we shall see – in touch with loyal people in the world of intelligence. All this was heavy with implications for the scenario of 1963.

Ward was as close to Bill Astor as he was to Bobbie, perhaps closer. Like Bobbie, Astor had had a miserable childhood. 'Though one of the most privileged children in the world,' observed John Grigg, a biographer of Lady Astor, 'he was therefore, in a sense, cruelly disadvantaged and deprived.' He had emerged from Eton and Oxford a shy, awkward man, by no means handsome, with a receding hairline and a baby-face complexion. In 1935, aged twenty-eight and pressed into politics by his mother – Lady Astor had been Britain's first female Member of Parliament – Bill won the Conservative seat of Fulham East.

During World War II, while in the Royal Navy, Bill Astor served in intelligence for three years. Though regarded as an intellectual lightweight, he ended his war with numerous connections to intelligence – links that were to prove very pertinent to the story of Stephen Ward and the Profumo Affair. Astor came home to a changed world and a changed situation for the family. His father had made over the Cliveden estate to the National

Trust under an arrangement that opened the place to tourists at certain times, while allowing the Astors to remain in residence. To his distress, meanwhile, Bill had been passed over as chairman of the *Observer* newspaper, which the family owned, in favour of his brother David.

As befitted the man who was to become master of the house of Astor, however, Bill in 1945 married Sarah, daughter of Baron Grantley, a prominent film producer, in the first lavish society wedding of peacetime. Lord Mountbatten, a family friend, had hosted Sarah's coming-out party, and the bride counted Prince Philip as a friend. She had also been close to Kathleen Kennedy – a sister of the future President – who had married the son of the Duke of Devonshire but died in an air crash after the war.

Bill's marriage did not last and ended in divorce in 1953, just after the death of his father made him head of the family and the new Lord Astor. Close at hand, and offering support, was Stephen Ward. Bill had gone to Ward years earlier for treatment following a hunting accident, and the two men became cronies. 'Bill fell into Ward's clutches,' his brother David said, 'at a time of great vulnerability and distress. Bill had difficulties in human relations. Ward gave Bill psychological support and introduced him to girls.' Lord Astor, for his part, gave Ward the keys to the social kingdom of Cliveden.

Many thought the world wars had sounded the death knell of the aristocracy. It seemed anachronistic, useless in a modern country. The aristocracy, however, did not go away. The 1950s saw great houses still open. To enjoy the company of lords and ladies was still the benchmark of social success. Seven years of Conservative rule kept them at the top of the hierarchy. This was the nobility's Indian summer, and Stephen Ward basked in its warmth. It began, for him, with dinner invitations to Cliveden.

'The Visitors' Book,' Ward recalled in his memoir, 'reads like *Who's Who*. After changing for dinner, the guests usually meet in the Long Drawing-Room. Champagne and cocktails are always served here . . . and the guests nearly always include at least one duchess. Dinner is announced by the butler, and the guests drift into the huge and ornate dining-room, once a room in Madame de Pompadour's hunting lodge. The flower decorations are superb and there are always dishes of grapes, nectarines and peaches, from the outhouses. Course follows course and wine follows wine, until the ladies leave and the men can draw their chairs together and pass the port and walnuts and, of course, tell each other the latest joke from White's or Boodle's . . .'

The Canford boy sat now among the dukes and duchesses, industrialists and politicians. Ward, who had a fund of dinner stories, liked to tell one about the young Winston Churchill having told an irate field marshal that he was entitled to wear a certain medal because his godmother had given it to him. The godmother in question, he explained, was Queen Victoria. There was also the yarn about a trick Picasso had played on a dealer who was pestering him to sell a picture. The artist waited until the dealer was asleep in the sun, drew very lightly on his chest and stomach, then roused him to say he had become the possessor of a genuine Picasso.

It was Ward's skill as an osteopath that made him *persona* very much *grata* at Cliveden. Lord Astor's widow, Bronwen, the last of his wives, would recall, 'Every guest, no matter who, on a Saturday night was asked, "Would you like a free session? Stephen's coming up, and if you've got any aches and pains . . ." Bill hunted nearly every Saturday, and part of his relaxation, especially if he had a fall or something, would be to have a massage.'

'In this way,' Ward wrote, 'I treated Duncan Sandys . . . a frequent visitor with his red dispatch-boxes from the Ministry

[Sandys held several different government portfolios] . . . and Peter Thorneycroft, later Minister of Defence in the Macmillan government, Lord Hailsham and several others.' Among the notables Ward saw during this period were the man who was to become Minister for War, John Profumo, and the actress Valerie Hobson, whom Profumo was to marry.

Lord Astor had first introduced Profumo to Ward in the late 1940s, when Profumo was still a bachelor and soon to stand as a parliamentary candidate for Stratford-upon-Avon. It was then that he invited young actress Hobson to make an appearance at the local fete. She fell for the 'boyish man', as she remembered him then – a man who enjoyed politics, but also practical jokes, society gossip and nightclubs. She later recalled, in a note to herself, that there had been 'an instant, electric sexual attraction. He's totally free sexually and in love with sex.' Profumo was shy of commitment, however, and it was she who instigated their affair.

Profumo noticed even then, after their first meeting, that there were 'a lot of pretty girls' around Stephen Ward's consulting rooms, 'a number of very young models, starlets. I also realised that Dr Ward had a receptionist who was quite remarkably glamorous.' He liked Ward, found him 'hugely charismatic', and went to one of the osteopath's cocktail parties.

That initial acquaintance was apparently only brief, and Profumo did not meet Ward again until 1956, when Lord Astor took him round to the osteopath's consulting rooms in Devonshire Street. At forty-one, Profumo, true to family form, was carving out a successful career. His grandfather, an Italian baron, had settled in England at the turn of the century, and he and his offspring had become English country gentlemen – with pretensions to being somewhat grander. Even after the scandal in 1963, John Profumo would style himself 'Fifth Baron of the late United

Kingdom of Italy' in his *Who's Who* entry. The family motto is 'Virtue and Work'.

Profumo had attended Harrow and Brasenose College, Oxford, where he distinguished himself as a horseman. The Profumos, a hunting family, would tow their horsebox to meets attached to an immaculate Rolls-Royce. He was born to Conservatism, the whole gamut – polo, horse shows, house parties and fetes. After Oxford, his barrister father had sent him around the world, to the Soviet Union, the Far East and the United States. He had met Bill Astor before the war, when – at the tender age of twenty-one – he became Chairman of the Conservative Association in East Fulham, where Astor was MP. When war came, Profumo went into the Army as a lieutenant and came out as a colonel with an OBE.

By the time he encountered Stephen Ward again in 1956, Profumo already had an impressive career behind him: governor of two London hospitals at twenty-four, Conservative Member of Parliament for Kettering at twenty-five and MP for Stratford-upon-Avon since 1950. He had been married to Valerie Hobson for two years. He already had the sharp features and the smarmed-back, receding hair that was to become so well known, for all the wrong reasons, in 1963. Until then, some thought him a potential prime minister.

In the fifties, he rose steadily in government: Secretary at the Ministry of Transport and Civil Aviation under Churchill, Under-Secretary of State for the Colonies, Minister of State for Foreign Affairs and finally, from 1960, Minister for War. In all of these posts, the prime minister under whom Profumo served was Harold Macmillan.

Profumo, who according to a Conservative Party official 'believed in the ruling class', ran his social life accordingly. He was a member of the Other Club, described as 'perhaps the most exclusive dining club in the world'. Founded by Churchill, its sixty members included Harold Macmillan, Selwyn Lloyd, Foreign Secretary in the 1950s, and Colin Coote, editor of the *Daily Telegraph* and the man who would one day introduce Ward to a Soviet spy.

Until the scandal that ruined him, little was known publicly about Profumo's love life. He was rumoured in the press to have had an involvement with 'a widowed member of the Royal Family', probably the then Duchess of Kent. Friends thought Profumo something of a blade, with a weakness for nightlife. 'Jack was the sort of chap,' his parliamentary colleague William Shepherd thought, 'who would go around the nightclubs with another chap who was in parliament, and who's now a peer. And they would like to sit with these hostesses, which I must say I found rather painful whenever I sat with them. I'd have wanted to be paid to sit with them. But this is what Jack liked . . .'

Profumo's son was to write that his father was attracted to 'decorative, fun-loving "available girls", and there was a certain fascination with the painted and, if not exactly the semi-professional, the obviously enthusiastic amateur.'

In only a few years, these weaknesses would spell ruin for Profumo. The clock was ticking, too, for Lord Astor. *Daily Express* owner Lord Beaverbrook, who was prone to vendettas, had had it in for the Astors since being criticised in the *Observer*, which was edited by David Astor. He ordered his reporters to dig for dirt on the family. An exposé of Lord Astor's homosexual half-brother Bobbie Shaw was pulled from the paper just before publication in 1958. If Beaverbrook had had second thoughts on that occasion, though, his hatred of the Astors had not gone away. The Profumo Affair, when it broke, would give him his revenge, in spades.

CHAPTER 6

The Cliveden Capers, and The Spooks

'I was in the motor boat,' Ward wrote coyly in his memoir, 'with a famous actress (the female lead in *The King and I* – I've forgotten her name), Lord Astor, and the second Lady Astor . . .' The female lead in the London stage version of *The King and I* was Valerie Hobson, in her late thirties the veteran of a string of films, including *Kind Hearts and Coronets*, *Great Expectations*, *Spy in Black*, *Unpublished Story*, *The Bride of Frankenstein* and *Lovers, Happy Lovers*. She was to become best known as the wife of John Profumo.

The day Ward went motor-boating with Profumo's future wife was the day he spotted Spring Cottage, a country hideaway that years later, even at the worst moments of the Profumo Affair, would still send him into raptures. It was larger than it sounds, with half-timbered walls, a turreted roof and a carved wooden balcony. In the grounds of Cliveden, to Ward's delight, were 'temples, statues and grottoes, caves, cliffs and streams. It was here, in probably the loveliest corner of all, and one of the most secluded, that my cottage lay . . .'

It became 'my' cottage when Lord Astor's second wife, Philippa, Harold Macmillan's god-daughter, noticed Ward's enthusiasm.

The cottage had long since been abandoned, and she persuaded Astor that Ward should bring it to life again and use it as a weekend place. Ward laboured long and hard to restore the house, much of the time with a young woman named Margaret Brown – perhaps the most beautiful of his many female friends – working alongside him. She was probably the last woman to hold his full attention, and she for her part would laud him at the time of the Profumo scandal as 'a wonderful person'. Brown, who went on to become a top model, and eventually marry the composer Jule Styne. 'She painted while I dug,' Ward was to say of their time together fixing up Spring Cottage.

Lord Astor allowed Ward his idyll at a peppercorn rent of £1 a year, on the understanding that he would provide his services as an osteopath virtually free. The generous Astor also lent Ward £1,000 – a significant sum in the 1950s – and that too was written off to occasional osteopathy.

The big house had become open house, and soon Ward was down at Cliveden nearly every weekend. After the gardening, Ward wrote, 'I always remember the rush to get the dirt off and change into my dinner jacket to get to dinner with Lord Astor . . .' Following the failure of his second marriage, Astor was lonely. Ward could help fill the loneliness his lordship felt in the stifling atmosphere of the big house at Cliveden, and the rigid social code to which he had to appear to adhere, with camaraderie, fun and young women.

Ward was now more than a gregarious osteopath – he was himself fashionable. 'The cottage is big enough to entertain Ward's friends,' drooled a national gossip columnist in 1958, 'and what a lovely line they can shoot at dinner parties . . . the Cliveden tag makes the Ward retreat unbeatable in the U-stakes!' 'U' was at the time slang indicating that a person or place was fashionable – and 'Non-U' was the opposite.

Cliveden's butler, Mr Lee, judged Ward 'an affable and friendly gentleman'. He did not fail to observe, however, the fact that Ward brought numerous young women down from London, and confided to Lady Astor's maid that he thought they were 'Windmill girls'. 'I treated them,' said Mr Lee, 'just as I would any other guests, and so far as I know – and I should have known if they hadn't – they conducted themselves properly when they were in the house.'

And when they were in the cottage? Woodrow Wyatt, then a Labour Member of Parliament, remembered walking by the river at Cliveden with Lord Astor one weekend. 'I let Stephen Ward use that house,' said Astor, pointing out Spring Cottage. 'Then,' Wyatt said, 'he giggled a lot . . .' Long afterwards, when Ward was dead and the place had been sullied by the memories of the Profumo Affair, Astor's widow said the cottage had taken on an 'evil atmosphere'. A later incumbent of Ward's weekend cottage committed suicide by drowning himself in the sink. So concerned was Lady Astor that she brought in a priest to perform an exorcism. Later still, it was handed over to the National Trust.

For a long time, there were men in England familiar with the sex games Ward orchestrated on the Cliveden estate. Some of them, once powers in the land, no doubt feared that long-ago indiscretions would be disclosed. Others, at whom accusations were levied, batted them away with denials – like Douglas Fairbanks Jr.

The American actor and producer, the star of now forgotten movies like *The Dawn Patrol* and *Sinbad the Sailor*, had never been a challenge to his famous father. Long an Anglophile with an entrée to high society, he had moved to live in England permanently after the war. He circulated, moreover, in the highest social stratosphere. His father had introduced him to the Mountbattens as a young man and he and his wife were among the few foreigners to have entertained the Queen and Prince Philip at home.

Fairbanks had long known Lord Astor – they had worked together during the war when the American served in Naval Intelligence. Fairbanks kept up his intelligence connections and, FBI files reveal, kept the US Navy representative in London briefed on interesting titbits he picked up. In 1957, one of his daughters had her coming-out party at Cliveden. 'I did, of course,' he told the authors, 'know Dr Ward, whom I went to for a serious bursitis attack. And I did meet him through the late Lord Astor.'

The osteopath never blabbed publicly about his famous friends, but could not control the tongues of the women around him. Mandy Rice-Davies, grilled at Ward's trial about activities at the flat she had shared with Christine Keeler, was asked whether she had had 'intercourse with any other man or men at Comeragh Road?' Her reply was crisp: 'Douglas Fairbanks.'

Though Fairbanks denied the allegation, Rice-Davies has since offered detail. 'I was seriously thinking of becoming an actress,' she said. 'It was one step on, I thought, from modelling, and making commercials had given me an idea of how to work with cameras and lights. I met Douglas Fairbanks Jr with his wife and daughter, Melissa, at Cliveden, and was able to talk to him about the film business. I was flattered by his interest when he telephoned me a few days later and invited me to lunch at the Dorchester.'

Rice-Davies was sixteen years old at the time. She went on: 'Even then, in his fifties, he was a remarkably good-looking man as well as being an amusing companion. After lunch he suggested we go upstairs . . . We went to bed. There were several of these little afternoon interludes. I was genuinely fond of him, and I imagined he felt something similar for me . . .'

Christine Keeler went further and described joining in 'a jolly threesome' with Fairbanks. It was great fun, she thought, to cavort with a star. According to Rice-Davies, she and Keeler posed for pictures taken by Fairbanks. Keeler, for her part, added a detail that would become significant. 'When Fairbanks was in action,' she would say, 'a camera was never far away.' In the late 1950s, Fairbanks had shown Lord Astor a Polaroid camera that produced instant black and white prints – a device almost unknown in England at that time. It may have been the use of that camera to take dirty pictures that, as a later chapter will suggest, eventually got the former movie star into hot water.

When matters came to court in 1963, Lord Astor himself was another famous casualty. His name surfaced when Mandy Rice-Davies was asked who had paid the rent at the Comeragh Road flat. Though at the time she had not yet met him, she truthfully answered 'Lord Astor'. Stephen Ward, who made the arrangements for the flat, had used a cheque Astor had given him as a loan. Later, when Ward took Rice-Davies along with him to treat Astor's wife's stiff neck, she did meet his lordship.

Rice-Davies went to bed with Lord Astor in November 1962, she said in testimony and in interviews, at Ward's place in Wimpole Mews. It was not, she maintained, a commercial exchange. Ward was in the other room while she and his lordship had sex in her bedroom. 'It's quite normal, isn't it?' she said perkily in 1963 to the startled trial judge. 'There's nothing wrong with it?'

Mariella Novotny, another of the young women around Ward, was a frequent visitor to Ward's cottage at Cliveden. Lord Astor, for his part, attended parties Novotny and her husband gave at their flat in Hyde Park Square. According to Novotny, there was a darker side to Astor's sex life – one that surely left him wide open to blackmail.

At first, Novotny wrote in an unpublished manuscript obtained by the authors after her death in 1983, Lord Astor simply took her out to dinner. 'Bill made a great fuss of me. We dined, gossiped leisurely . . . he could be an amusing partner when he forgot to be pompous. Then he said he could show me something really exciting if I wanted a special scene.' Astor then took her, she said, to a Mayfair brothel that catered for sadomasochists.

In an elaborately equipped torture chamber, Novotny wrote, 'Every type of whip and cane was neatly displayed. Bill selected a cat-o'-nine-tails with fine thongs of leather, and showed me how to manipulate it . . .' A young black woman was selected from several candidates and strapped to rungs set in the wall. 'I tentatively lashed her buttocks,' Novotny continued. 'Bill told me I was just playing at it. He provoked me with derogatory comments. The girl's gasps of pain and Bill's derisory remarks got me going. I lashed her backside with all my strength . . . I ignored the blood running down her legs, and her shrieks simply made me more and more sadistic. Finally . . . Bill grabbed the whip and said I'd gone too far – he had to pay fifty pounds instead of the usual ten.'

This episode, Novotny said, occurred in 1960 when she was eighteen and Lord Astor fifty-four. Is it true? Novotny certainly did within a year or so become deeply involved in sadomasochism. She was to preside as hostess at the infamous 'Man in the Mask' orgy, which will be described later in this book. A female witness at the Ward trial, an Austrian identified during the case only as 'Miss R.' – in fact Ilya Suschenek – testified that Ward asked her 'to go to a party given by a woman, Mariella . . . he said that at this party I would see girls being tied up and whipped'.

Did Mariella Novotny tell the truth about Lord Astor? A roman-à-clef entitled *The Last Temptation*, published in 1984, would suggest – given its provenance – that she did. It features a character named 'Lord Asterisk' and contains the following conversation between two men at a party:

Man 1: Well, certainly I was warned about Bill Asterisk and all the boots and spurs and things. But I didn't expect to have to dress up as a policeman.

Man 2: Policewoman, surely, darling.

Man 1: No. That is the whole point. *Not* a policewoman, a police*man* with a helmet and a truncheon . . .

The Last Temptation is a thinly veiled account of the life of Guy Liddell, who was Deputy Director of MI5 in the late 1940s and had been close to the traitor Guy Burgess. It drew on Liddell's journal 'Wallflower', so-named for security reasons, which was seen by various fellow officers – following his death – and eventually published in censored form. It is the identity of *The Last Temptation*'s author, however, that provides a firm link to Lord Astor. He was David Mure, a former World War II Army Intelligence officer who had served in the same units as Lord Astor. Mure, whose memory was legendary, had headed the 31 Committee in Beirut, which specialised in double-crossing the enemy.

Astor had extensive involvement with intelligence, professionally and personally. As the naval intelligence representative to the 31 Committee, he had had regular contact with MI5 and MI6 officers in the Middle East. Later, in London, he had continued to work in intelligence at the Admiralty. His first wife, Sarah, had been a translator at Bletchley, where Germany's Enigma code was broken. His second wife, Philippa, was the daughter of Lieutenant-Colonel Henry Hunloke, MI5's man in Jerusalem during the war.

Astor's service colleague Mure used pseudonyms to describe his intelligence contacts in both *The Last Temptation* and in another book, *Practice to Deceive*. In both books, he referred to the wartime MI6 station chief Charles Dundas as 'Fergie', and in *The Last*

Temptation to Guy Burgess as 'the Duchess'. 'Fergie,' Mure wrote, 'frequently attended the Duchess' parties with his friend, Lord Asterisk, the prominent whipman.' In 1955, after the defection to Moscow of Burgess and Maclean, Lord Astor declared in the House of Lords that he had never met Guy Burgess. Did his old comrade Mure spin a vicious lie? Or did he tell the thinly veiled truth?

Stephen Ward, for his part, had his own strange connections to people in the worlds of diplomacy and intelligence. He and royal photographer Baron used to visit the Gargoyle Club, where Burgess and Maclean regularly got drunk. As noted earlier, he consorted with the homosexual diplomat Sir Gilbert Laithwaite and with Monsignor Montgomery, whose brother was Anthony Blunt's lover. Ward was also close in the 1950s, according to Robert Harbinson, to two remarkable women who had served in intelligence during the war – Gwen le Gallienne and Princess Dil de Rohan.

Gwen le Gallienne, an accomplished portrait painter, was a lesbian who wore her blond hair cropped short and on occasion sported a monocle. She had been the lover of Louise Bullitt, sometime mistress of the socialist journalist John Reed, one day to be portrayed in the film *Reds*, and wife of the first US ambassador to the Soviet Union. The Bullitts socialised with the Astors.

Harbinson, who knew them all, said, 'Ward hated to be thought gay, except in the company of Gwen le Gallienne, when it was all chaps together. There were terrible scandals about her, which Ward was fascinated by. Stephen, of course, was a mine of information on all this.'

Princess de Rohan, who was also lesbian, worked for the British wartime Ministry of Information. She had arrived in London, following life as a Berlin hostess in the 1930s and marriage to a homosexual German prince. Both de Rohan and le Gallienne worked with Tomás Harris, a left-wing associate of Burgess, Blunt and Kim Philby. De Rohan later lived at the home of the painter Sir Francis Rose, a former close friend of the leader of Hitler's Brownshirts, Ernst Röhm – Rose had himself met Hitler.

Rose was close, too, to Italy's celebrated pioneer frogman, Prince Doria. In 1953, when he came to England, Doria stayed at the home near Windsor of his relative, the Duchess of Newcastle. There, too, was the ubiquitous Stephen Ward, providing his osteopathic services – and taking a great interest in both Doria and underwater warfare.

Sir Francis Rose's 'soulmate' in London, Harbinson said, was British World War II frogman hero 'Buster' Crabb, who disappeared in 1956 while on an operation to examine the hull of the Soviet cruiser *Ordzhonikidze*, then on an official visit to the UK. The Crabb operation had been ordered by naval intelligence, with the connivance of MI6, contrary to the wishes of Prime Minister Anthony Eden. Ward, said Harbinson, was a fund of information on the Crabb episode. As late as 1962, according to Mandy Rice-Davies, he was still deeply interested in submarine warfare. Was this interest, odd perhaps in a society osteopath, entirely casual?

MI6, as reported elsewhere in this book, was interested in Ward from the early 1950s. According to the agent who monitored Ward's activity, MI6 concluded, moreover, that its sister service, MI5, used Lord Astor and his estate at Cliveden for 'honeytrap' operations – operations designed to entrap intelligence targets by compromising them sexually. Lord Astor, an MI6 officer said, was 'on friendly terms with senior members of MI5, and was happy to help them, and in his view the country, when asked to do so . . . When they needed to make use of Ward, to provide suitable women for visiting heads of state, they went through his friend Lord Astor.'

Given Lord Astor's connections, which British intelligence

service was doing what at Cliveden? Given the rivalry between the two agencies, there is no easy answer. MI6, certainly, has pandered to the sexual needs of visiting dignitaries. Greville Wynne, who was contact man for Soviet traitor Oleg Penkovsky, revealed that MI6 had high-class whores on call, available for the use of chosen guests. Norma Levy, a call girl and leading lady of a later sex scandal, the 1972 Lord Lambton Affair, said she entertained foreign diplomats at the behest of a 'Mr Whitehouse of the Foreign Office'. The Foreign Office is responsible for the activities of MI6. If Cliveden was indeed used for honeytrap operations, was it coincidence that Stephen Ward, purveyor of female bait, was on hand?

Lord Astor's third and last wife, the former model Bronwen Pugh, did not like Ward. 'I knew about him already, from another model girl,' she told the authors, 'and when I heard that he had a cottage on the estate, I was just horrified. I could sense who was taking my husband for a ride, and when it was innocent and not so innocent. I felt that Ward was manipulating Bill, and I was there to marry Bill not to manipulate him. The whole beginning of my life at Cliveden was marred by the presence of this man.'

Ward was a guest of the Astors at Christmas 1960, enjoying dinner at the big house alongside Astor's family, Lord Palmer of Huntley & Palmers biscuits, and the young Lord Gowrie, who later became Margaret Thatcher's Minister for the Arts. Astor's friend Maurice Collis, who was also there, thought Ward amusing, 'quite at home in good society'. Lady Astor did not approve of his being there, and banned him from future dinners. Ward continued to be available to give massages, however, and – as indicated by the bedroom frolic with Mandy Rice-Davies – Lord Astor continued to see the osteopath behind his wife's back.

The columnist Godfrey Winn sized Ward up having observed

him at a bridge party. He remembered him as 'this tallish man, with a face free of fat to match his thin body. I suspected he was already in his forties, though his manner was consistently more youthful, at times almost coquettish' – Ward was in fact nearly fifty – 'tough in an entirely masculine way. His facile smile turned on and off like a light in a dark room – in momentary repose, the skin of his face had a peculiar emanation of deadness; above all, his elaborate attentiveness gave the impression of someone who, though eager to please through not being absolutely sure of himself, yet at the same time had an equal desire to manipulate the company, even to command.'

Some people, Lady Astor included, were troubled by the fact that Dr Ward manipulated not only bodies but also human lives. It was already too late, though, to have such qualms. Besides, the rich men Ward cultivated had no wish to part company with him. Without him, after all, how in the world would the chaps get a bit on the side?

CHAPTER 7

A Recipe for Scandal

'Nowadays,' Profumo's friend William Shepherd said in the mid-1980s, 'if you go to the best places you are quite likely to meet the worst people . . . There are one or two places left . . . there's the Stork Room and there's Eve's, a place Jack Profumo used to go to quite a bit – but nobody who's anybody ever goes to them now.'

Shepherd was ruminating on the melancholy state of things – from the standpoint of his generation – before the first edition of this book was published. Nightlife in the capital in the 1950s and 1960s was a phenomenon of the era. 'London was a much smaller place in those days,' Jon Pertwee remembered. 'The social scene was a mixture of the characters of London. Something to do with the war bringing everybody down to a certain level . . . I mean, today, people who go to Tramp would never dream of going to Stringfellow's, or wherever, downmarket. The social scene in our day ranged right across from the Berkeley to the Nuthouse and Boogie Woogie . . .'

Stephen Ward's post-war London club scene was a melting pot. There were idle aristocrats, Members of Parliament playing hookey during an all-night sitting, and actors winding down after the last curtain. New to the ranks of the clubbers, though, were a more raffish type, nouveau-riche millionaires, art dealers and salesmen with money to burn. By now not everyone who made the scene

59

spoke with a public-school accent, though many affected one. What they had in common, of course, was lust.

'An older man,' said Pertwee, 'had absolutely no problem in finding a pretty young lady to accompany him. A Bentley, an old banger of a Bentley I mean, or an old sports car, and your fifty-year-old would have no problem getting his twenty-year-old girl.'

Stephen Ward entered middle age in the 1950s. The teeth were false, but smiled agreeably. The blue eyes of the boy from Canford School had not dulled much, and the soft baritone, practised at seduction, survived. He always had a sports car parked around the corner – probably on hire purchase, but who was to know? In the clubs, Ward not only cultivated his upper-class cronies but also made friends of the new sorts who showed up. Some of them were amusing, in a bohemian sort of way, and could be useful. One such was Horace – 'Hod' to those who knew him – Dibben.

Eighty-two when interviewed for this book, Dibben was proud of his roguish past. The son of a Southampton ironmonger who was a member of the Plymouth Brethren, he had a religious background that predisposed him to rebellion in matters involving sex. In the 1930s, when locked in a dull job and a dull marriage, he stumbled on something strangely exciting. One night, during a furtive approach to the home of a female associate, Dibben peered through the curtains to get a glimpse of her. She was with another man, and she was whipping him.

Soon, Dibben was tied to a tree in the woods himself, being flogged with briars until the blood flowed. Pleasure followed pain, and Dibben went on to become an ardent sadomasochist. A record of his interview with the Denning inquiry would note that, 'In addition to his interest in black magic, he had a tremendous appetite for sex so long as it was perverted enough . . . Dibben was allegedly a man of fathomless depravity with cunning, in whose hands Ward was clay.'

In old age, as an old man in a dirty cardigan with gold chains and an Egyptian medallion dangling round his neck, he cheerfully acknowledged his bizarre preferences and provided a stream of ancient gossip. Gossip, someone once said, is history, and Dibben appeared to the authors to be truthful.

Like Ward, Dibben had been something of a Pygmalion. He was an acknowledged art restorer and expert on eighteenth-century antiques. At war's end, on being demobbed from the Royal Air Force, he had placed an advertisement in the papers that went something like: 'Intelligent young girl required for antique business. Must have knowledge of art.' The one problem with the applicant he chose, a sixteen-year-old grocer's daughter named Patsy Morgan, was that she had a provincial accent. Not right for the showrooms, so Dibben sent her to a finishing school run by the Countess of Devon. A year or so on, duly tutored, Morgan joined Dibben at Lytes Cary Manor in Somerset. The aristocracy – and the not-so-smart – began flocking to the parties they threw. 'The sweet life,' as one magazine put it, 'had begun.'

In London, 'everyone' soon knew Dibben and his girl Patsy. Dibben went bankrupt, but that did not cramp his style or hers. Patsy, who went on to run a publicity agency in London's West End, was forever in the newspapers, attending first nights, being photographed – heavily made-up – in the fashionable nightspots. By the mid-1950s she was running one herself, the Torch Theatre Club, dubbed Esmeralda's Barn. She said it was the 'place where everybody went, the Duke of Kent, jazz singer Josh White, Lord Suffolk, the Earl of Warwick, and John Huston'. And, sure enough, Lord Astor, accompanied by Stephen Ward. Patsy, whom most assumed to be Dibben's daughter, was ever present, smiling her painted smile and calling everyone 'Sweetie', be they peer or jumped-up commoner.

There were perks for Dibben. 'Hod was a voyeur,' said Michael

Mordaunt-Smith, old Etonian nephew of Lord Oranmore and Browne. 'The only thrill he got was from watching other people screw. He would sit in the corner of a semi-darkened bedroom and . . . just watch.'

Then Patsy disappeared for a while. When eventually traced, to the home of an Argentine millionaire in the Bavarian Alps, Patsy said she was in hiding from someone. She had left behind a diary, press stories reported, containing 'notes about love affairs with high-placed personalities, the names and peculiarities of so-called refined people, and tales of narcotics and degenerate impulses'. Her lawyer's advice, Patsy said, was to stay abroad. Seven years later, when Christine Keeler in turn headed for Spain, people would again wonder what was being hushed up. Dibben had lost his Patsy, but there were more where she came from. One, indeed, was to be directly relevant to the Profumo Affair.

Stephen Ward had known Dibben for years by the time Patsy moved on. 'He came to supper every Thursday,' Dibben said. 'It was a regular thing. He had often been to the Thursday Club during the day. Later, we saw him mostly at Cliveden. John Profumo was a regular visitor.' Ward's Thursday dinners with Dibben took place at the Belgravia home of a mutual friend, gynaecologist Dr Edward Sugden.

'Teddy Sugden had a paralysed face,' said Jon Pertwee. 'He was horrific-looking, one side of his face was permanently down. And he kept alligators and lizards and snakes in his surgery . . . When you went to see him you saw these horrifying animals all crawling around in their cages. He was weird, but a most loved man. His morals were not quite as people would expect them to be, but he was generous and nice . . .' Dibben agreed: 'You couldn't have met a nicer man.'

There were things about Sugden that certainly were not nice. He liked female companions to simulate sex with one of his pet snakes. On a visit to China in the 1920s, according to an acquaintance, he had filmed the torture and rape of a group of Russian ballet dancers who had fallen into Chinese hands. The footage pleased Sugden so much that he had several frames reproduced as stills – to show his friends.

Sugden's main line of business in the 1950s was abortion. Abortion did not become legal until 1967, and – unlike poorer women, who tried to deal with their problem with gin and knitting needles – women with connections and money went to the likes of Dr Sugden. Sometimes he helped women free of charge, and could afford to do so. According to several sources, he was performing up to fifteen paid-for abortions a day at up to £200 a patient. The Messina brothers, notorious Sicilian pimps of the day, sent their prostitutes to him when they got pregnant. Meanwhile, Sugden gave interesting parties.

'At the end of every week,' Dibben said, 'Teddy used to go round to the wine merchants and load up his huge Bentley with drink.' 'Teddy had a house on an island in the middle of the Thames, near Ham I think,' Pertwee said. 'He was a great nudist . . . everybody used to go down and wander around in the nude in the sun. It was quite jolly.'

The most exotic parties were held at a place known as 'Teddy's hut', which, Dibben recalled with glee, 'was next to Windsor Castle's sewage department . . . a bungalow on the banks of the Thames, and he enclosed it completely with a very high fence . . . We would take off all our clothes when we got there, and didn't put them back on until we had to go back. People tried to bore holes in the fence to see what was going on.'

'Teddy had an unlimited supply of girls,' Dibben said, 'because all the actresses and models in London came to him for their abortions, and then he'd ask them down to Windsor . . . Teddy's wife never let him join in – he could only watch.' One of the partygoers was an actress – just starting out then – who went on to win many international awards for her film and television roles. She cannot be named here because she is still alive.

Dibben recalled how, having squared things with the local police force, Sugden invited an officer to one of the parties. 'We asked him in and gave him some whisky,' Dibben said. 'He was lying on the grass watching the naked bodies cavorting about when one woman popped her head up and said "Hello!" It turned out that she was his daughter . . .'

'The first time Stephen Ward came,' according to Dibben, 'he arrived by boat – he'd borrowed one from the Astors. He brought a load of girls with him, four girls. They had just arrived from Australia and were coming to work as models, and Stephen had just met them at Southampton. He had taken them to Cliveden and brought them on to Teddy's. Three of the girls were absolutely delighted with what they saw – a load of naked guests – but the fourth left and went straight on back to Southampton . . .' Ward, for his part, kept his clothes on at the Sugden parties. He even had his clothes on when once, at the Cliveden cottage, Dibben blundered in on him in bed with a well-known model.

On rainy weekends, the Star Tavern in Belgravia was a favourite haunt. 'London Lotharios pulled their sports cars up to the door to display their latest girls,' recalled an American who knew Ward at the time of the Profumo Affair. 'Dr Ward invariably showed up with the envied beauty.' The Star was in those days a hang-out for the better class of criminal. They included 'Dandy Kim' Caborn-Waterfield, a former lover of actress and self-styled sex symbol Diana Dors, who also reportedly associated with Stephen Ward, and 'Chelsea Scallywag' Bobbie McKew. McKew generated funds for the notorious Dr Emil Savundra, said to have perpetrated the biggest car-insurance fraud of all time, and who pursued sex as avidly as he did money. Savundra liked blondes and redheads 'with long legs and very white skin', and McKew introduced him to Ward – and Ward obliged. The evidence of one of those blondes was to cost Ward dear at his trial in 1963.

The next phase of this saga is the sorry story of three teenaged girls, three virginities lost, and three trips to London that took the girls into the orbit of Ward and his friend Dibben – and eventually to starring roles in the Profumo scandal.

CHAPTER 8

Christine, Mandy and Mariella

One day in 1957, a girl in Staines, Middlesex, went to the lodgings of a Ghanaian student, a sweeper in the dress shop where she worked, to help him with his homework. The Ghanaian told the girl how lonely he was, and she listened. When he began kissing her, she did not object. When he asked her to get into bed, she said it was time she was leaving – and then gave in. 'Of course,' she said later, 'once he started he went the whole way. I was not very stimulated . . . On the train home I began to feel guilty and full of secret shame for what I had done.'

The girl was Christine Keeler, and she was fifteen. Her father had left home long ago, and much of her childhood had been spent with her mother and stepfather in a converted railway carriage. Keeler loathed the stepfather, which led her mother to take her to see a psychiatrist. The stepfather had molested her early on, she said, and – at twelve or thirteen – she had seen him and her mother making love. 'I was afraid,' she said, 'that what went on might happen to me.'

Once it had happened to her, Keeler no longer had much time for home. At sixteen she was hanging around a pub called the Angel, picking up American GIs from the several US bases in the area. She had a preference, one that was to prove durable, for black men. Soon she was in a swanky American car, heading for the NCOs club at Langley airbase. There were bottle parties, a first encounter with marijuana – not yet a common indulgence in England – and a second lover.

This was a hard-faced black sergeant – she remembered him as Jim – about twenty years older than Keeler. He became the first man to enjoy her favours for a whole night. When Jim was long gone back to America, she discovered she was pregnant. 'I then did all the usual things,' Keeler wrote in her book *Nothing But* . . . 'gin and hot baths, castor oil, and finally the horrible self-probing with the knitting needle.' In a horrendous way, it worked. The baby arrived, damaged, when Keeler was alone in bed. 'A slimy mauve and red head, there, not there, and there again. Mum heard my call and cycled away for the doctor.' The child – it was a boy – died six days later in hospital.

In the summer of 1959, not long after her seventeenth birthday, Keeler stole a car – by slipping a piece of silver paper into the ignition – and headed for London and a job as a waitress. Then a woman named Maureen O'Connor told her there was good money to be made at Murray's Cabaret Club in Soho. Soon Keeler was being introduced to Percy Murray, a pseudo City gent in spectacles and a double-breasted suit. Murray's boast was that most of Europe's nobility had sat at his tables, and that Winston Churchill had been a customer during the war. Princess Margaret had favoured Murray's with her presence, and King Hussein of Jordan was a regular. A mix of aristocrats and commoners would gather amongst the potted palms to drink, watch the costumed dancers and flirt with the 'showgirls', who performed topless.

Keeler, who was hired as a showgirl, teetered on to the stage for the first time wearing high-heeled shoes, a shiny cache-sexe and an assortment of feathers and sequins. She was red-haired and slim, and more amply bosomed than met the eye when she was clothed. It was the profile that gave the beauty the public would later see in myriad press photographs. 'She had the face of Nefertiti,' a female friend would say.

Like other Murray's girls, Keeler sat with male customers between acts, encouraging them to buy more drinks. Each order brought her a commission, and there were also tips. Murray's had a 'no sex with customers' rule, which – according to Keeler – existed to protect not the girls but the reputations of the customers.

Percy Murray himself set the real tone. 'He used to bed me once or twice a week,' Keeler claimed, 'and there was always an extra fifteen quid in my hand afterwards.' 'I think I would divide the girls between those who did and those who didn't,' said former MP William Shepherd, an habitué of Murray's. Keeler, one of those who did, was soon a hit with an old Etonian and ex-Guards officer called Michael Lambton, a cousin of the Lord Lambton who was to figure in a later sex scandal. Michael Lambton, a wealthy young publisher, had a problem with drink. He was prone, according to one of Keeler's friends, to saying, '"Pass the potty, dear" – and one would lean over to get the baby's pot kept in the back seat of the Bentley like an aircraft sick bag.'

One night another of Keeler's friends came into Murray's, a wealthy Arab she remembered as Ahmed. With him came a film starlet and a second man, Stephen Ward. Ward's opening gambit was supposedly, 'You were delightful in the show. Will you dance? What are you doing later?' Keeler claimed she at first tried to avoid him. Much to his Arab companion's irritation, however, he wormed her phone number out of her. Then Ward wished everyone a very good night and departed with the starlet.

He called Keeler three times the following day. She fobbed him off, she claimed, but he turned up one weekend at her home in Staines to charm her mother and stepfather – Ward made a habit of cultivating his girls' parents. Then, on their second date, Ward asked her to move into his flat.

In spite of the age difference between them, Ward had much to offer. Keeler felt highly vulnerable in London, a lonely bird of paradise in the big bad city. Ward, for his part, offered an undemanding sort of friendship. Unlike most men, he did not pester Keeler for sex. The few passes he made seemed only half-hearted. They occasionally slept in the same room, but never had sex. Soon, she would recall, they were living 'like brother and sister'. 'I felt,' she said later, 'that there would always be Stephen.' Keeler could not know then just how much, as long as she lived, there would always be Stephen.

Sex, though not with Ward, was all around. Stephen Ward derived amusement from introducing his young discovery to upper-class sex orgies. He confided that he found himself impotent at sex parties, but liked to watch. He took Keeler to swapping sessions in Maida Vale, then hosted one of his own at the cottage on Lord Astor's estate. Keeler looked on in youthful surprise as a husband and wife – she referred to them pseudonymously as 'Bertie' and 'Mary' – had sex with other partners in each other's presence. The husband's main concern, she thought, was that his wife should enjoy herself as much as possible.

Ward explained the theory on which he based such diversions. Group sex, he thought, did not cause upset and unhappiness in marriage but stimulated relationships. 'It makes you think, little baby,' he mused, 'perhaps that's what it's all about.'

Keeler became a regular weekend guest at the Astors' cottage. On one occasion they were joined by another young woman, whom Keeler has called 'Barbara', and whose sexual preference was bondage. She lay tied to the bed shrieking hysterically, laughing one moment, crying the next. 'Leave her there,' Ward said as solemnly as possible, 'that's what she deserves.'

The flat Ward had in London at that time was small, and he wanted to move. He had a friend in property, a man who had all varieties of accommodation on his books. This was Peter Rachman, one day to be exposed as a property racketeer on the grand scale. 'Rachmanism' was eventually to enter the *Concise Oxford Dictionary*, defined as 'exploitation of slum tenants by unscrupulous landlords'. The man himself was an expatriate Pole, aged forty-one in 1960, who had started his career in Britain as a scorer at Solomon's billiard hall in Soho. Rachman got into the property business by locating rooms for prostitutes, then helped the Messina brothers – the pimps who funnelled females to Dr Sugden's abortion clinic – in the capacity of 'investment consultant'. The police in London did not give him trouble – his money looked after that.

Rachman became a property mogul in Notting Hill and Bayswater at the right time, during a wave of immigration from the West Indies. He supplied overcrowded accommodation at extortionate prices. Rachman owned clubs as well as accommodation, and hired thugs enforced his rule. Slum rents alone raked in £78,000 a year for him – a fabulous sum by late 1950s' standards.

By 1960, Rachman was telling a friend he would soon be 'one of the richest men in England'. He would achieve it 'honestly', by transferring properties to surrogate owners and taking a stake in property slated for the construction of the M6 motorway. He had been tipped off to the project by Members of Parliament, including Ernest Marples, the Minister of Transport – a man who kept his shares in his road-construction business despite the conflict of interest. He was later to flee the country at dead of night to live abroad, to avoid prosecution for tax fraud.

Ward and Rachman shared a mutual friend in Dennis Hamilton, Diana Dors' husband. Hamilton had a 'fish book', listing women available to service him and his friends in London, at his flat in

Bryanston Mews, or at his country place. The country place featured cameras to film orgies, tape recorders hidden under beds, and a two-way mirror in the ceiling through which guests could watch others having sex. The flat was in time acquired by Rachman, who in turn eventually rented it to Stephen Ward.

While Ward and Keeler were looking for a new place, Rachman invited them to dinner at the El Condor, a trendy joint patronised by Princess Margaret, the Duke of Kent, and a coterie of nobility and former military men. The invitation was a chance for Rachman to tell Keeler he fancied her. She was tempted by the overture, coming as it did from a millionaire, but knew to accept would be to let Ward down. She packed her bags, however, and moved to Rachman's flat. He thenceforth had her daily, usually after lunch. 'Sex to Rachman,' Keeler said, 'was like cleaning his teeth and I was the toothbrush . . .'

Ward was furious, for a reason that in hindsight is laughable. Keeler's reputation would suffer, he said, from being seen in the company of a man like Rachman. Keeler was soon to get bored with the property racketeer anyway. There would now be fresh adventures, with a new female friend – one who, conveniently, would look after Rachman as she had done.

Mandy Rice-Davies was to say she was 'slower than most finding out about sex. I knew about horses. I had read *Forever Amber* and believed fervently in the agony and ecstasy of love – red, violent and blood-splashed.' She was sixteen in 1960, still known as Marilyn , the name given to her by her Welsh parents – the change to 'Mandy' would come later. Her father was an ex-policeman who worked for the Dunlop tyre company, her mother a miner's daughter. As she entered her teens, she had been interested in a pony called Laddie and Roman Catholicism. At fifteen, she was modelling mink for fashion shows at a Marshall & Snelgrove department store not far from her home in Solihull – and flirting with a trapeze artist in a visiting circus.

Before turning sixteen, she lost her virginity – 'in the room over the sweet shop next to the Odeon cinema' – to a Trinity College, Dublin, graduate. 'I was an enthusiastic participant,' Rice-Davies said, 'in what struck me as a perfectly pleasant way to spend an afternoon. I had expected, afterwards, to feel in some way fundamentally changed by my experience, but in this respect was disappointed. "Oh, so that's it," I thought, as I set off home.' Soon after, following a meeting in the street with a talent spotter, she was in London, posing as a model at the launch of a then new car called the Mini. The pay for the week was £80, and there was no keeping Rice-Davies in Solihull after that. She gave her notice at Marshall & Snelgrove, said goodbye to her parents and boarded the train for Paddington.

So it was that an advertisement in the London *Evening Standard* brought her in turn to Murray's Cabaret Club, to take a job as a dancer – her costume, to the extent she had one, was that of a American Indian squaw – and a meeting with a twelve-month veteran, Christine Keeler. 'It was dislike at first sight,' Rice-Davies recalled, and Keeler felt the same. Nevertheless, in part because they went to the same parties, the two became companions. Keeler thought they functioned well together because Rice-Davies had a good head for money, which she did not.

It was also a satisfactory partnership in the bedroom. Threesome sex sessions with men became something of a speciality, one that – Keeler thought – excited the men so much that they forgot any desire they might have had for a two-woman lesbian show. Neither of the girls, she said, was bothered by group sex – it was amusing, and brought in money for clothes and partying.

Unlike Christine Keeler, who looked better in photographs than face to face, Rice-Davies was to survive the coming scandal still looking 'fresh as a milkmaid'. Her face, one observer said, was 'very pretty' if somewhat hard and 'cat-like'. She found wealthy admirers during her two months at Murray's, starting with Aziz, an Arab friend of Keeler's Ahmed. Then she discovered Walter Flack, a partner of property magnate Charles Clore. Flack wined and dined Rice-Davies but never propositioned her. Clore, on the other hand, paid Keeler to go to bed with him.

Eric, the 3rd Earl of Dudley, showered Rice-Davies with flowers, sent her a case of pink champagne and took her off in his ancient Jaguar. He told Rice-Davies how to address the Queen – should they meet – and took her to dinner with the woman who had missed becoming Queen, the Duchess of Windsor. Lord Dudley proposed to her at one point, then quarrelled with her over Aziz and went off to marry Princess Grace Radziwill. Next in line was Robert Sherwood, a married millionaire machine-tool manufacturer from New York. 'This is no place for you,' he told Rice-Davies one night at Murray's. 'Go back before it's too late.' She did return to Solihull, but only for Christmas.

On New Year's Eve, Rice-Davies and Keeler moved into a flat on Comeragh Road, in unfashionable Baron's Court, courtesy of rental arrangements made by Stephen Ward and Lord Astor. Ward's cousin Tim Vigors, a Battle of Britain fighter pilot, made a play for Keeler at the house-warming party. Keeler's cast-off boyfriend Rachman, who was also present, moved in on Rice-Davies. As her lover on and off for almost two years, he became the fount of all good material things – and money seemed a very good thing to the sixteen-year-old from Solihull.

And then there was the third woman who entered the story while still in her teens. Mariella Novotny.

She was born Stella Marie Capes near Sheffield in Yorkshire, according to her birth certificate. The certificate named her mother as Constance Capes, a shorthand typist, but did not identify the father. There is no record of her having attended schools in the area. To fill the gaps, we must fall back on Novotny's own account, a handwritten draft manuscript put together before her death in 1983, on interviews with her future husband and her mother, and on the fragmentary official record.

In an interview with a reporter when Mariella made her debut as a topless dancer – at the London nightspot Latin Quarter – she and her mother indicated she was the offspring of a relationship – perhaps a marriage – between Mrs Capes, who was part Spanish, and a Czech named Anton Novotny, who was serving at the time at a Lincolnshire airbase. Mariella would say later that her father had been 'a Czech in the RAF'.

According to Mrs Capes, they had all travelled to Czechoslovakia after the war. She had returned to England in 1948, when the communists seized power, while her husband – who she said was in the anti-communist underground – attempted to follow two years later with nine-year-old Mariella. According to Mariella, she reached Germany with her father but, after they became separated, she spent months in a camp for displaced persons. To prove it, she would produce a childhood photograph of herself standing in a breadline. She said she was later reunited with her mother in London.

Who exactly Mariella's Czech father was has never been fully resolved, and – given the Cold War security issues that would be at the core of the Profumo Affair – it may be very relevant. Novotny said he was 'first cousin' to President Antonin Novotny, the Khrushchev protégé who came to power in Czechoslovakia – as it then was – in 1957. While a document the authors found shows that he was refused a visa to enter Britain after the war, Mariella's mother said he was eventually admitted. Her husband 'acted very strangely' after his arrival, according to Mrs Capes.

'Mariella has grown up in an atmosphere of intrigue . . . What my husband's secrets were I don't know . . .'

Whatever the elusive truth about Mariella Novotny's father, her link to the Profumo case began shortly before Christmas 1959, when she met Stephen Ward's friend Hod Dibben. He was by this time a nightclub boss again, running a Mayfair joint called the Black Sheep. It would, he said, cater for 'black sheep from the titled families'. His clientele included among others the Duke of Kent, Antony Armstrong-Jones and Douglas Fairbanks Jr. When eighteen-year-old Novotny came his way she was already something of a veteran of London nightlife.

She had started as a hat-check girl at the Pigalle, then graduated to topless dancing. Told there were no dancer vacancies at the Black Sheep, she settled for a job as a waitress and met the boss, Hod Dibben. He was fifty-four years old to her eighteen, but they were married within a month. That came about, supposedly, because – though sensationally good-looking – she could hardly see the customers she was serving in the gloom of the nightclub. When one manager threatened to fire her, she rushed up to Dibben in tears, begging him to help. 'How about if I marry you?' he is said to have replied. Novotny stopped crying and said, 'I will.'

'Hod, of course, was an antique compared to Mariella,' recalled Matt White, a journalist who observed the touching scene, 'but when he put a pair of black-rimmed glasses on her she said, "I still love you. And I can't wait. Let's get married right away."' She took the plunge, Novotny said years later, to get away from her mother.

The couple married in January 1960, with abortionist Dr Sugden as best man, and Dibben found himself within hours facing an unaccustomed hurdle. The new wife he hardly knew was still a virgin. The process of 'de-virginization', as she later put it, took a month to achieve. The deed once done, Novotny recalled, she thought: 'What a fuss people make of so little! . . . I suspected there must be more to it, set about finding out, and am still discovering fresh games to play.'

According to Dibben, his wife's 'first time' occurred in the course of a threesome – he watched from the sidelines, high on amyl nitrate and attired in a leather bondage suit, as a friend had sex with Novotny. If so, she started as she was to continue. 'Possibly my slow, late start as a promiscuous girl,' she wrote in her unpublished memoir, 'urged me to taste more than most . . . Hod made it clear from the start that I could be as permissive as I liked . . . The endless parties that I went to were extravagant, and I met many famous names.'

At one of those parties, Novotny met a friend of her husband who not far in the future would become notorious around the world – Stephen Ward. The party was, she recalled, 'a turning point', one that soon took her to New York and sexual adventures for pay – including, according to her, an encounter with John F. Kennedy.

CHAPTER 9

The Kennedy Connection – Mariella in New York

The party that brought Stephen Ward and Mariella Novotny together was thrown by the American oilman, filmmaker and philanthropist billionaire Huntington Hartford. Hartford, who was Douglas Fairbanks Jr's stepson, reputedly had sex with thousands of women. He kept an apartment in London's Curzon Street solely for assignations with women. They would be delivered – on occasion two or three of them a day – by pimps responding to his every whim.

Also present, and showing that he was much taken by Novotny's good looks, was a show-business impresario named Harry Alan Towers. Soon after, over tea at Claridge's, he came out with an enticing proposition. He said, Novotny remembered, 'He could make me into a television model for commercials, in America.'

Harry Towers had been a leading figure in the founding of commercial television and become a senior executive of ATV. He would eventually go on to success as a producer of movies – they included *Venus in Furs*, *Marquis de Sade: Justine* and *Eugenie . . . The Story of Her Journey into Perversion*. At the time he met Novotny, however, one of his companies had gone into liquidation, owing £48,000 to creditors.

Towers' secretary in 1960, Margaret Van Beers, thought him 'a genius in many ways' but 'a pig' in others – including sex. She recalled with disgust 'the times I left his flat and office and met some sleazy tart on the way up'.

When Towers invited Novotny to his flat, ostensibly merely to meet his mother and several Americans, he apparently had other activity in mind. One of the Americans, having asked her into another room to speak privately, promptly stripped off his clothes. 'I was anxious to do well in New York,' she wrote, 'so I shrugged and decided to do whatever was necessary . . . Neither Towers nor his mother gave any indication of knowing what we had done on our return to the drawing-room . . .'

As for the trip to the States, Towers told the authors he simply asked Novotny, 'Do you want to come to New York and have a laugh?' She agreed, he said, and he bought her a plane ticket. 'The day before I flew to America,' Novotny said, 'Stephen Ward came to dinner and drew three sketches of me.'

Towers and Novotny offered divergent accounts of what happened in New York. She was to tell the FBI, 'Towers took me to the Great Northern Hotel . . . The following afternoon Towers brought a prostitution date to me, ------- ---------- [name redacted in FBI release], who paid me $40 to commit a sexual act. Thereafter I entertained prostitution dates regularly and earned approximately $400 a week. I gave Towers about $300 of this money.' Later, Novotny told the FBI, 'Towers was present when prostitution acts were committed' at a Manhattan apartment. She provided detailed lists of madams and prostitutes who had arranged dates or taken part in threesomes with her – all of them, she claimed, introduced to her by Towers. One of the customers, whom she named, paid for what was in those days a peculiarly British speciality. 'They desired to be whipped with cat-o'-nine-tails.'

Towers told the authors: 'I had an affair with her and didn't know she was a hooker. Our total involvement was that she joined me in New York and lived with me in a couple of hotels . . . I got into trouble through my own stupidity.' Towers dismissed Novotny's accounts as 'fantasy'.

Reality for both Towers and Novotny came the day in March 1961, three months after Novotny's arrival, when police raided Towers' apartment. An anonymous caller had told the District Attorney's office that Novotny was working as a prostitute at that address. Officer Thomas Flood later told a court how he had posed as a customer, waited until Novotny was half naked, then identified himself as a police officer.

'I was in the other room writing a screenplay,' Towers recalled. 'She'd asked if she could come up to meet somebody. I was busy working when she rushed in, naked, and said there was a policeman in the other room.' Novotny, in her memoir, remembered it differently: 'Towers was hiding in a walk-in cupboard. They hauled him out . . . He denied knowing me . . .'

Towers and Novotny were both arrested. He was charged with having imported a woman for prostitution, and Novotny was held as 'a wayward minor'. Bail for Towers was set at $10,000, for Novotny at $500. The Assistant District Attorney who prosecuted the case, Alfred Donati, remembered Novotny as having been 'confident, pretty, with a sense of humor. She looked like a model, not like a whore . . . she made no great denial of the charges.'

Donati was troubled by two elements of the case. Novotny had told him, as had the FBI, that she was related to President Novotny of Czechoslovakia, part of the communist bloc. He said he realised, moreover, that 'It was not just a prostitution case. It would be high profile. I thought celebrity names would be brought in.' At a further court hearing, Donati asked that Towers' passport be confiscated and a higher bail set. He spoke of information that 'a large number of men and women of prominence and very substantial financial means were customers or otherwise involved in the defendant's procurement business. The trial, of necessity, would expose a number of people to a great deal of unwanted publicity, so that – should some or all of them desire to make their resources available to the defendant to induce him to leave the country – there would be nothing to lose except the sum of $10,000 bail presently imposed.'

Judge Matzner, a recent federal appointee, did not grant the request. He asked the FBI to watch Towers and Novotny, but was told that was not possible. Assistant DA Donati was therefore not surprised, shortly afterwards, to learn that Towers had flown the coop. He had left the country – destination unknown. Not long afterwards, Mariella Novotny also got away, having boarded the ocean liner *Queen Mary*, bound for England, under the name "Mrs R. Tyson". She had managed to get aboard without a passport, probably by pretending she was seeing someone off, and was not discovered until the liner was at sea. The ship duly arrived at Southampton, and – in spite of having no passport – Novotny disembarked without difficulty.

'One faction,' Novotny wrote later, 'sighed with relief when I left . . . I had become a political pawn . . . Three authorities, the state police, the FBI and Immigration, were all claiming I came under their jurisdiction, but the most popular theory is that the CIA made my escape easy . . .'

Later, in London, Stephen Ward discussed Novotny's return from America with Mandy Rice-Davies. 'He said,' she recalled, 'that one night the CIA or something had picked her up, literally, from her apartment, and eventually put her on a boat, and that was that. Stephen said it in a matter-of-fact sort of way.'

'Marie [*sic*] Novotny was obviously aided by persons unknown to leave the US as she didn't have the brain power or the money to execute her departure . . .' an FBI official would state in a report obtained by the authors. Who was behind her improbable escape, and who were the 'persons unknown' who wanted her out of the country?

Novotny's account of her American adventure was published soon afterwards in the *News of the World* in the form of a rambling account that told much of her arrest and escape, but little of what she had actually been doing while in New York. In an interview with the authors, however, the newspaper's then chief crime reporter, Peter Earle, revealed that the full story Mariella poured out had been withheld – for diplomatic reasons.

What Novotny had told the paper – and Earle had believed her – was that Harry Towers had arranged for her to have sex both with the man who was about to be inaugurated as President of the United States, John F. Kennedy, and his brother Robert, shortly to become Attorney General.

Shortly after her arrival in New York, Novotny wrote in her unpublished memoir, she had been squired to a series of lunches and parties. She was introduced as 'the new import from swinging London'. The first lunch date, she recalled, had been at the venerable Lüchow's restaurant on East 14th Street, and 'there I met Peter Lawford, one of the leaders of the Kennedy clan . . . Then I was shot into the whirl of parties and was introduced to JFK, the President-elect. I heard several stories of his escapades, and met some of the girls he had had affairs with . . .

'The first time I met JFK was at a large party held at the Hampshire House. Vic Damone, the singer, was the host . . . The suite contained a number of rooms,' Novotny wrote. 'JFK was simply called the Senator and we were shown into an empty bedroom . . . it seemed quite natural to be taken aside for a quiet talk. He talked about England briefly, but locked the door and undressed as he chatted . . .'

Novotny recalled a hurried sexual encounter, followed by a discreet return to Vic Damone's party. The gathering abruptly broke up, she recalled, when Damone's Asian girlfriend locked herself in a bathroom and slashed her wrists. 'I have never known a party finish so quickly. JFK disappeared with a group of close associates – I was bustled out among a crowd of nervous guests . . .'

In a second document, apparently written later, Novotny corrected what she said was an error. Her initial meeting with John Kennedy, she said, had been at an apartment in New York's Gracie Square. It was the first encounter involving sex, she explained, that had taken place at the Hampshire House, and the tryst had been arranged by English actor and Kennedy brother-in-law, Peter Lawford.

Was Novotny's story true?

These days, only the most devoted keepers of the flame deny that John F. Kennedy was a chronic philanderer. 'He had the most active libido of any man I have ever known,' said his close friend and confidant Senator George Smathers. As another politician put it, 'Travelling with him was like travelling with a bull.' Kennedy, who was forty-three when he allegedly bedded the nineteen-year-old Novotny, had no qualms about paying for his pleasure on occasion. In the months that followed, a White House staffer was to recall how he was once turned away by a Secret Service agent with the explanation, 'The President has got a hundred-dollar hooker with him right now.' (In the early 1960s, that was expensive.) A Los Angeles District Attorney's investigator got used to requests from Secret Service colleagues to 'find a woman for the President'. Sometimes the order would be for two young women at a time.

Peter Lawford, who Novotny said was her first contact with the Kennedys, was married to Kennedy's sister Patricia. He was himself a debauched figure, a devotee of group sex and something of a masochist, a trait that may have made Mariella Novotny seem especially interesting. One former female associate recalled that, rather than making love, Lawford 'wanted me to bite his nipples till they bled'. 'I saw Peter,' Dean Martin's former wife Jeanne told one of the authors, 'in the role of pimp for Jack Kennedy.'

The time frame in which the escapade with Novotny allegedly occurred is plausible. Kennedy was elected to the presidency in November 1960 and inaugurated on 20 January 1961. He stayed at the Carlyle hotel, his usual base when in New York City, during the first week of January. As has been well established, Kennedy had his own escape route from the hotel, a series of tunnels that connected the Carlyle with nearby apartment houses and other hotels. Novotny had arrived in New York in December, and did not leave the country until the end of May.

The alleged encounter at the Hampshire House aside, Novotny also recalled an occasion on which she took part in a group sex game with Kennedy. The scenario played out involved two other prostitutes who pretended to be nurse and doctor to Kennedy as patient. It was again Peter Lawford, Novotny claimed, who had recruited the prostitutes. They duly arrived, 'an attractive blonde with a stern face . . . and a younger girl with a kind, fresh look'. One of the women said she had indeed studied medicine at the University of California. After a teasing session with the girls in hospital uniforms, they all had sex together. Subsequently, according to Novotny, she not only visited the President at a house in Washington but also had sex with the President's brother Robert.

While it is possible Novotny fabricated her story, it is not inherently implausible. John Kennedy had long been ill with chronic back and glandular ailments, and had Addison's disease – a condition of the adrenal glands that reduces the ability to resist infection. (It has been suggested that the medication he took for the disease contributed, as it did in other patients, to heightened sexual desire.) Kennedy was no stranger to hospitals, and if he was to have a fetish, a nursing scenario seems as likely as any. Anecdotes of his sex life, from women and from law-enforcement sources, leave little doubt that he enjoyed group sex. Robert Kennedy, meanwhile, though long regarded as a sexual puritan, did have some extramarital dalliances.

In her contacts with the FBI before slipping out of New York, Mariella Novotny produced an address book containing a list of names of men from the worlds of politics, law and business who – she said – had been her clients. According to the Bureau, the address book was later destroyed, as was the FBI's New York file on Towers and Novotny.

The Kennedy brothers, of course, were dead long before the first edition of this book was published. Mariella Novotny died young, in 1983. As for Harry Towers, he pleaded guilty twenty years after the event to a lesser charge of bail-jumping and contempt of court. The prostitution charges were dropped, and he was able to resume his business activities in the United States. He died in 2009.

Following his escape from the US back in 1961, Towers turned up in Moscow. 'The most inaccessible place I could think of was to do a tour of the USSR,' he told the authors. 'It took an awful long time to live it down, and all I did was spend four or five months in the USSR, Czechoslovakia and Hungary . . . It was immediately assumed on top of everything else that I was a communist spy . . .'

The Assistant DA who originally handled the Towers/Novotny case, Alfred Donati, was asked in 1982 whether it had involved espionage. 'I can't comment on that,' he replied. 'Things get back to confidentiality between the District Attorney and the FBI.' Asked whether the case had merely been a vice matter, he responded, 'If it were just an open-and-shut case I could certainly comment on it. Right? You understand what I'm saying? I cannot be more specific . . .'

It is not certain that Mariella Novotny's New York activity in early 1961 involved only Towers. She wrote in her memoir, and he told the authors, that he spent a good deal of his time away from New York. Meanwhile, Novotny's nominal husband – Stephen Ward's friend Hod Dibben – had arrived in Manhattan. Interviewed for this book, Hod Dibben said he visited New York at that time 'to see Mariella and to buy antiques at [auctioneers] Parke-Bernet'.

Dibben said he attended the Hampshire House party at which Novotny allegedly had her first sexual encounter with John Kennedy. He remembered the President-elect being bundled out of the building when it was discovered that a young woman had slashed her wrists in the bathroom. Novotny later told him of her encounters with the Kennedys, and he had believed her. And there was something else.

In her memoir, Novotny recalled having received 'a special delivery letter from Douglas Fairbanks Jr' during her stay in New York. 'Stephen Ward had told him to get in touch . . . Hod and I went to see him and were amused at his prominent display of photographs of the Royal Family. I found him almost a caricature of himself, but he was fun for a while . . .'

In his interviews, Hod Dibben also described how he and Novotny had been to see Fairbanks – he remembered specific details of the Fairbanks apartment. Fairbanks, for his part, told us, 'Although I am very interested in your letter, I am sorry I cannot help you, because I don't remember meeting or even knowing anyone by the name of Mariella Novotny . . . If I did meet Miss Novotny it must have been in a group . . .'

Fairbanks did know Stephen Ward and, as reported earlier, not one but two of Ward's young women claimed to have gone to bed with him. The actor had also, moreover, been a patron of Dibben's Black Sheep Club in London.

Novotny recalled that in early June 1961, back in England following her curiously easy escape from the New York authorities, 'Stephen Ward was the first to contact me . . .' She was soon with Ward at the cottage on the Cliveden estate, on her way to a new career as London's premier orgy hostess. It appears, too, that she was soon to be asked to play a role in an effort to entrap a Soviet agent using diplomatic cover.

Back in Washington DC, Novotny's most famous sex partner was now President – and had doomsday worries on his mind.

CHAPTER 10

A Ploy in a Time of Peril?

John F. Kennedy's friends and family noticed a change in him that summer of 1961. The jaunty young man who had taken office just months earlier seemed worn, preoccupied, would fall into deep thought at social events. One night, sitting up late in the White House, the President telephoned Paul Fay, Secretary of the Navy and an old wartime friend. 'Have you,' he asked, 'got around to building that bomb shelter yet?' 'No,' Fay laughed, 'I built a swimming pool instead.' 'You made a mistake,' Kennedy said quietly.

The presidency had begun with a disastrous skirmish with Fidel Castro, when a US-sponsored invasion of Cuba went down to humiliating defeat at the Bay of Pigs. Now a far greater confrontation was looming – with the Soviet Union. Soviet leader Khrushchev was trying to force the West to relinquish its occupation rights in West Berlin. The giants were wrestling, in a bout that would not end till the Cuban Missile Crisis in late 1962. Then, the world would tremble – more than ever before or since – in the shadow of nuclear war.

The way the world heard the political thunder was through the bombast of politicians: Khrushchev banging his shoe on the desk at the United Nations, Kennedy's defiant cry of 'Let them come to Berlin!' The real doomsday clock ticked down more quietly, in private places where diplomats talked alone: the Rose Garden of the White House, at Chequers, the British Prime Minister's country mansion, and at meetings unknown to anyone but the participants – the secret assignations of spies. Huddled in hotel rooms and restaurants, at airports and border crossings, these men and women spun the thousand threads of the tapestry of information that would eventually determine the decision between peace and war. In 1961, Dr Stephen Ward became part of that tapestry.

Two years later, at the height of the Profumo Affair, Prime Minister Macmillan would ask Lord Denning, the senior judge of the Court of Appeal, to inquire into the security aspects of the scandal. His brief was to 'examine the operation of the Security Service . . . and to consider any evidence there may be for believing that national security has been, or may be, endangered'. What had British intelligence been up to? Had there been a security leak? Those were the questions being asked in Parliament, questions that mattered far more than who had slept with whom.

The 343 numbered paragraphs of the Denning Report, submitted three months later, managed to obscure the very issues it set out to investigate. Its conclusions, almost lost in verbiage, were that British intelligence had correctly decided that 'there was no security interest in the matter', that there had been no security leak.

The reality was that there was a very real security issue, and excellent reasons – from the point of view of the government and of British intelligence – for covering it up. The espionage-related part of the story, Denning suggested, had begun only because Stephen Ward – by then dead and unable to respond – wanted to go to Moscow. Ward, according to the Report, was therefore introduced by the editor of a national newspaper to Captain Yevgeny – or, in the name's English rendering, Eugene – Ivanov, an assistant naval attaché at the Soviet embassy. Then, according to Denning, events tumbled one upon another, by chance rather than design. Ward met Ivanov, who met one of Ward's young women, Christine Keeler. Ivanov and Keeler met Minister for War John Profumo at Lord Astor's swimming pool. The Minister went to bed with Keeler, and the seeds of scandal were sown.

The actual evidence bears throughout the fingerprints of British intelligence – manoeuvring against Soviet intelligence, groping to please its counterparts in the CIA. These were events that developed on the espionage battlefield, the murky backdrop to the world-shaking events of 1961 and 1962. It all supposedly began, however, with a tiresome case of lumbago.

The man with the supposed bad back was Colin Coote, managing editor of the staunchly Conservative *Daily Telegraph*. According to Coote, in his published memoir, a friend suggested he visit Stephen Ward for osteopathic treatment. It worked, and a grateful Coote invited Ward to his home for bridge. Ward played a 'quite passable' game, and the two men got to know each other. It was Coote who brought Ward and Soviet attaché Ivanov together.

In January 1961, Stephen Ward had hurried up the stairs of the Garrick Club, a few minutes late for the lunch that would in the end lead to his downfall. Waiting for him were Coote, David Floyd, the *Telegraph*'s specialist on communist affairs – Floyd had once worked briefly for MI6 in Eastern Europe – and the Soviet assistant naval attaché. 'Sir Colin is a great gourmet,' Ward recalled in his memoir. 'The food and wine were excellent. So was the conversation, and I listened with fascination as Floyd and Eugene Ivanov argued backwards and forwards on issues which I had never heard discussed before in an intelligent and informal manner.' After lunch, Ward and the Soviet diplomat went from the Garrick to Ward's consulting rooms in Devonshire Street, pausing en route to visit the impresario Jack Hylton on Savile Row in Mayfair. Hylton played the piano, and the spy and the osteopath talked. 'I realised for the first time,' Ward wrote, 'that this ought to happen more often – a frank discussion of points of view between ordinary Russians and Englishmen. We arranged to meet again.'

There were further meetings, and they were to have momentous consequences. But why did Colin Coote introduce the pair in the first place? Coote said later that he did so as a favour to Ward. He claimed that, aware of Ward's talent as an artist, he had hired him to go to Israel to draw scenes at the trial of the Nazi war criminal Adolf Eichmann. Subsequently, while again treating Coote for his back ailment, Ward said he was having trouble getting a visa to travel to the Soviet Union, where he hoped to draw Khrushchev. It so happened, according to Coote, that he had met Ivanov a few days earlier during a visit by a group of Soviet naval officers to the offices of the *Telegraph*. Thinking that Ivanov might be able to help Ward get a visa, he therefore set up the luncheon at the Garrick.

The Denning Report was to deal with this entire episode, the beginning of the Profumo Affair, in just nine lines. Coote's own account, published within two years of the Affair, is a jumble of inaccuracies. Ward indeed covered the Eichmann trial for the *Telegraph*, but not until months *after* Coote had introduced him to Ivanov. Stephen Ward himself, in his memoir, said flatly: 'There is no truth in the suggestion that I befriended Ivanov because I wanted to draw Khrushchev.' Colin Coote had suggested he join the lunch party because he thought Ward would find Ivanov 'fascinating'.

David Floyd, the only man who had been at the lunch who was available for interview by the authors, said he was 'drawn into it by Colin Coote, who wanted someone to translate'. There was no translating to do, however, for 'Ivanov spoke very good English'. Floyd said he attached little importance to the lunch at the time.

Coote, in his memoir, poured venom on the dead Ward. The osteopath's political views, he said, referring to Ward's interest in a continuing dialogue with Russia, 'would have seemed ludicrous to a mentally deficient child . . . I should doubt,' he went on, 'whether a more trivial person has ever seriously embarrassed a government.'

Yet Ward was a man whom Coote had chosen as a bridge partner and dining companion. And there was something else. Contrary to the impression Coote gave – that he had met Ward not long before the Profumo Affair began to develop – Ward himself referred to Coote as 'a friend of mine for many years . . . it was this friendship which led me into the limelight over the Profumo Affair'.

Coote seems to have been strangely keen to distance himself from Ward, to suggest that the actions by him that triggered the contact between Ward and the Russian were entirely inadvertent. Nowhere in his memoir did he mention a second Ivanov visit to the offices of the *Telegraph* that Ward referred to in his manuscript. Rebecca West, a perceptive observer of political affairs, was perplexed by the explanation of the Garrick lunch that was given to the public. 'The story,' she mused in her book *The Meaning of Treason*, 'is already odd.'

At the height of the Affair, just before a key debate in the House of Commons, Prime Minister Macmillan sent Coote a letter:

Dear Colin,

I think I ought to let you know that in my speech . . . I shall refer to the fact that as it happened Captain Ivanov was first introduced to Mr Ward by you. I shall say expressly that there was nothing whatever *unusual or reprehensible* [authors' italics] in this introduction. It is only that it forms part of my narrative.

Yours ever,
Harold Macmillan

Coote and Macmillan were both Balliol alumni, old friends from pre-war days, when both had opposed appeasement. Macmillan was known in political circles as the 'Old Actor-Manager', and the note may indicate that there was something unspoken, that he was ensuring that everyone got the story straight. A look at Coote's background may be instructive.

Coote had served with distinction in World War I, then as *The Times*' Rome correspondent in the twenties and thirties. During that period, he had had a second role – as controller of an intelligence network run by Sir Desmond Morton, the number-three man in the Secret Intelligence Service – MI6. In World War II, Coote headed the Public Relations department at the War Office, and was involved in propaganda operations. In the years leading up to the Profumo Affair, he was a close friend and golfing partner of Roger Hollis, the Director General of MI5. He was introduced to Ward by Sir Godfrey Nicholson, who recommended the osteopath to him. Nicholson, a Conservative MP, would later be involved in negotiations with the Soviets.

British intelligence has always used journalists, and there was a time when '*Times* correspondent' was almost synonymous with 'intelligence agent'. As late as 1975, the *Washington Post* reported that some journalists on all London dailies were in the pay of British intelligence. Kim Philby, the double agent and traitor to

Britain, used the *Observer* and *The Economist* as cover in the 1950s. A list of alleged 'agent' journalists published by the Soviets was probably supplied to them by Philby. It included the name of Michael Berry – later to become Lord Hartwell – owner and editor-in-chief of the *Daily Telegraph* and thus boss of the man who set up the meeting between Ward and Ivanov. The *Telegraph*'s foreign editor, S. R. 'Pops' Pawley, is known to have been the paper's principal liaison with the security and intelligence services.

Why would British intelligence contrive such a meeting? For various reasons, some justifiable, some less so, straightforward reporting about British intelligence is notoriously difficult. Writers must obviously make careful judgements as to whether to reveal the identity of agents, who might be personally damaged by disclosure. Using the Official Secrets Acts, meanwhile, the government has gone to ludicrous lengths to prevent former intelligence officials from publishing their memoirs, and to protect secrets that need no longer be secret. From this point on in this book, although sources will always be named if possible, a number must remain anonymous. We ask the reader to bear with us as we investigate British intelligence operations following Yevgeny Ivanov's arrival in Britain.

CHAPTER 11

A Net for an Agreeable Spy

Ivanov had taken up his post as an assistant naval attaché at the Soviet embassy in March 1960, ten months before the fateful introduction to Stephen Ward. He held the rank of captain, second rank, in the Soviet Navy, equivalent to a commander in the British service. He was thirty-seven, dark and tall, unusual in a man who claimed Mongol ancestry. Colin Coote deemed him 'an agreeable personality', while Christine Keeler was to think him a 'huggy-bear of a man'. He was well mannered and more sophisticated than most of the Soviet diplomats Moscow sent abroad in those days. He enjoyed socialising, and seemed to be free to meet with foreigners – as at the Coote luncheon – without a Soviet colleague tagging along. There was something different about Ivanov, and MI5 had noticed.

MI5's D Branch, responsible for counter-espionage, quickly identified Ivanov as a Soviet intelligence officer using diplomatic cover, a common practice worldwide. According to one source, part of Ivanov's mission may have been to supervise Soviet penetration of Britain's naval base at Portland in Dorset. Portland, the development base for several of Britain's most secret submarine and radar projects, had in the late 1950s been the target of

Soviet spy Gordon Lonsdale, who in turn controlled Harry Houghton and his girlfriend Ethel Gee, who worked at the base. MI5's surveillance of the Portland spy ring had continued for more than a year until arrests were made in January 1961 – the month of Ward's introduction to Ivanov. Whether its interest in Ivanov involved Portland or not, MI5 had by early 1961 built up a dossier on him.

In April that year, three months after Coote's luncheon with Ivanov and Ward, one of the most important episodes in the history of espionage took place, at dead of night, at London's Mount Royal Hotel. The chief delegate of a Soviet trade delegation slipped out of his room and proceeded to a suite on the floor above. The suite had been specially prepared for a major intelligence debriefing – tape recorders, encoding machines, radio equipment, and a special phone link to the CIA in Arlington, Virginia.

The team waiting to talk with the Russian included MI6's leading Soviet specialists, Harold Shergold and his assistant Michael Stokes, and – from the CIA – Joseph Bulik and George Kisvalter. Kisvalter, known as 'Teddy Bear', was the lead interviewer. The Soviet traitor about to be questioned was for Allied intelligence the 'single most important spy' ever to bring his country's secrets to the West.

He was Oleg Penkovsky, nominally a senior civilian member of the State Committee for Coordination of Scientific Research, in fact a colonel in the GRU – Soviet military intelligence. Contrary to a popular notion, it was the GRU, rather than the internal security apparatus the KGB, that was responsible for most Soviet intelligence successes. The GRU had considerable independence, and GRU officers considered themselves the professional superiors of their KGB counterparts.

Colonel Penkovsky had fallen into MI6's lap in November 1960, after he approached an official at the Canadian embassy in

Moscow. The contacts matured during the London visit in the spring of 1961, as he sat in the Mount Royal Hotel pouring out Soviet secrets. So much was there to discuss during the nocturnal exchanges that MI6 kept a doctor on hand with drugs to keep Penkovsky awake. His nickname became 'Sleepless Nights' and the resulting material was code-named 'Alexander'.

The 'Alexander' dossier produced information directly relevant to MI5's interest in Captain Ivanov. Penkovsky, using his access to the GRU's central registry – and thus to the personal files of numerous GRU officers – was able to provide much detail on GRU personnel at the Soviet embassy in London. They included station chief Nicolai Karpekov – case officer for the homosexual Admiralty spy William Vassall – his deputy Anatolij Pavlov, and assistant naval attaché Ivanov, who had attended the same training school as Penkovsky.

Usually, when a new Soviet diplomat arrived in town, Western intelligence had little more to go on than a name, a rank and another taciturn foreigner in an ill-cut suit. The rest was a blank requiring investigation. From Penkovsky's information, passed on by MI6, and from its other sources, MI5 was now able to put features on the Ivanov blank.

His relations by marriage were significant. A sister-in-law was married to the former Soviet air attaché in London, who was also a member of the GRU *rezidentura*, or local station. His father-in-law was Alexander Gorkin, Chairman of the Soviet Supreme Court. Ivanov was a drinker and womaniser, and Gorkin had once had to intercede to save him from dismissal following an arrest for drunkenness during a posting in Norway. The man who had tried to fire him was the current head of the GRU, General Ivan Serov, a veteran of SMERSH and the KGB, of which he had been head in the mid-1950s.

MI5 thus knew that Ivanov, connected by marriage to a man

high in the Moscow elite, had – whatever his professional talents – risen through the bureaucracy thanks to family patronage. Ivanov, by now known in London diplomatic circles as 'Foxface', had brought with him his wife, a shy, petite former teacher. As MI5 had not failed to observe, the attaché liked his alcohol, and regularly left his wife to cool her heels at home. He drove a black Austin A40, and bought his clothes at Barkers in Kensington High Street.

By 1961 standards, Ivanov was a somewhat different sort of Russian. As the Coote lunch had shown, he was trusted to meet Westerners on his own. MI5 wondered: was he a dedicated GRU man doing his job, or was he – just maybe – susceptible to an approach? The regime of Ivanov's boss, General Serov, was extraordinarily corrupt, even in a system in which corruption was a way of life. Historically, this was a period when a few GRU officers voluntarily made contact with Western services and provided useful information. Those contacts, however, had been made with US intelligence, and MI5 was keen – almost desperate – to develop its own Soviet sources.

Might it be that, adroitly handled, Ivanov could prove a useful source? Was there even a possibility that, in intelligence parlance, he could be turned? Was he potentially that ultimate prize, a traitor in place, or perhaps a valuable defector?

The Denning Report would state tersely that there had come a point when 'a thought occurred to the Security Service that . . . it might be possible to get Ivanov to defect?' Denning would be in a quandary, however. He had to go through the motions of showing he had looked into the performance of the security services, because that was his brief. The very idea of such an investigation, however, was a contradiction in terms. The Security Service in Britain was built on the principle that it must remain secret. Its very existence was not mentioned in the Official Secrets Acts, the legislation governing national security. In 1963, an Establishment under attack had no interest in rocking the boat of the Service, a creature of the Establishment staffed by Establishment officers born and bred into the same class as the Conservative Prime Minister and his ministers.

Lord Denning was able to report that he had made two visits to MI5 headquarters and had interviewed its chief, Roger Hollis. MI5 even gave him some documents for publication, the first and only time such material had been provided by British intelligence. 'I had complete access to their files, memoranda, correspondence,' Denning was to say in 1986. A senior MI5 officer, however, speaking unattributably, said flatly, 'Denning had wool pulled over his eyes.'

Peter Wright, the MI5 officer at the centre of a 1987 row over publication of his memoirs, was to say of his own case, 'None of the files will be released. The Director has supreme power . . . what they do is, they cook the files for an enquiry.' Wright, who had served in MI5 at the time of the Profumo Affair, sounded as though he spoke from experience. MI5 did not willingly cooperate with Denning – to the extent it did so, it acted on the instructions of the Prime Minister. It seems that high MI5 officials – including, according to Wright, Director General Hollis himself – showed Denning files that had been doctored, or 'sanitised'. At best, MI5 did not lie – it simply did not tell the whole truth, and certainly not about its plans for Ivanov.

The notion of Ivanov defecting did not just 'occur' to MI5. The turning of an important defector is a matter as sensitive as the hooking of a trout in an especially difficult pool. The right lure must be selected, the cast well made, the right moment chosen to strike. Should the lure be taken, the fish must be played with skill and patience before it ends up in the landing net. A false move during the first stages of the process, and the prey is gone.

So it is in intelligence. MI5 would happily have devoted months, even years, to the turning of an Ivanov.

On 18 January 1961, FBI files reveal, the ideal sort of information for such an operation reached MI5. A few months earlier, Ivanov had attended a party at the home of a US naval attaché at which he 'drank too much, was boisterous, made passes at wives'. A photograph that appeared later showed him in a friendly embrace with the assistant naval attaché's wife. So it was that Britain's Director of Naval Intelligence sent a report on Ivanov to the Foreign Office. Ivanov's 'character weaknesses,' he wrote, 'are apparent when he is under the influence of alcohol, notably his lack of discretion and loss of personal control, his thirst for women and his tactless bluster'.

The best guess is that MI5's operation began that same month, January, at the Colin Coote luncheon. Stephen Ward, perhaps unwittingly at that point, was the lure. One MI5 source has said that the service became interested in Ward only months later, on account of Ivanov's visits to his flat. The claim is less than convincing. The source claimed Ward was identified only by matching his name to his address – 17 Wimpole Mews – on the Electoral Roll. The authors found, however, that Ward's name did not appear in connection with that address in 1961 – or in any other year. (In fact, the Service had initially approached the wrong 'Ward'!)

More likely, British intelligence was aware of Ward *before* the planning for the Ivanov operation. A former MI6 source says his service was briefed on the plan, and that MI5 knew about Ward through his friend Lord Astor, himself a former naval intelligence officer with experience in manipulating enemy agents. The decision to put Ivanov and Ward together was made following Ivanov's visit to the *Daily Telegraph* offices as part of a Soviet naval group. After that, it would not seem contrived for editor Colin

Coote, a personal friend of the head of MI5, to invite Ivanov to lunch.

Astor and Coote both knew Ward well, and knew he fitted the bill as a lure for Ivanov. Ward could appear soft on the Soviet Union – he was forever talking about dialogue between nations and seeing the good side of communism. He was a social gadfly likely to be glad to roam the London social scene with a real live Russian in tow. Ward, moreover, would give Ivanov a good time. As Astor – and a large number of wealthy men in London – knew, Ward could always be relied upon to provide a 'popsy'.

The elements were there for, at a minimum, a reconnaissance. Perhaps, just perhaps, there might be a successful operation, using a woman to target Ivanov. The Soviets themselves had long been exponents of the honeytrap ploy, but – by the early sixties – Western agencies were also interested in it. Alert to this, KGB and GRU officers were taught to beware of women in bars and nightclubs because they might be in the pay of a hostile service. Sexual liaisons outside Soviet embassy communities were forbidden.

Ivanov, the Russian target now under consideration, was not only a trained agent but also – and it might make him less vulnerable – a married man. However, as Denning would report, he also 'drank a good deal, and was something of a ladies' man'. Using Ward might be a way to get him into the company of a female who was not a common prostitute, to catch him off his guard. A honeytrap might work. In any case, an introduction to Ward was a way to bring the Soviet attaché into the orbit of men who were not only Ward's friends but also close to MI5 – without scaring him off. It might work.

So it was that, following lunch at the Garrick, Stephen Ward came to take a stroll through London with Ivanov, then invite him to visit the cottage on Lord Astor's estate at Cliveden.

Without special permission, Soviet diplomats were not allowed to travel more than twenty-five miles outside London. Happily, however, Cliveden was just inside the red circle that marked the limit on the map the attaché kept in his car. Ivanov drove down to the cottage that very weekend.

Ward was to write: 'We all chip in there with the work, chopping wood, washing up, cooking and cleaning. [Ivanov] joined in with gusto . . .' Ivanov was soon a regular guest. 'We used to ramble in the lovely woodland, and picnic on the lawn,' Ward recalled. 'He used to heave rocks about as I built my rock garden, and we constructed a flight of steps which we christened the Steppes of Russia.'

Back in London, Ivanov started to spend time at the Wimpole Mews flat in Marylebone. Ward and the Soviet played bridge, a game Ward loved and of which Ivanov knew the rudiments. As his bridge improved, he began to meet Ward's friends. 'He used to come round at any time,' Ward wrote, 'usually bearing vodka or some rare and undrinkable liqueur from some remote part of Russia.'

There was talk about politics. 'Many were the arguments and discussions we had, some heated, always ending in a draw,' according to Ward. New acquaintances got over their misgivings about hobnobbing with a Russian. People discovered, Ward thought, 'that Russians could be very human, and that it was possible that there was another side of the question. I seldom saw disapproval . . . there was curiosity and interest.'

At Cliveden, Ivanov was 'obviously fascinated' – as Ward put it – by the idea of visiting Lord Astor's mansion, just half a mile from Ward's cottage. The Russian seemed convinced that the aristocracy still played a key role in Britain, and he may not have been entirely wrong. On his visits to Wimpole Mews in London, meanwhile, he was only rarely accompanied by his wife. Ivanov encountered several of Ward's girls – including Christine Keeler.

* * *

That spring of 1961, Ward the artist was busier and more successful – in august company – than ever before. In January, the month he had met Ivanov, his work had been exhibited at the Leggatt gallery in Jermyn Street. This was an honour, the first time the gallery had shown the works of a living artist since its foundation in 1820. According to the broadcaster Walter Harris, Ward's ability as an artist got the attention of the Prime Minister, so much so that he gave permission for Ward to draw Parliament in session at the House of Commons.

Macmillan himself sat for Ward, and in little more than a year so did Sir Winston Churchill, Home Secretary R. A. Butler, former Chancellor of the Exchequer Derick Heathcote-Amory, Speaker Sir Harry Hylton-Foster, Leader of the Opposition Hugh Gaitskell and, from overseas, Canadian Prime Minister John Diefenbaker and Cypriot leader Archbishop Makarios.

Former Foreign Secretary Selwyn Lloyd, who was now Chancellor of the Exchequer, sat for Ward, for the second time, in March 1961. On that occasion, the artist-osteopath took the opportunity to add a mischievous little crack about the government's unpopular current national 'Pay Pause' – he sketched in, behind the Chancellor's ear, a minute hammer and sickle. He mentioned to Lloyd, too, that he had friends at the Soviet embassy and thought Soviet diplomats should be cultivated.

Lloyd emerged from the sitting uneasy about Ward's attitude and background, and – back in his office – inquired what information MI6 might have on Ward. The letter of introduction that had originally led him to see Ward, meanwhile, was sent to MI5. That Lloyd took this action was to be suppressed by the government after the Profumo scandal broke, 'lest,' wrote Prime Minister Macmillan, 'it be known to the press that enquiries about Ward had been instituted as early as 1961 and ignored'.

This episode, however, should not be taken to mean that Ward was not being manipulated. Just weeks later, he would be on his way to Israel for the *Daily Telegraph*, to sketch Nazi war criminal Adolf Eichmann at his trial in Jerusalem. With him on the trip, to write the story, was the Earl of Birkenhead, brother-in-law of *Telegraph* editor Coote, and a veteran of political intelligence.

The editor of the *Illustrated London News*, Sir Bruce Ingram, meanwhile, was so impressed by Ward's skill as an artist that he commissioned him to do a series of sketches of the Royal Family. The fact that Ingram had been close to the Queen's grandfather, George V, oiled the approach to Buckingham Palace. Between March and July, Ward sketched eight royals: the Queen's sister Princess Margaret and her husband Antony Armstrong-Jones, the Duke and Duchess of Gloucester, the Duke and Duchess of Kent, Princess Marina – and Prince Philip.

As he scurried from sitting to prestigious sitting, Ward continued to see Soviet assistant naval attaché Yevgeny Ivanov. The authorised history of MI5 claims that the service learned in May 1961 that Ward was seeking to impress Ivanov by boasting of his society connections. If he did, it was very clearly no idle boast. According to the authorised history, it was now that MI5 decided to make a direct approach to Ward.

Did MI5 fear that Ivanov might, through Ward, get access to or information on people at the very highest levels of the British Establishment – even at the level of the Royal Family? Or did it now see its opportunity to entrap the Soviet spy?

Ward's 9 June 1961 audience with Prince Philip at Buckingham Palace went well. Ward thought the Queen's husband 'a wonderful sitter, still as a rock, but relaxed'. The sketching session, though, was not quite the same as those with other members of the Royal Family. As the sitting began, the Prince exclaimed, 'By

Jove! You're the osteopath. I never connected you with this appointment.' He had not realised that the artist Stephen Ward who had come to draw him was one and the same as the Dr Stephen Ward he had met back in the 1940s. Before he left the Palace, Ward recalled, he and the Prince 'discussed the old days'.

'The old days' – the years of the Milford Haven debauches – were not a topic the Prince would relish becoming a public talking point. Had he had an inkling of the scandal that was to break around Ward, he would not have been so relaxed.

CHAPTER 12

Dr Ward is Recruited

On Sunday, 4 June 1961, at the start of a broiling summer, President Kennedy flew into England and drove through the streets of London in an open car, cheered by the crowds, Prime Minister Macmillan at his side.

Kennedy knew England well. He had spent time here as a young man before World War II, when his father was American ambassador. Then and on subsequent visits, he had enjoyed himself amongst the elite of British society. He had met the Astors and the Cliveden set, controversial at the time for their efforts to keep Britain out of the war. The President was even linked by marriage to the British leader he was now visiting – Macmillan had married a daughter of the 9th Duke of Devonshire, while Kennedy's sister Kathleen had married a son of the 10th Duke.

On this London trip, the President was staying at the Georgian townhouse near Buckingham Palace of his sister-in-law, Princess Lee Radziwill, whose daughter's christening at Westminster Cathedral he was to attend. Kennedy's chronic bad back, recently wrenched during a tree-planting ceremony, was giving him severe pain – at a time of great international tension.

Kennedy had flown into London following a gruelling summit meeting with Khrushchev. The Soviet leader had taken the two great powers closer to military confrontation over Berlin. Sixteen years after World War II, he declared, it was intolerable that West Berlin should retain its separate status as an island, accessible to US troops, inside East Germany. That East Germany and its borders remained unrecognised, moreover, was also intolerable. Khrushchev had told Kennedy he planned within months to sign a treaty with the East that would cancel Allied occupation rights. The intention was to force the withdrawal of Allied troops from West Berlin and replace them with a Soviet force.

Khrushchev said the proposed changes would bring peace. Kennedy saw them as an ultimatum. What Khrushchev wanted would disrupt NATO, give Moscow the ideological initiative in Europe and demoralise West Germany. The West would be humiliated, the balance of power shifted. Existing plans in the event of trouble over Berlin assumed a US military response, and the possibility of World War III – nuclear war.

Now, in London, the President consulted Harold Macmillan. Charles de Gaulle, in France, and Chancellor Adenauer of West Germany were urging a show of strength against the Soviets. Over drinks at Downing Street, Macmillan told the young President to avoid making Khrushchev feel trapped. Driven into a corner, the Soviet leader might indeed resort to violence. The President listened, then flew home. His wife Jacqueline stayed on, to dine next evening with Jakie Astor, brother of Stephen Ward's friend Lord Astor.

At that very time, the US ambassador David Bruce received a request from Sir Bruce Ingram – the *Illustrated London News* editor who had also arranged for the Royal Family sittings – asking him to sit for a portrait by Ward. He did so a few weeks later, and Bruce and the artist-osteopath got on well.

Back in the United States, President Kennedy flew to Florida to rest for a few days and nurse his bad back. He had seen specialists during the European trip and – according to one source – Stephen Ward may have been one of them. Averell Harriman, who had accompanied the President to Europe as an adviser, had – while ambassador to London after the war – been one of the first of Ward's famous patients. Another, more recently, had been former President Eisenhower. When his successor arrived, suffering agonies from back pain, Ward would have been a natural choice.

Later, Ward recalled a prophetic conversation he had with Yevgeny Ivanov during Kennedy's visit to Europe. 'What,' Ward asked the Soviet attaché, 'would happen to a Russian in Moscow who had an Englishman for a friend?' 'Oh,' Ivanov replied, 'he'd be visited pretty soon by the Secret Service, just like you will be here.' 'Nonsense,' Ward replied. 'Oh yes you will,' retorted Ivanov.

He was right. Within a week, on 8 June, Ward received a telephone call from the War Office, asking the osteopath if he would mind meeting 'our Mr Woods' for 'a little chat'. 'Woods', we now know, was Keith Wagstaffe, an MI5 officer working for DI(a) Operations, a section of the counter-intelligence branch. Wagstaffe in turn then called Ward, giving his address as Room 393 at the War Office – MI5's front address. Before calling, Wagstaffe had read an informant report noting that Ward 'was a difficult sort of person, inclined to be against the government. This attitude stemmed from the war years, when the Army refused to recognise his American medical degree . . . At some time or other Ward had been declared bankrupt, and he is also believed to have been involved in a call-girl racket.'

Ward agreed to meet with Wagstaffe, and the two men lunched together in Marylebone. In Ward's account of the meeting, in his draft memoir, he recalled Wagstaffe as having been 'charming, well-dressed, obviously an army officer in plain clothes'. Wagstaffe openly acknowledged his affiliation to MI5. He said his people had 'noticed' Ward's friendship with Ivanov. When Ward asked whether they had any objection, Wagstaffe replied, according to Ward, 'None at all. In fact, we like the Russians to meet ordinary people in this country.'

Wagstaffe wanted to know what sort of questions the Soviet attaché had been asking, Ward recalled. 'I put his mind at rest at once. Ivanov had never sought any guarded information.' Wagstaffe told him, 'If anything should happen that you feel we should know about, I want you to contact me immediately.'

As later supplied to Lord Denning by MI5, Wagstaffe's contact report read:

> Ward, who has an attractive personality and who talks well, was completely open about his association with Ivanov ... Ward asked whether it was all right for him to continue to see Ivanov. I replied there was no reason why he should not. He then said that, if there was any way in which he could help, he would be very ready to do so. I thanked him for his offer and asked him to get in touch with me should Ivanov at any time in the future make any propositions to him ... Despite the fact that some of his political ideas are certainly peculiar and are exploitable by the Russians, I do not think that he is of security interest, but *he is obviously not a person we can make any use of* [authors' italics].

Is that last sentence credible, or was Wagstaffe's report doctored for publication in the Denning Report? There is reason to think it was indeed doctored – to distance MI5 from Ward. Colin Coote's role in introducing Ward, and information from intelligence sources, indicate that Ward was deliberately brought together with the Soviet attaché. MI5 was now risking a direct approach to Ward, not least because it would seem the natural development, the one Ivanov had in fact predicted. Not to have contacted Ward at this point would, indeed, have seemed a suspicious omission.

Ward saw Ivanov within days of meeting with Wagstaffe, to ask him whether he could arrange for the Soviet Minister of Culture, Yekaterina Furtseva, who was about to visit London, to sit for a portrait. Ivanov did arrange it, and the portrait duly appeared in the *Daily Telegraph*. Surprisingly, the *Telegraph* acquiesced to a Soviet plea that an account by Ward of the talk he had with Furtseva should not be published. She was a powerful figure in Soviet politics, of whom it was said, 'What Furtseva thinks, Khrushchev says . . .' Furtseva's daughter was married to Deputy Prime Minister Frol Koslov, who was considered a possible successor to Khrushchev.

Furtseva's talk with Ward had covered a wide range of political topics and – published or not – may have been passed to Colin Coote's friends in intelligence. Why, though, was Ward granted this unusual opportunity to talk privately with a senior Soviet minister? As MI5 watched Ivanov, and as the Berlin Crisis developed, what was Soviet intelligence up to?

The week before Furtseva sat for Ward, the *Daily Express* – a paper that contained some good reporting in those days – had carried a story about Soviet sexual entrapment and blackmail of foreigners. The writer, the star correspondent Chapman Pincher – who specialised in espionage stories – was drawing on an MI5 source he identified to the authors as Michael McCaul. McCaul told Pincher that British intelligence was concerned about the potential risk to British nationals attending the forthcoming Electronics Trade Fair in Moscow. An article on past cases, the MI5 officer suggested, would serve as a timely warning to businessmen not to fall for sexual approaches made to them in the Soviet Union.

In the event, a Conservative MP named Anthony Courtney did walk into such a trap at the Fair. Courtney, who had campaigned in Parliament for a reduction in the number of Soviet embassy personnel in London, succumbed to seduction by an Intourist guide who was in reality a 'swallow', a female KGB agent with special training. The Soviets then successfully used photographs of Courtney and the woman, in various states of undress, to cause him disgrace at home. He duly lost his seat at the next election.

Also in Moscow that spring was Greville Wynne, an MI6 agent on a vital mission. Posing as a businessman, his task was to renew contact with Colonel Penkovsky, the Soviet who had passed on important information – including details about attaché Ivanov, identifying him as a GRU officer – during his recent visit to London. By way of deception on the Moscow trip, Wynne was to pass low-grade technical data to Penkovsky in order that Penkovsky could claim – as cover – that it was he who had recruited Wynne. A Soviet 'swallow' tried to get Wynne into bed during the visit, but the Englishman – a trained agent, alert to such possible tricks – rebuffed the advances.

In London, the *Daily Express* article on such Soviet practices had drawn a sharp response. The Soviet press attaché, Anatolij Strelnikov, ranted on at reporter Pincher for having published the story, then offered a bribe if he would reveal his sources. Pincher duly reported the episode to his contact in MI5. This was a time of honeytrap and attempted honeytrap, of trick and counter-trick.

Stephen Ward was never publicly linked to any Soviet official other than Ivanov. We discovered, though, that Ward was in contact with at least two other Soviet officials. Following Ward's death in 1963, discovered amongst his possessions were ten 35mm colour transparencies, taken by Ivanov, outside the Cliveden cottage and at the Soviet embassy. Details in the pictures suggest they were taken in the summers of 1961 and 1962 – and two of them feature press attaché Strelnikov, the Soviet who tried to recruit Chapman Pincher.

What to make of this additional Ward contact with the Soviets?

Had he merely met the diplomat socially, in the course of his acquaintance with Ivanov? Or was there more to it? And why is there no mention of this evidence in the Denning Report, which was set up specifically to examine the security angle?

We may never know now who was playing what game. The Soviets, suspicious about Coote's introduction of Ivanov to Ward – and knowing or guessing at Coote's connections – may have sought to turn the situation in their favour. MI5, on the other hand, had been hoping to obtain evidence that would get Strelnikov expelled from the country. They would have had it when Strelnikov tried to bribe *Daily Express* reporter Pincher, had not Arthur Christiansen, the paper's editor, refused to complain to the Foreign Office for fear of endangering his correspondent in Moscow. Had MI5 hoped, through Strelnikov's contact with Ward, that he would compromise himself again?

Following the rebuff by Pincher, Strelnikov went on to turn his attention to Betty Boothroyd, who in the distant future – as a Labour Party MP – would become the first (and so far only) female Speaker of the House of Commons. Back then, early in her career, she had served as legislative assistant to a US congressman, then returned to Britain to work as an aide to senior Labour Party politicians. MI5 monitored the Soviet operation against Boothroyd. Did it, though, fail to realise the Soviets were trying a honeytrap operation against a far more significant target?

Also found in Ward's pocket after his death was a calling card that bore the name 'Evgenij Beliakov'. Beliakov had been a first secretary at the Soviet embassy – but only until mid-1962. It stands to reason, therefore, that Ward had met Beliakov many months before his death in mid-1963. Until now, no one appears to have realised the significance of that calling card.

The authors can reveal that Beliakov was a senior KGB officer who specialised in honeytrap operations. Earlier, while serving with Ivanov in Norway, he had taken part in an attempt to compromise Werna Gerhardsen, the wife of that country's prime minister. By using her and her influence over her husband, the Soviets hoped to undermine Norway's ties with the United States. KGB officer Beliakov was good-looking, with a charming personality, and reportedly had managed to seduce Gerhardsen. Compromising photographs had been taken, according to a Soviet defector. The Norwegian press finally reported in 2013, based on newly released Russian files, that Gerhardsen did pass secret NATO information to the KGB.

The purpose of later posting Beliakov to London, according to Russian sources, was to carry out a specific honeytrap operation. The new target? Sources suggest it may have been Minister for War John Profumo's wife, Valerie Hobson. Once Profumo himself was compromised and open to potential blackmail, however, there would no longer have been any point in targeting Hobson. This may explain Beliakov's departure from London in mid-1962.

Why, though, at his death in 1963, was Ward carrying the card of a Soviet agent who had left Britain a year earlier? Why, moreover, is there no reference to Beliakov in either the Denning Report or in any known MI5 report?

A report by Ward's MI5 contact Wagstaffe did, however, contain a significant aside. 'More than once,' it read, 'Ward assured me that if Ivanov . . . showed any inclination to defect, he would get in touch with me immediately.' Once again – as published in the Denning Report – that sentence has an odd ring to it. As Ward had no reason to imagine that Ivanov would consider defection – the osteopath's memoir shows that the Soviet struck him as a dedicated communist – it would seem highly unlikely that *Ward* brought up the possibility of defection. The evidence indicates, however, that in June, immediately after the Wagstaffe meeting, Ward began setting a honeytrap for Ivanov.

He started by trying to capitalise on the return from New York of Mariella Novotny, fresh from the brush with the law that had followed her encounters with President-elect Kennedy. Ward got in touch within days of her arrival at Southampton on 4 June, according to Novotny. 'He pestered me almost daily,' she wrote in her memoir, 'to meet Eugene Ivanov.'

By her account, though, she was unwilling to be the would-be seductress of a Soviet diplomat. 'After my strange experience in the States,' she wrote, 'I vowed to avoid politicians of either side. I had been warned by a responsible lawyer that I should be careful whom I mixed with in the political scene. I appreciated this sound advice . . . [Ward's] most pressing invitations to attend Soviet Embassy parties etc. were all rejected . . . But Ward was not to be put off, he pressured me to have lunch one Sunday at Cliveden . . . he gave me his assurance Ivanov would not be present . . .'

Her concerns thus assuaged, and driving the Mercedes sports car she had acquired, Novotny drove down to Cliveden. Ward had told her to come before other lunch guests arrived so he could show her Lord Astor's famous gardens. 'He took me straight into the cottage,' she said. 'A man stood with his back to us, looking from the window onto the river . . . It was Ivanov – Ward introduced us quickly and rushed from the room . . . Ivanov talked well, and said that he was aware I had avoided meeting him . . . His manner was so nice it was difficult to fault . . . Ward brought drinks in, explained he had had no idea Ivanov was coming, and left us alone.'

According to Novotny, Ivanov tried to play on her missing Czech father, hinting that he could help arrange a visa to Prague – a trip Novotny had always assumed would likely be fraught with problems. 'The temptation was great, exactly what I had hoped for one day,' she wrote. She was suspicious and afraid, nevertheless, and cut Ivanov short 'before he could tell me what was expected on my part. I left him alone and joined the other people arriving for lunch.' 'She realised she was being set up' her husband Hod Dibben said she told him.

'My controversial American involvement was of special interest, I was later informed,' Novotny said years later, referring to her sexual encounter with John F. Kennedy. She did not say just who told her this had been what Ivanov especially wanted to know about, but such information would obviously have been of interest to any Soviet agent. Ward, she said, had been describing her to all and sundry as 'the girl who made such an impact in America with the Kennedy clan'.

Novotny had no doubt the meeting with Ivanov had been orchestrated. She felt, too, 'that Bill Astor had a hand in the matter. From evidence I later saw, it was obvious Astor gave Ward his orders and controlled him to a great extent . . .' Ward's role as procurer for his wealthy friends was continuing, and in parallel to his efforts on behalf of MI5. Soon, Novotny noticed, Ward was trying to pair her off with one John Profumo, Minister for War. 'Profumo was another friend of Ward's I did not take to . . .' Whether that was the truth or not – it would surely have been unlike Novotny to be so choosy – Ward was busily putting the finishing touches to another young woman, one he had been grooming since their first meeting: Christine Keeler.

That summer Novotny's husband told her of an odd evening spent at Ward's flat in Wimpole Mews. 'Hod watched Christine [Keeler] serve dinner. Ward had finished training her, but – to test her ability – instructed her to cook, lay the table correctly, and eat with them. Hod related to me her lapses, and how Ward told her not to sprinkle salt on her food . . . Several such mistakes were criticised by Ward – he wanted to impress Hod with his teaching technique.' What was Ward, in his Pygmalion role, preparing Keeler for?

MI5 officer Keith Wagstaffe and Ward had not parted immediately following their first meeting, the lunch in early June 1961. Instead, Wagstaffe had accompanied Ward back to Wimpole Mews. There, according to Wagstaffe's report as published by Denning, 'he introduced me to a young girl, whose name I did not catch, who was obviously sharing the house with him. She was heavily painted and considerably overdressed, and I wondered . . . whether this is corroborating evidence of the allegation . . . that he has been involved in the call-girl racket.'

The girl was Christine Keeler. She served tea, and – Wagstaffe was to acknowledge later – he was greatly impressed by how lovely she was. If MI5 was hoping to set a honeytrap for Ivanov, Keeler fitted the bill as the honey.

Exactly a month later, two bees would be buzzing about the honey. One of them was Ivanov. The other would be John Profumo, the British Minister for War. And that, assuredly, was not part of MI5's operational plan.

CHAPTER 13

A Screw of Convenience

'The first time I met Jack Profumo he was in a dinner jacket and I was clutching a towel around me. My hair was hanging in strings, water was pouring off me – and I was acutely embarrassed.' Thus, two years later – her embarrassment alleviated by payment of a huge fee from the *News of the World* – did Christine Keeler describe her fateful encounter with the Minister for War beside Lord Astor's swimming pool in July 1961.

High summer that year brought little relaxation for world leaders. In the United States, it was then that President Kennedy advised a friend that he should be building a bomb shelter. As the crisis over Berlin rumbled on, British Prime Minister Macmillan was trying to unite the European allies. 'It is quite clear,' he declared, 'that we cannot countenance interference with Allied rights in Berlin. This is an issue on which the peoples of the Western World are resolute. It is a principle which they will defend.'

There was pressure on John Profumo. It was his task to honour promises that Britain would increase its troop numbers in Germany, and that was virtually impossible. Not enough soldiers were available, and Profumo was responsible for recruitment. There were serious problems, too, with a current operation in the Middle East. Six thousand troops had been sent to shore up the beleaguered oil emirate of Kuwait, then, as it would be in the future, under threat from neighbouring Iraq. Unprepared for conditions in the Persian Gulf, the rescue force did not perform well, and Profumo got the blame.

On Saturday, 8 July, in spite of these worries, Britain's War Minister took a weekend off. Accompanied by his wife Valerie, he headed for Cliveden, where Lord Astor was playing host to some thirty guests. The Astor house party included Lord and Lady Dalkeith, several Tory MPs, the Profumos and the guest of honour, the President of Pakistan, Field Marshal Ayub Khan. Khan was en route to Washington for talks on Berlin and the role of the non-aligned nations.

Two years later, when the Profumo scandal broke, the fact that Khan had been at Cliveden that weekend would cause a secondary frisson of alarm. Khan was a close friend of Sir Gilbert Laithwaite, who had earlier served as British High Commissioner in Pakistan. Laithwaite, as we mentioned earlier, was a homosexual intimate of Lord Astor's half-brother Bobbie Shaw, and had had involvements with numerous Foreign Office officials scattered around the world as senior diplomats. Laithwaite and Shaw both had Stephen Ward to thank for introductions to homosexual partners, and both had visited him at his Cliveden cottage. When the Profumo Affair broke, they would rush in panic for advice from Lord Astor.

Although what occurred that infamous weekend has been described many times, the whole truth may not have surfaced. The facts may have been adjusted – to protect the Astors and their distinguished guests. What follows is the best reconstruction now possible.

Ward, who was at his Cliveden cottage that weekend, had several guests. They included, notably, Paul Mann, a bridge-playing friend, Gerry Wheatman, who rented the garage at

Wimpole Mews, Christine Keeler, her sometime boyfriend Noel Howard-Jones, an Iranian friend named Leo Norell, and a young woman Keeler and Norell had picked up on the way at a bus stop – Ward had asked Keeler to find an additional female for the weekend. It was warm, about seventy degrees, and Ward had a standing invitation from Lord Astor to use the swimming pool.

According to Keeler and others, including Lady Astor, Ward and his party headed to the pool from the cottage late that evening, between 10 and 11 p.m. Up at the mansion, dinner was finishing. The guests, some of the gentlemen in evening dress, some of the women wearing tiaras, were chatting. For the men, it was time for brandy and cigars.

An Astor staff member remembered the episode somewhat differently. 'The one thing they never told straight,' she insisted, 'was that Dr Ward and Miss Keeler were up at the house already. Then people set off for the pool together.' If that version is correct, it would suggest the story was altered later to dissociate the Astor party from the Ward group, to cover the fact that Ward and Keeler had been socialising with the VIPs present.

Whatever about that, the beauteous Christine Keeler ended up at the pool. She recalled first picking out one of the swimming costumes that Lord Astor provided for guests. It was not very comfortable, and – Keeler said – Ward laughingly suggested that she take it off. A moment later, naked, she was diving in. Long afterwards, she remembered how grand it felt, plunging nude through the dark water. The sound of splashing and laughter drifted up from the pool, according to the traditional account, and some guests decided to wander down and take a look. Two of the men, Lord Astor and Profumo, walked ahead of the others. By now, Ward had found a spotlight and was shining it on Keeler.

'In came two figures in dinner jackets,' Keeler recalled. 'One was Bill [Lord] Astor, and the other Jack Profumo. I'd met Bill before of course. I didn't even know who the other fellow was at that moment. All I knew was that I was naked as the day I was born – and I swam to the far end of the pool. It was then that Stephen played another of his little jokes. Laughing his head off, he tossed my costume clean into the bushes . . . "Now you're for it, little baby," he chuckled. I jumped out, and grabbed a towel.'

It was then, as she stood there dripping, that Astor said, 'Christine, I'd like you to meet Jack.' Then more guests arrived at the pool – and it was, ironically, Profumo's wife Valerie who offered Keeler a swimsuit. 'So,' as Keeler put it, 'the first time I met her husband, I also took her bathing costume.'

In a book about the former minister, Profumo's son, David, recalled his father saying he had met Keeler before the episode at the pool. 'I knew she was a call girl,' he said, 'because earlier I met her in a nightclub [the club was Murray's]. I probably had a drink with her.' Initially, he said, he did not recognise her at the Astor swimming pool, 'didn't put two and two together'.

'It was totally innocent high jinks,' Lady Astor told the authors. 'You couldn't see that the girl had nothing on . . . I was expecting my first baby, and I went early to bed.' While Lady Astor slumbered, however, the high jinks continued. Ward and his companions were asked back up to the big house, where John Profumo and Keeler paired off – ostensibly to tour the vast mansion.

Profumo, Keeler was to say later, was 'a type I find hard to say no to . . . I didn't terribly mind being alone with him . . . There were some suits of armour in one room and, on a dare, I let my companion dress me up in one. He paraded me in front of the others. Everybody laughed like hell. I am quite certain that the guests forgot their problems for a few hours that evening. Lord Astor invited us to return the next day for an afternoon swim.'

Sunday dawned fine, warmer than the previous day. Keeler, who had returned to nearby London overnight, set out for Cliveden again, this time accompanied by two other young women.* Photographs taken that weekend – of Keeler, the two other women, Ward, and of Keeler and Profumo – were to vanish when the scandal was about to break.

Also at the estate that day was Yevgeny Ivanov. Ward and the young women made straight for the pool when they arrived, and the working girl from Staines now enjoyed more fun with the rich, the powerful, and the Soviet spy.

'Ivanov and JP had a race down the pool,' Ward recalled. 'We started it off with a countdown, "Three, two, one, fire!" in Ivanov's honour. And although no legs were to be used, John Profumo shot ahead – using his legs.' Having won the race by cheating, he joked: 'That'll teach you to trust the Government!' Everyone, the Soviet agent included, was then invited up to the house.

The Soviet attaché was a happy man. 'There it all was,' wrote Ward, 'all his dreams come true. There was the Minister, the President of Pakistan and the Pakistan High Commissioner, duchesses, peers, and even officials of oil companies. Well, of course it was difficult to explain that this was not the hatching of any dreadful plot concerning oil, the Far East, and all points west . . . I could see the sort of report that was going back to the Embassy.'

Christine Keeler did not have international relations on her mind. 'I liked Ivanov,' she recalled. 'He was a *man*. He was rugged with a hairy chest, strong and agile. But somehow when we decided to have a water piggy-back fight, it was Jack Profumo's shoulders I climbed on . . .'

'Once or twice,' Keeler was to say, 'I caught sight of Stephen's wicked, twinkly grin as he noted Jack and Ivanov vying for my attention. Ivanov certainly saw Jack's hand accidentally brush

---

* The two other women were Sally Norrie and Grundie Heiber.

against my calf . . . I was lying by the side of the pool when, with Jack's back turned for a moment, he came up to me and touched me . . . It was all very pleasant.'

Surreptitiously, Profumo asked for her telephone number – and she replied that he should ask Stephen Ward. That evening, though, it was with Ivanov that she drove back to London. The Russian had apparently made no advances down at Cliveden. What happened next remains the subject of controversy.

Keeler's first public account today reads somewhat quaintly, redolent of a different era:

> He had a bottle of vodka with him. We sat on the green divan at Stephen's Wimpole Mews flat. I knew that if he came for me I wasn't going to resist overmuch . . . Suddenly he was kissing me, rolling his dark curls into my neck . . . I dropped my glass . . . I was surprised as I was pleased. Gosh. I'd always wanted him, why shouldn't I admit it? He came at me again. I half rose, and the obvious happened. We fell clean off the divan. There was a wild thrashing about, a real Russian romp! We crashed across the room. A little table went flying. He pinioned me in a corner by the door. I relaxed. Because he was just kissing me with all the power of a man in a frenzy of passion . . . Our very impetus carried us through the door, and we half fell into my bedroom. From that second I threw all reserve to the winds . . . we had been together, Russian man and English girl . . .

True or false? Keeler said she told Stephen Ward next morning what had had happened. Ward, on the other hand, wrote in his memoir, 'She said she would *like* to have intercourse with him. I have always believed myself she never did. I think, like a lot of people, she tells a story often enough and comes to believe it and does tell lies.' Mandy Rice-Davies, who was close to Keeler at the time and often saw Keeler and Ivanov together at Ward's flat, says she was unaware Keeler had had sex with the Russian. 'She didn't tell me at the time, and Stephen never mentioned it. Something always puzzled me about this. The first time I heard about it was in the *News of the World*.'

Lord Denning interviewed Christine Keeler twice, but said he remained uncertain. If there was sexual intercourse with the Russian, the judge thought it had been a solitary incident, never repeated. Yet, in a first account for the *Sunday Pictorial*, never published, Keeler spoke of 'having an affair' with Ivanov. Perhaps that was a newspaper euphemism for 'having had it away', as Keeler usually described sex, just once. On oath at Ward's trial, she said she had gone to bed with him – and continued to say as much far into the future. Ivanov, for his part, wrote in his 1992 autobiography that he and Keeler had indeed had sex.

Whether Keeler fooled around with the Soviet spy, went to bed with him once, or had a full-blown affair, does not matter much. What matters is that she saw him frequently, that he was a regular visitor at the Ward flat, at a time when she was sleeping with the British Secretary of State for War. And that affair is not in doubt.

Two years later, when John Profumo confessed that he had earlier lied to the House of Commons, he would merely admit to there having been 'impropriety' with Christine Keeler. The Denning Report covered the matter in two paragraphs, acknowledging that there had been an affair.

Following the initial meeting at Cliveden, the Minister for War did not waste time. Though he knew Ward, it was Lord Astor he asked to pass on word that he 'had been much taken with Miss Keeler, and would like to meet her again'. A tryst was arranged, by telephone, almost certainly on the Tuesday after the weekend encounter.

According to Keeler, 'I got a phone call from Jack. He said, "What about a drive?" I replied "Hi! Nice to hear from you again." . . . The upshot was that he came round to the flat while Stephen was out – meeting with Ivanov. We drank, chatted, and mucked about in general. I didn't think he was handsome, but his ways appealed to me . . . But then, as was so often to happen in our future meetings at the flat, I had to say, "Stephen will be back very soon", and – as always when Stephen's name was mentioned – Jack got up and said that he had better be going.'

'Jack Profumo and I became lovers,' Keeler said, 'the third time that he came around . . . We started laughing and talking as usual, and then suddenly we both stopped. There was one of those electric, potent silences and then without a word we were embracing, and he was kissing me, and I was returning his kisses with everything that I suddenly felt for him. That was how it all started.'

Lord Denning, who interviewed Profumo twice, stated in his Report that the Minister had indeed had sex with Keeler at the Wimpole Mews flat. If there was anyone else there, Denning noted, 'he would take her for a drive until the coast was clear'. 'Our meetings were very discreet,' Keeler said. 'Jack drove a red Mini car. We never once dined out, or had a drink in a pub, or went anywhere . . . He was worried about the press finding out about us. And above all he was worried about Valerie.'

The notion that Profumo was concerned about his wife was likely a Keeler exaggeration. According to the couple's son David, their marriage was going through a rocky stage in 1961. Valerie already suspected her husband might be having an affair. Keeler, for her part, was aware Profumo had dalliances with women other than herself. Privately, Valerie drew up a list of positives and negatives about her husband. The negatives included his 'reluctance to discuss – or even mention – sex. Not "ours," but any erotic or interesting sexy things.' She also objected to Profumo's flirting, his 'casing the dance', and the way he kissed women he 'hardly knew'.

For her part, Valerie was herself becoming intimate with a married man not her husband – the authors were told by a member of the Profumos' circle that this eventually led to a sexual relationship.

John Profumo took his mistress Christine Keeler back to the family home he shared with his wife, a grand Nash house in Regent's Park. 'It was late,' Keeler said. 'The butler and the rest of the staff were in bed, and Jack let us in with his own key. We crept around the lovely rooms. And then we got to *their* bedroom . . .'

Keeler described Profumo's house to the police, giving details that left no doubt she had actually been there. 'I went up some steps,' she told the police, 'into a square hall where there are two large ornamental animals . . . The stairs bend to the left and on the wall is a picture . . . all the things that Valerie likes and dislikes, including pigeons and jewellery. From the top of the stairs is Jack's office, with a drinks cabinet inside. I noticed a strange telephone and he said it was a scrambler. Next door is the Profumos' bedroom with an adjoining bathroom . . .'

The couple had sex on the marital bed, Keeler said. Profumo, she thought, exuded power. She felt, as she put it, the way other women might feel about 'fucking Marlon Brando'. The same night the couple went to the Profumos' home, Keeler said, they drove to Chelsea to see Profumo's friend – a former Secretary of State for Air – Viscount Ward. The Viscount was a brother of the 3rd Earl of Dudley, the Ward friend said recently to have proposed to Mandy Rice-Davies. He told the authors, however, that he had 'never met Stephen Ward'.

Once, Keeler said, Profumo borrowed a 'big black car. It had a silver hare on the bonnet as a mascot.' This was a Bentley that belonged to another Profumo friend, Minister for Labour John Hare. Hare, who later became Viscount Blakenham, was initially to deny having lent the car to his colleague, only to acknowledge later that he had.

Profumo took astonishing risks. At Ward's trial on prostitution charges in 1963, a Major James Eynon would admit he too had had sex with Christine Keeler on several occasions, for money. Once, he told the court, he arrived at Wimpole Mews only to find another man already there. When Eynon 'arrived at the door,' Keeler recalled, '. . . I had to let him in, and introduce him to the War Minister . . . Jim obviously recognised him, but behaved in true Army fashion; no names . . . Jack nearly died.' Mariella Novotny's husband Hod Dibben also encountered Profumo at Ward's flat. 'I was at Stephen's flat when he came to pick her up one night,' he told the authors. 'He didn't come in. He waited at the door.'

On 3 August 1961, Profumo would much later tell his son David, he and Keeler had sex in front of the television set in the living room at Ward's flat. One of Keeler's woman friends walked through while they were at it.*

Sometimes, Keeler told *News of the World* chief reporter Peter Earle, she and Profumo had sex in his car. Once they did it in the open air – near his home in Regent's Park. He gave her gifts, including a Flaminaire cigarette lighter, and – at least once – money. 'She said her parents were badly off,' Denning observed, so Profumo 'gave her twenty pounds for them, realising this was a polite way on her part of asking for money for her services.'

Profumo also gave Keeler a bottle of Femme perfume – his wife's favourite fragrance – thinking perhaps that its smell would mask his infidelity. Eventually, when Valerie discovered what he

---

* Sally Norrie.

had been up to, she poured her own bottle of Femme down the lavatory and never used the perfume again.

Christine Keeler's relationship with the Minister for War, as she was to put it, was 'a very, very well-mannered screw of convenience; only in other people's minds, much later, was it "an affair".' The authors also refer to the relationship as an 'affair' – it is the convenient description of the episode. How long the affair was to last, and what it meant in the context of national security, hung on two factors not yet considered – the role of Stephen Ward, and the continuing role of MI5.

CHAPTER 14

A Nuclear Question

On the morning after the night before, Monday, 10 July 1961, Stephen Ward and Christine Keeler had discussed the eventful weekend at Lord Astor's place. Keeler told Ward she had been to bed with Ivanov. He, knowing that Profumo was also keen to see her, exclaimed, 'My goodness! What with Eugene on one hand and your new friend on the other, we could start a war . . .'

Ward made a joke of it, but he was worried. Keeler later spoke of having had 'an argument with Stephen', a row so fierce that she stormed out of the flat.

Manipulating human beings, playing with their lusts and emotions, had backfired, and Ward had reason to be troubled. A Profumo-Keeler-Ivanov triangle was obviously potential dynamite. Ward must have seen at once how perilous it was, how easily the situation could spiral out of control. Boosting this fear was something Ivanov had asked Ward, something that made the sexual imbroglio yet more worrying. That same Monday, Ward called his MI5 contact, Keith Wagstaffe. They met within forty-eight hours.

Ward, according to MI5, wanted to share his views on Soviet policy. Wagstaffe, however, was more interested in hearing Ward's description of what had occurred at the house party at Cliveden. Profumo, Ivanov and Keeler, Ward said, had all been at the house party. The MI5 officer was keen to know more about the Russian. Ivanov, Ward said, was attracted to Keeler, and – he noted – the pair had drunk two bottles of whiskey between them at Ward's flat on the Sunday evening. Ward observed, too, that the Minister for War was a fairly close friend who on occasion visited Wimpole Mews – information that caused alarm at MI5 headquarters. Ward did not say Keeler was having an affair with Profumo – it had not started yet.

Wagstaffe reported that his assessment of Ward had not changed. 'I do not think he is a security risk in the sense that he would be intentionally disloyal, but his peculiar political beliefs combined with his obvious admiration of Ivanov might lead him to be indiscreet unintentionally.' That comment, almost certainly, arose from something else Ward had reported. Ivanov, he had told MI5's man, 'had asked him to find out when the Americans were going to arm West Germany with atomic weapons'.

That question, as we shall report in detail, was of key interest to a Soviet agent in 1961. In reporting it, Ward was doing exactly what Wagstaffe had asked him to do, to get in touch 'should Ivanov make any propositions'. So far as the record shows, however, Ward would receive no thanks for having done the right thing. So far as the public were concerned, he was to be smeared as a suspected traitor.

In 1963, as the scandal began to break, Christine Keeler told the police that 'on one occasion when she was going to meet Mr Profumo, *Ward* [authors' italics] had asked her to discover from him the date on which certain atomic secrets were to be handed to West Germany by the Americans'. Keeler told *Sunday Pictorial* reporters much the same thing and, speaking with the *News of the World*, also said: 'One night a friend asked me directly to find out from Jack when Germany was going to be armed with atomic weapons, but I refused. I felt instinctively and deep down that this was spying. I also knew that even if I were capable, which I wasn't, I couldn't do it. Jack and I were just not that way. He never talked to me about business and affairs of state. How could I possibly ask him such a thing when all he wanted with me was to relax?'

Several years later, however, she told the story differently. There was a night, she said, when she shared a bed with Ward – as they occasionally did, not for sex but companionship. They were lying in bed, according to her, when 'Stephen asked me if anyone had mentioned to me anything about the bomb . . . What bomb? At the time I was totally innocent of world affairs, since I never read the papers or watched the news.' Ward replied, 'The bomb America is giving to Germany . . . you could easily find out about it if you tried.'

Keeler said she was baffled, and responded, 'But no one would discuss anything like that with me.' Ward then laughed and said he was 'only joking'. She replied uneasily that it all seemed 'so funny to me, you and the other two . . .' The other two, of course, were Ivanov and Profumo. Then Ward changed the subject, and they went to sleep.

This was apparently not the fiction of a young woman who was being paid too much money for her memoirs. In an interview for this book, Mandy Rice-Davies recalled a 1961 visit with Keeler to London Zoo. As they strolled between the cages, chatting about men, Keeler spoke of her affair with Profumo. Then she said, as Rice-Davies remembered it: 'I've got to tell you something. Stephen has asked me to ask Profumo about "bomb-heads", or "missile-heads", for West Germany.' Astonished, not sure whether her friend was serious, Rice-Davies asked, 'What are you going to do?' Christine replied, in all gravity, 'I would never betray my country . . .'

There is on the face of it a massive contradiction here, one that was barely noted, let alone resolved. On the one hand, as recorded in the Denning Report, we have Ward – asked a question on a sensitive matter by a Russian spy – promptly reporting back to his MI5 contact, as he had been asked to do. On the other hand, we have a plausible report that Ward deliberately tried to get Keeler to worm the answer out of Profumo. Was Ward loyal citizen or would-be traitor? Or did he try to serve two masters? Denning and Ward were for once at one in the way they explained away Keeler's allegations.

Ward, in his memoir, made the whole thing sound light-hearted. When Ivanov asked him to get information on nuclear warheads, he claimed, he said he might if Ivanov were to respond by arranging a visa for Ward to go to Moscow – to draw Khrushchev's portrait. As for the sinister-sounding request to Keeler, Ward passed it off with: 'I did joke with Keeler at the time of her affair with Profumo. I cannot remember my exact form of words. But it concealed my genuine anxiety. It was something like this: "All it needs now is for me to get the information that Ivanov wants, and we would have a real set-up here."'

Lord Denning accepted the 'joke' version. He thought there had been 'a good deal of talk in [Keeler's] presence between Stephen Ward and Captain Ivanov about getting this information. And Stephen Ward may well have turned to her and said, "You ought to ask Jack about it." But I do not think it was said as seriously as it has since been reported.'

Christine Keeler took it seriously, though, and still did so long afterwards. While making a tape recording of her experiences for Robin Drury, who acted as her business affairs manager at the time of the scandal, she baulked at discussing the 'bomb-heads' issue. 'Christine asked me to turn off the tape recorder,' Drury recalled, 'because what she had to tell me was too dangerous . . . it was the touchiest item in the whole scandal . . .'

Remembering the incident years later, Keeler said Ward had

looked deadly serious – and anxious. The public knew only what Denning had to say on the subject and – as so often when he dealt with a knotty problem – what he said was diffused across different sections of his Report. If he knew how Christine Keeler had recalled the episode, or if he knew Mandy Rice-Davies corroborated it, he did not say so. Yet there is no dodging Keeler's account. It is too specific to have been fabricated, let alone by a teenager – she was only nineteen at the time the incident occurred – and totally ignorant of politics. Stephen Ward clearly did ask her to pump Profumo. Why?

It might seem to make no sense for Ward to have asked Keeler to question Profumo *after* having warned MI5 that Ivanov wanted the information. Even if he fancied himself as a double agent, that would have been to invite serious trouble. The answer to the riddle lies in MI5's scheming, in the nature of the question itself, and above all in its timing.

In early July 1961, as the crisis over Berlin deepened, Soviet traitor Penkovsky was back in London again, pouring out further important information. Ensconced with him at Coleherne Court, a venerable block of flats off the Old Brompton Road – where the future Princess Diana would one day live – Western intelligence officers milked the Russian for information on the Soviet rocket programme. Penkovsky had arrived in London carrying two rolls of microfilm, data about troop movements and Khrushchev's plans for the treaty with East Germany to alter the status of Berlin. Khrushchev, Penkovsky had learned, had ordered his ambassador in London to report on Britain's likely response to confrontation over Berlin.

As vaguely related in the Denning Report, Ivanov had asked Ward 'when the Americans were going to arm West Germany with atomic weapons'. Elsewhere, this became 'American intentions to provide the West Germans with the Bomb'. Put that way, the request was almost laughable. There never was any question of letting West Germany have the nuclear bomb.

In fact, Keeler told a friend in 1962, the question as it was passed on to her was about something much more specific: '*nuclear warheads*'. Rice-Davies, an intelligent woman with excellent recall, remembered Keeler telling her – in their talk at the Zoo – about a request regarding 'bomb-heads' or 'missile-heads'. Whichever it was, the *heads* part stuck in Rice-Davies' mind. As a subject of Soviet interest in 1961, that makes much more sense.

Just a week before the party at Cliveden, there had been press reports that the United States was planning to increase the firepower of West Germany's army. The Bundeswehr might soon be supplied with the Davy Crockett, a jeep-mounted artillery missile, and the Sergeant, a medium-range ballistic missile. The Crockett was a small weapon that could be deployed on the battlefield with a three-man crew; were the United States to give it to the Germans, Washington would be abdicating a degree of control. The Crockett and the Sergeant were both, according to *Jane's Weapons Systems*, 'capable of carrying either a nuclear or a high-explosive warhead'.

It is hard now, unless one lived in those post-war years, to comprehend the gravity with which the Soviet Union viewed German rearmament. Far into the future, Moscow's propaganda would still be voicing the possibility that Germany might again be an aggressor. The Soviet political and military leaders of 1961 were men who remembered both world wars, conflicts in which the Soviet Union – with some twenty-nine million casualties – suffered far more than any other nation. This was the Soviet psychology that long insisted that Germany remain divided and that no German finger should ever rest on a nuclear trigger. Khrushchev's concerns were very real.

In 1960, on a European inspection tour, members of the US

Congress' Joint Committee on Atomic Energy had observed US fighter aircraft 'loaded with nuclear bombs sitting on the edge of runways with German pilots inside the cockpits and starter plugs inserted'. The sole indication of American control was 'an American officer somewhere in the vicinity with a revolver'. The American congressmen were appalled. Khrushchev, too, has to have been aware that some degree of the control of nuclear weapons was beginning to pass to the Germans.

The West German Defence Minister in 1961 was the pugnacious right-winger Franz Josef Strauss. In early summer that year, he publicly demanded 'atomic armament for the Bundeswehr'. Delay in delivery of tactical nuclear weapons to West Germany, he asserted, would have disastrous consequences for military morale and the political fortunes of the Adenauer government. 'There can be no second-class allies,' Strauss would say, where defence was concerned. Opinion in the United States and in some NATO countries, however, was that deployment of nuclear missiles in Germany would probably make their use in a possible Soviet invasion virtually inevitable – and trigger full-scale nuclear conflict.

Strauss' demands were eventually to lead to full-blown political upheaval and his resignation the following year. In summer 1961, however, he was still in office and demanding that West Germany be supplied with both Crockett and Sergeant weapons systems, with *nuclear warheads*.

In the midst of the ongoing crisis over Berlin, then, the Soviets urgently needed to know whether Strauss would get what he wanted. Would the United States send the missiles to West Germany, and would West German commanders have control of them? If the missiles were to be supplied, when were they due to arrive? Most important of all, would they carry conventional or nuclear warheads? Against that scenario, Ivanov's question to Ward makes absolute sense.

In 1963, many would scoff at the notion that Christine Keeler could ever have been used as a Mata Hari, and doubted whether John Profumo would have known the status of the missiles in any case. In fact, Keeler could have put the question, perhaps in a conversation in which Profumo's young mistress – though blatantly ignorant on current affairs – asked her eminent lover to give her the gist of the ongoing crisis over Germany. The question about the missiles, after all, had featured in the newspapers – the difference being that, in the Minister for War, Keeler had someone who might know the answers.

'What atomic secrets,' asked former Prime Minister Macmillan as late as 1980, 'could Jack Profumo possibly have known?' The War Minister was not privy to all 'secret' material, but – Cabinet papers released in 2007 reveal – he regularly attended meetings at which sensitive matters concerning atomic weapons were discussed. Profumo was also on the Defence Committee, and the British Rhine Army was a major part of his brief. There was close cooperation between the US, West German and British forces, and the Secretary of State for War certainly did know – as Macmillan would later concede to the journalist Chapman Pincher – whether and which battlefield weapons were to be conventional or nuclear.

It is a documented fact that, some time before the 1963 scandal broke, Profumo came close to resigning during a debate over the Blue Water missile, a weapon capable of carrying a nuclear warhead. Just three days before the Cliveden weekend, Profumo had been asked in Parliament about nuclear weapons policy. He had declined to reply, in order not to 'disclose information which might be useful to a potential enemy'. Ivanov not only had every reason to ask the warhead question, he had reason to believe Profumo would know the answer. And, as we shall see, there was a way that MI5, briefed on the question in advance by Stephen Ward, could turn it to their advantage.

Probably in the same period, troubled by Ivanov's persistent talk about the United States rearming West Germany, Ward took the Soviet spy to see the man who had originally brought them together, *Daily Telegraph* editor Colin Coote. Soviet intelligence, Ivanov told Coote over lunch, thought Washington had already decided to supply West Germany with the controversial weapons systems. This was correct. It is now known that the Crockett weapons system was delivered to the US 3rd Division in West Germany in late 1961. The Sergeant missile would be deployed by American forces in the spring of 1963 and – the following year – by three West German battalions.

Neither the Denning Report nor Coote in his memoir would mention the lunch with Ward and Ivanov, or Ivanov's accurate prediction.

Two days after Ivanov, Profumo and Keeler had met at Cliveden, Soviet cosmonaut Yuri Gagarin – the man of the hour for having been the first man in space – arrived in London to attend the Soviet Trade Fair at Earls Court. A Sputnik was on display, the Soviet satellite suitably sanitised of any secret equipment. One of the Soviet officials showing off the exhibits was assistant naval attaché Ivanov, and a young woman named Christine Keeler was among the visitors.

Throughout the week after the Cliveden episode, as Gagarin made his triumphal way from ministerial reception to Buckingham Palace luncheon, the crisis over Berlin worsened. Khrushchev fulminated about nuclear war. Refugees from the East rushed to freedom in West Berlin, afraid – rightly – that it might be their last chance. And the Soviets moved more troops into East Germany.

CHAPTER 15

An Operation Botched

Before Gagarin left London, there was a glittering reception at the Soviet embassy. Stephen Ward was there, making sure he had his photograph taken with the cosmonaut. The Minister for War was there, and of course Ivanov – as one of the Russian hosts. 'I passed on into the reception room,' Ward recalled, 'and ran at once into John Profumo and Valerie, his wife. And at that moment up came Ivanov, splendid in a gold and beaded uniform with several medals. We chatted for a moment, and we went off to get vodka for Valerie.' It was the second time in a week that the Minister and the Russian spy had met – a week in which both had been dallying with Christine Keeler.

When Profumo arrived at the Wimpole Mews flat for his first date with Keeler, she said, Ward had been on his way out. He and the Minister waved to each other. Soon Keeler was off with Profumo on a drive to the War Office and Downing Street in his 'long shiny black car'. When he dropped her off at home, Ward was there 'lolling about', waiting, with a raised eyebrow, a languid 'Well?' and a request for a full account of the excursion. On Wednesday of that week, the Denning Report tells us, Ward sat down with MI5's Keith Wagstaffe to tell him that Keeler, Profumo and Ivanov had all met at Cliveden, and that Keeler had spent an evening getting drunk with Ivanov.

According to the Denning Report, there was no reference at this meeting to any goings-on between Keeler and Profumo. Lord Denning claimed, indeed, that MI5 was to know nothing of that until January 1963, when the scandal began to break. That is what MI5 Director General Hollis had told Denning, but it was not true. It was, rather, an MI5 officer was to say later, a 'brazen lie'. In fact, MI5 had a six-page dossier of the Ward/Keeler/Profumo/Ivanov relationship – held on a need-to-know basis.

'It seemed to me that Jack was behaving foolishly,' Ward told his close friend Warwick Charlton shortly before he died, 'so I reported the matter to Mr Woods [MI5 man Wagstaffe's code name] . . . He told me he would deal with the matter . . .'

Ward's memoir makes it clear that – not least because of Ivanov persistently bringing up the subject of German rearmament – the osteopath felt he had to tell MI5 what was going on. 'This was in the summer of '61,' he wrote. 'It was around this time that JP met Keeler – you can possibly now understand my anxiety about this relationship . . . I felt that I must inform the security people of the friendship which had developed . . . I sought to be as practical as possible as I broached the delicate subject . . . I had got it off my chest.'

At the end of July, according to the Denning Report, MI5 asked the Metropolitan Police Special Branch to 'get more information about Ward's establishment and about Christine'. Special Branch reported that neither had a criminal record and that the Wimpole Mews address was not known to the Vice Squad as a 'disorderly house' – a reference to the earlier suggestion that Ward might have been 'involved in the call-girl racket'.

Two sources indicate there was surveillance of Ward's flat in July 1961. Robin Drury, Keeler's business adviser in 1963, quoted his client as saying that 'MI5 took a picture of a man leaving the flat. They thought it was Ivanov, but when it was developed it turned out to be Profumo.' According to a second account, the surveillance was bungled.

'Mr. Profumo was followed by security men,' ran a report in the *Daily Telegraph*, 'when he met Miss Keeler at Dr Ward's London home . . . Captain Ivanov was watched by security men at the same time, and I understand that one night security men watching Mr Profumo had an encounter in Wimpole Mews with security men watching Mr Ivanov.' The source of that story, according to the report, was Ward, who presumably either witnessed the farcical episode or learned about it from his MI5 contact. The mix-up probably resulted from a failure in communication between MI5 and the police Special Branch with which it liaised.

The same *Telegraph* article stated that British intelligence 'had a record' of Profumo's meetings with Christine Keeler. According to Stephen Ward, Profumo visited Keeler at his flat five times while he was away at the Cliveden cottage. 'Christine has told me of those visits,' Ward wrote. 'Intercourse took place on each occasion – Christine has told me intimate details that leave no doubt in my mind that this is so . . . When I realised that was happening, I contacted Mr Woods [Wagstaffe] of MI5 . . . I also mentioned to Woods at this time that she was in some relationship with Ivanov. I used these words: "Please do not make an official report on this matter. I have no wish to damage Mr Profumo, but you will see that I am in a very invidious position here."'

Ward's memoir says he then arranged for Wagstaffe to get a second look at Christine Keeler, a statement she corroborated. During her affair with Profumo, she was to say, 'Stephen had a visit from MI5 . . . I remember the man coming. I opened the door to him . . . I don't know what he said to Stephen as I didn't stick around. They didn't seem to want me to.' Keeler made it clear that this MI5 visit occurred after she had started meeting Profumo, and that Ward did tell Wagstaffe about her and the Minister.

'Afterwards,' Keeler said, 'Stephen told me that it was perfectly all right. It was just that they were checking up on who I was, because Ivanov was also a frequent visitor to our flat. After that, Stephen and I used to get up to jokes on the telephone. We suspected our line was being tapped. So we would ring one another up and say curt things like, "Is it all right? Have you got the plans? Right!"'

While people who think their phone is tapped are usually imagining it, Ward and Keeler were probably not. If security personnel were watching the flat and taking photographs, they were likely also tapping the phone. There would have been little difficulty in obtaining a warrant to intercept calls – and indeed electronic surveillance has sometimes been carried out without a warrant.

On 31 July, three weeks after the Cliveden weekend, MI5 chief Sir Roger Hollis spoke with Cabinet Secretary Sir Norman Brook. Brook was one of the most powerful insiders in government, an éminence grise who had been the confidant of four prime ministers. Anthony Sampson, author of *Anatomy of Britain*, described him as 'caught up in an intricate, secret world . . . the central cog in the British Government . . . When in fifty years' time the official secrets are revealed, the name of Brook will certainly feature a good deal in the making of decisions.' Of all the prime ministers he served, Brook was closest to the incumbent, Harold Macmillan. He had long experience of liaison with MI5.

Hollis contacted Brook, according to Denning, with two things in mind. He wanted Profumo to be warned to be careful what he said to Ward – Ward was a chatterbox who might repeat snippets of information to Ivanov in casual conversation. The Director General's second point was central to MI5's real purpose. He suggested, Denning reported, 'that with Mr Profumo's help it might be possible to get Ivanov to defect. Mr Profumo might be a "lead-in" to Ivanov.' Hollis wanted Profumo to become part of the honeytrap.

Brook talked with Profumo just over a week later, on 9 August, and passed on MI5's messages. They had quite a conversation, one that was probably conducted in that understated fashion in which a British gentleman ought to discuss a sensitive matter with another.

Profumo, whose stomach must have been swarming with butterflies, thanked Brook for warning him to be careful around Ward. He assumed, as well he might, that MI5 had learned of his affair with Christine Keeler. Brook's visit, he guessed, was a polite way of telling him to stop seeing her. Very delicately, however, the Cabinet Secretary moved on to MI5's request for assistance. 'Was it possible,' Brook asked, for Profumo 'to do anything to persuade Ivanov to help us?'

MI5 now knew, from Ward and its follow-up surveillance, that both the Minister and the Soviet spy had been intimate with Keeler. Junior MI5 officers had indeed schemed to entrap Ivanov, but so far had not succeeded. Profumo's amorous adventure had not been part of their plan – and now threatened to derail the operation at a crucial stage. Unless, Director General Hollis proposed, Profumo either dropped Keeler or agreed to become a co-conspirator. It was a pivotal moment for all concerned.

Before Brook's meeting with Profumo, MI5 must have decided just what it was they wanted the Minister to do for them. We can hazard a guess as to what it was – a ploy, perhaps, that would make sense at last of Ward's odd request to Keeler to get information out of Profumo on missiles in Germany. At the height of the crisis over Berlin, British intelligence may have hoped to pull one of the most effective and time-honoured tricks in the intelligence book: to mislead the Soviets with false information. Disinformation, swallowed whole by an enemy, can change the course of history. It sows confusion at the very least, and that in itself is almost always useful.

Profumo's sudden intrusion into the ongoing honeytrap operation could be turned to their advantage, Hollis may have theorised. If Ward could just get Keeler to ask the question to which Ivanov wanted an answer, and if Profumo was primed into giving her an answer – a *phoney* answer – the Soviets might be fooled. It was a matter of whether this could be stage-managed.

Whatever Hollis' precise suggestion was, some officers thought the notion of embroiling a minister of the Crown in the operation 'outrageous', a gross misjudgement. Hollis himself appears to have realised this was a misstep and – according to Peter Wright – was to remove a relevant letter from the file that went to Lord Denning.

Fortunately for Hollis, according to the Denning Report Profumo turned down MI5's request, 'thought he ought to keep well away from it'. Convinced that he had been caught out indulging in his foolish sexual adventure, his mind must have filled with foreboding – ruined career, marital misery, the whole catastrophe. To help MI5 in the way proposed was a complication Profumo could do without. So the Minister for War plumped for self-preservation, and – sportingly enough – suggested colleagues might be warned so as to avoid the predicament in which he found himself. A number of other men in Ward's circle, including another minister, he told Brook, should also be warned. The second minister, who was cautioned, has never been publicly identified.

That same day, within hours of the difficult talk with the Cabinet Secretary, Profumo sat down to write to Christine Keeler – on War Office notepaper. She kept the letter, so we know it read:

9/8/61

Darling,

In great haste and because I can get no reply from your phone –
Alas something's blown up tomorrow night and I can't therefore
make it.

I'm terribly sorry especially as I leave the next day for various
trips and then a holiday so won't be able to see you again until
some time in September. Blast it. Please take great care of yourself
and don't run away.

Love J.

PS I'm writing this 'cos I know you're off for the day tomorrow and
I want you to know before you go if I still can't reach you by
phone.

Profumo spent most of Parliament's summer recess with his family
on the Isle of Wight. The ambiguous letter to Keeler lay in a
drawer in her bedroom in London, a paper time bomb. Did the
affair with Keeler end with that letter, and did Profumo stick to his
refusal to cooperate with MI5? Profumo eventually told Denning
that he stopped seeing Keeler in August. Earlier, however, in
Parliament, he said he saw her again as late as December. Keeler
also said they met in December. The Denning Report noted that
she 'adopted this date, evidently following him'.

There is no special reason to accept the December date as
truthful – the statement in which Profumo offered it was the one
in which he lied to Parliament and said there never had been an
affair. Two witnesses told Denning that the affair continued into
1962. One was a later Keeler lover, 'Lucky' Gordon. The other,
never properly identified, was 'a man called Hogan' who claimed
he took the couple tea in bed together at the Dolphin Square flat
Keeler used in 1962. There is further evidence on this, to be
reported later in these pages.

It seems extraordinary that Profumo would even have considered seeing Keeler again following the frightening encounter with Cabinet Secretary Brook. Yet his letter of 9 August merely postponed their next meeting. It seems, too, that there were more letters. Keeler referred to as many as four, though there may have been more. Two were left with her friend Michael Lambton, who, she thought, returned them to Profumo, and two disappeared. One, written after the meeting with Brook, made an arrangement for a further meeting.

There came a day, Keeler said, when Profumo suggested that he would provide her with a flat and maintain her as his mistress. According to her she declined the offer, saying she was content with the situation as it was. 'But darling,' Keeler quoted her lover as replying, 'I won't be able to go on seeing you while you live here with Stephen . . .' She harboured the thought, though, that Profumo hoped to turn her into a sort of call girl – on permanent call to his political friends. Keeler did, in December 1961, move to new accommodation in Dolphin Square.

While the date and contents of Profumo's second letter are unknown, Keeler has referred to the essence of the last one. In it, she said, he told her 'that if I wanted to see him again, I could get in touch . . .' Keeler claimed that she did have a further meeting with him, at Murray's Club, in late October. She was having trouble with one of her black boyfriends from Notting Hill, and was considering Profumo's offer to set her up in a flat. In the event, they wound up having sex again – in Profumo's car.

If Profumo did continue seeing Keeler after the warning from the Cabinet Secretary, was it the ultimate in foolhardiness? Or did he perhaps, after all, do so under pressure to help MI5, as British intelligence pressed ahead with the scheme to get Ivanov to defect? The one sure thing is that the Minister for War was at that stage highly vulnerable to pressure from anyone with knowledge of the affair with Keeler.

'What is certain,' wrote Lord Kennet, a former Labour minister who authored a book on the Profumo case:

'is that the triangle Profumo–Keeler–Ivanov laid Profumo wide open to blackmail. The scandal which broke when it was finally discovered, and the degree of ruin which overtook him personally, can hardly have surprised Profumo. The extent to which he expected them is the measure of his vulnerability to blackmail. In the market of these things, big scandal equals big hush payment, and big hush payment may be made in big secrets. We should probably know if Profumo had been unsuccessfully blackmailed by the Russian intelligence service; he would probably tell us about it if he had stood up to them. But we do not know, and we shall never know, whether he was successfully blackmailed in the nineteen months between August 1961 and March 1963; we only know that the Russians had good leverage on him . . . It cannot be assumed that a man who has lied to conceal adultery from the House of Commons will not lie in order to conceal a breach of security from Lord Denning, any more than it can be assumed that he will . . . when you have a real hold over a man there is no longer any reason to complicate the channel with cut-outs, whether conscious or unconscious . . . the risk was high.

'Whether there was a breach of security at any time,' Harold Wilson, the Labour leader and future Prime Minister, told Parliament, 'whether there was a leak of information, is something we shall never know . . . There is no means now of finding out . . .'

For two years, until he resigned, Profumo was indeed open to manipulation – not only by the Soviets, but also by anyone with knowledge of the extent to which he was compromised. Ivanov, for his part, would remain an entrapment target for a further eighteen months – until he left London in January 1963.

Stephen Ward, it later became clear, remained the tool of MI5. A book on MI5 by Nigel West, an author with excellent intelligence sources, contained sensational insights into the Profumo Affair – in spite of government attempts at censorship even two decades later. Following up, *Sunday Times* reporters Barrie Penrose and Simon Freeman succeeded in extracting information from former MI5 officers who had been directly involved in the Ward operation: Graham Mitchell, who had been Deputy Director-General of MI5 in 1961, Keith Wagstaffe, Arthur Martin and his assistant Mrs Clarke. What they had to say amounted to the rehabilitation of Stephen Ward.

Speaking on the basis of anonymity, the officers said Ward's call-girl contacts had been 'the very qualities MI5 thought valuable'. Ward was approached in 1961, the *Sunday Times* reported, because British intelligence had earmarked attaché Ivanov as a potential target for entrapment. Ward was told it would be 'helpful' if the Soviet were to become friendly with Ward's young women friends – making it possible for MI5 to exert pressure on him. Re-interviewed, Christine Keeler admitted that 'it was Stephen Ward who encouraged me, nudged me, towards Ivanov'.

Keith Wagstaffe was asked whether Ward was encouraged to see himself as a patriot spying for his country. 'Exactly. This is so,' the former officer replied. Two colleagues described him as having been 'a very nice, very pleasant chap' who 'did his very best for us'.

'Nowhere in the Denning Report,' Graham Mitchell noted, 'does it say that Ward was acting under our instructions. That is very unfortunate.' Lord Denning, asked to comment as he headed into retirement, would say only that he would 'prefer to stay out of this'.

Ward did not finger his masters in British intelligence even when he was made a scapegoat. Perhaps he was afraid to, or perhaps he was simply loyal. Ward did hint at the attempted honeytrap operation in his unpublished memoir, writing of Ivanov, 'There can be no doubt that he was marked. I was, of course, the means by which this was done. Did I do wrong? . . . I personally think that it is tragic that such portentous matters should have been dealt with in this amateur fashion . . .' British intelligence not only played Stephen Ward for the weeks in 1961 that were to make him infamous. It pushed him around the London square of the political chessboard until the scandal broke two years later. He revelled in it – at the time.

On 2 August 1961, as tension built between Moscow and Washington, Lord Astor wrote to the Foreign Office suggesting that if officials wanted the Soviet embassy to be correctly informed on Allied intentions, then Ward's relationship with Ivanov might prove a useful back channel.

The following day, Ward the artist was interviewed in the London *Evening Standard* for an article that would go unnoticed during the Profumo Affair. The subject of the interview was his sketching of famous subjects, and his hope that he would be able to travel to Moscow to draw Khrushchev for the *Daily Telegraph*.

'Dr Ward became nervous,' the *Standard* reporter wrote, 'when he talked to me about Berlin. He has friends in the Soviet Embassy. One of them has warned him to watch out for "big trouble" in the autumn. Said Dr Ward, "He said he thought America would give West Germany the bomb, and if they did China would have the bomb within five minutes."'* Dr Ward, the reporter noted, was 'frankly worried by the situation'.

Everyone had cause to worry. Ten days later, before dawn on

---

* The rift between the Soviet Union and China did not become serious until the following year, 1962.

13 August, East German troops began erecting barbed-wire barriers between East and West Berlin – the first step in the building of the obscene cinder-block divide that became the Berlin Wall. By late that month, American and Soviet tanks would be confronting each other 'eyeball to eyeball' across the line. President Kennedy, however, resisted calls for actual military action.

Odious though the Wall was, some in the West welcomed its appearance. While it enabled Khrushchev to cut off the embarrassing haemorrhage of refugees streaming to the West, its very existence discredited communism. The Soviet leader, meanwhile, withdrew the six-month deadline he had set for the enforcement of new border arrangements. The crisis between the superpowers eased temporarily, and the Soviet tone softened.

Behind the scenes in London, assistant Soviet naval attaché Ivanov asked Stephen Ward to carry messages to the British government. Ward jumped to oblige. On 2 September, Lord Astor wrote to the Foreign Office suggesting that his friend Dr Ward might act as intermediary between the government and the Soviet embassy. A fortnight later, Ward was interviewed at the Foreign Office. Then he turned to a man he had known for twenty years, his friend – and patient – senior Conservative Member of Parliament Sir Godfrey Nicholson. Having seen the Foreign Secretary, Lord Home, Nicholson in turn passed the Ivanov messages on, through Ward, to the Foreign Office. Then he sent Ivanov three Foreign Office-approved letters, entrusting delivery to Ward – Lord Home had probably told Nicholson to avoid any direct contact with the Soviet agent.

'A series of suggestions were made through me,' Ward recalled in his draft memoir, which 'had the sanction of the FO and had been passed by security. These I gave to Ivanov, except the last and probably most important, which I delivered myself to the Soviet Embassy, since Ivanov was temporarily back in Russia for a holiday.'

An improbable courier, it seems, may actually have delivered the letters. On three occasions, Keeler wrote in her auto-biography, Ward sent her off to the Soviet embassy carrying letters for Ivanov. He gave her to understand they were invitations to play bridge, or apologies for missing one of the Russian's social occasions. Much later, Keeler said, she remembered that the envelopes had been too bulky to have been mere notes.

Ward's role as intermediary – then and later, during the Cuban Missile Crisis of 1962 – has been used to suggest he was a Soviet agent of influence, or at least a fellow-traveller. A number of people got that impression. One of his patients, whose husband moved in Ward's circle, told the writer Rebecca West she thought he 'had been a convinced communist for about seven years, from about 1955 or 1956 . . .' The entertainer Michael Bentine, who had known Ward for years, thought him 'extremely left-wing', as did the sports broadcaster Max Robertson, who got to know the osteopath following treatment for a tennis injury. Lord Denning described Ward as 'without a doubt a communist sympathiser . . . a potential danger'.

Sir Godfrey Nicholson, who was as much a part of the London approaches as Ward, was no left-winger. Lord Denning called him 'a most loyal Englishman'. Though Nicholson declined to discuss the detail of his role in the back-door diplomacy of 1961 and 1962, he wrote to us in staunch defence of Ward: 'The side I saw was generous and compassionate, and I liked it . . . He was, I am quite certain, a patriotic British citizen, and he would, I am sure, never have done anything harmful to this country.'

Perhaps, though we do not know this, Nicholson acted in 1961 and 1962 with the knowledge we have only now, that Ward had long been acting on behalf of British intelligence. If, as MI5 officials told us, he cultivated Ivanov at their request, it would certainly have been necessary for him to express sympathy for the Soviet point of view. On occasion, however, Ward was not afraid to argue with Ivanov.

On 15 September, during the Ward-Nicholson diplomacy, a military clash over Berlin seemed a distinct possibility. In the disputed air corridor over Germany, Soviet MiGs buzzed US civilian airliners. Foreign Secretary Lord Home, at the United Nations that month for high-level talks on the crisis, said, 'One false step, one failure in communication, even one failure in comprehension, might mean war.'

In London, Ward took Ivanov to task over the Soviet provocations. 'Why,' he asked the Russian, 'when you talk of a gesture, do you do this?' Ivanov had no answer – his ambassador was away. 'It brought home rather vividly,' Ward went on, 'that none of them would express an opinion unless they had been briefed.'

His own overall view of international politics, he wrote, was that 'the real sin in the world is failure to try to understand the views of others, and to respect them as genuine, however different from our own. The culmination of our present way is to try to destroy an idea with a bomb.'

As the global crisis stuttered on, Ward celebrated his forty-ninth birthday. When his ego was not being pumped by contacts with the high and mighty, what was left for him?

CHAPTER 16

The Man in the Mask

'The trouble with Stephen,' a female friend was to say, 'is that he has a Peter Pan complex.' He still had his charm, but the fabric of life was threadbare. The partying, however, continued.

One night in December 1961, as Christine Keeler and Mandy Rice-Davies were sitting around at home, Ward called. 'There's a party over at Mariella's,' Keeler told Rice-Davies. 'He wants us to go over.' Soon the two girls were ringing the doorbell to the flat in Hyde Park Square Mariella Novotny shared with her husband Hod Dibben – in time to join a party that was to keep the rumour mill going for years to come.

On her return from America, Novotny was to recall she had 'started to give lavish dinner parties in London, and weekend parties in Hampshire. Since my name was linked with extremely erotic activities, I decided to entertain on a large scale ... I chose to concentrate on exotic food and fascinating personalities. This combination stunned my friends when my sexual games completed the dinner parties. Within weeks my parties became the subject of gossip among the élite in London . . .'

Some of the entertaining was quite innocent. 'I normally arranged for twenty-four to dine, and served about seven or eight courses . . . The sort of friends I invited were not dumb. Among them were Walter Flack, Charles Clore's partner, Bill Astor, Sir William Emrys-Williams, Chikie Moss, Sheila Scott, Count Manfred Czernin, Beecher and Bobbie Moore, Eustace Chesser, Douglas Fairbanks Jr, Felix Topolski, Lord Belper, Lord Spencer, and many others.'

Some on this Novotny guest list have already featured in these pages. Of the rest, Sir William Emrys-Williams was Secretary of the Arts Council and a Trustee of the National Gallery; Chikie Moss was golfer Henry Cotton's stepdaughter; Sheila Scott was the flying ace; Lord Spencer was a member of the Advisory Council of the Victoria and Albert Museum – and grandfather of the future Diana, Princess of Wales. Those on the list from the art world were presumably invited to Hyde Park Square because of Hod Dibben's work as an antiques dealer.

While many of her guests took no part in what Novotny called her 'games', others attended – as she put it – 'both kinds of parties'. The goings-on, she wrote, 'amazed' psychiatrist Eustace Chesser, then a renowned authority on sex. As Novotny put it, 'some strange incidents developed . . . The bizarre became normal for me . . . My sadistic nature was no secret. I became humorously known as the Government Chief Whip.'

Of Stephen Ward, who was a frequent guest at the parties, Novotny noted that he 'had a strong fetish for shoes with high stiletto heels . . . These he pressed over his nose and mouth without any physical sexual activity.'

Lord Denning and his staff were preoccupied by Novotny and Dibben. The inquiry's secretary, Home Office official Thomas Critchley, was present when Novotny was interviewed. 'A beautiful blonde of Czech origin,' he noted, 'she had grown up witness to the horrors of the turbulent post-war years in Europe, and experiences of rape and torture that twisted her nature into something vile and deformed.' She had a character 'as hard as nails, and taste in sexual matters that by this time . . . had degenerated into extreme forms of depravity.'

It was Lord Denning himself who was to call the occasion in December 1961 'the Man in the Mask Party'. Those who claimed to know all about it called it 'the Feast of the Peacocks'. According to Novotny, it was one of a kind.

Though virtually over when Rice-Davies and Keeler got to Hyde Park Square, the party still managed to shock Rice-Davies: 'Stephen met us at the door, wearing nothing but a sock. I thought it was a joke. Everyone was in déshabillé, and Mariella was there wearing a kind of black corset and carrying a whip. Naked people were everywhere, draped over chairs, or standing around laughing and joking. But the real orgy had finished, nothing was going on – everybody was weary if not fainting . . .' Keeler, however, said she observed Novotny on a bed, simultaneously entertaining no less than six male guests.

'I didn't know where to look,' Rice-Davies says. 'After all, I *was* only seventeen, even if I had been around. I remember spotting this plate of tangerines – they were a rarity in winter in those days – and I attacked those tangerines and some chocolates until I felt sick. We must have spent about twenty minutes there. Then we left, with Stephen . . .'

The only person to have offered a detailed account of what had gone on earlier that evening was hostess Mariella Novotny herself. She devoted several pages of her unpublished manuscript to the party. A man, she wrote, had been 'strapped between wood pillars. A flail or whip was in front of his naked figure. As each guest arrived they gave him one stroke, then left the man to join the party. When he was released before dining, he was ordered to remain beneath the long table, out of sight . . .' Novotny continued:

I cooked a pair of young peacocks for the main dish, skewered their necks and heads in position, and added the colourful tail feathers of older birds. When they were carried to the table, a girl became hysterical and screamed that they signified death. She created havoc and had to be sent home, before she ruined the party . . . Badgers were another unusual animal I cooked . . . I object to my parties being called vile and revolting. Had they been unpleasant, the clamour to be invited would not have been so enormous.

The man in the mask was a masochist and asked me to treat him as my 'slave'. I willingly agreed, and caused him mental and physical pain. This was what he wanted – I did nothing against his wishes. The humiliation he underwent was extreme, but was the dream of his life. Under the table he obeyed any order I gave him to please my guests . . . Everyone went home well satisfied.

What people wanted to know eighteen months later, of course, when the Profumo scandal broke, was just who the 'satisfied' guests at the party had been. Rice-Davies had noticed among the guests 'some well-known actors and a politician . . . There was one well-known barrister . . .' Novotny, in her manuscript, identified only one alleged participant, Conservative MP William Rees-Davies.

Who, though, was the Man in the Mask? Rice-Davies and Keeler were to say Ward gave them the impression it was then Minister of Transport Ernest Marples. In his testimony to Lord Denning, Ward denied ever having said that – he thought the girls must have misconstrued something said in jest. The rumour spread, nevertheless, in Ward's social circle. Marples, whose nefarious financial activity has been described in a previous chapter, was indeed said to have often used prostitutes – and Cabinet colleagues became alarmed. When the rumours reached Marples himself, he took out a bizarre form of insurance against being dragged further into the scandal: he sought Cabinet authority to have a bug installed in his home.

Those best qualified to say who the masked man was, of course, were hostess Novotny and her husband Hod Dibben, both of whom were interviewed by Lord Denning. Denning reported that they told him the masked man's identity and that he interviewed the man – who declared himself 'grievously ashamed of what he did'. Neither he nor any of the guests, Denning said, had been a 'Minister or any person prominent in public life'.

When the authors asked Hod Dibben who the masked man had been, he stuck to his own code of honour. 'I promised the person in question I would never reveal his name and I never will, even though the man is dead.' Dibben was, though, prepared to say the man had not been Transport Minister Marples. His wife Novotny could not be questioned – she died in 1983 – but the manuscript she left behind contained information on the identity of the Man in the Mask.

'I lied to Lord Denning,' Novotny wrote, 'but not about a politician – my lies were to protect someone from ruin and a criminal charge . . .' Elsewhere, in brief notes written later – probably in the mid-sixties – Novotny named the masked man. He 'was not a politician,' she wrote. 'He was a peer of the realm . . . it was Lord Asquith.'

This seemed at first to the authors to be a bizarre calumny. Formally speaking, 'Lord Asquith' was at that time Julian, the 2nd Earl of Oxford and Asquith, grandson of the Liberal Prime Minister, and a diplomat. In 1961, on the heels of a posting in the Caribbean, Asquith was appointed Governor of the Seychelles. There is no reason whatsoever to think he attended the Feast of the Peacocks, or any sex orgy. At the time of the Man in the Mask Party, he was thousands of miles away. Hod Dibben, moreover, dismissed the suggestion that he had been the masked man.

Another Asquith, however – a man who was *known* to some as 'Lord' – turns out to have been a candidate for the role of Man in the Mask. This was the Honourable Anthony Asquith, youngest son of the former prime minister, the 1st Earl of Oxford and Asquith. Following education at Winchester and Balliol College, Oxford, Asquith had gone on to success as a director of movies – including *Pygmalion*, *French Without Tears*, *The Winslow Boy*, *The Millionairess*, *The VIPs* and *The Yellow Rolls-Royce* – and became president of the Association of Cinematograph, Television and Allied Technicians, a fellow of the British Academy and a governor of the British Film Institute before his death in 1968.

Anthony Asquith – 'Puffin' to close friends – had been dubbed 'Lord' by his film technicians. Fifty-nine in 1961, his talent had not been matched by happiness in life. The son of a domineering mother, he never married and struggled with alcoholism. The truth was that he was a sad, repressed homosexual in an era when open homosexuality was utterly unacceptable. This son of an aristocrat was sometimes to be found at weekends serving up food in a lorry drivers' café near Catterick in Yorkshire. The actors Michael Denison and Dirk Bogarde, who worked with him, saw parallels between him and Lawrence of Arabia, whose life Asquith once hoped to bring to the screen – he would say that Lawrence, who had been a friend, was a 'not practising' homosexual. 'His recurrent trips to Joe's Café at Catterick,' Denison said, 'seem to me very like T. E. Lawrence's escape into anonymity.' Lawrence, of course, was a masochist.

'Puffin,' said another friend, Pierre Rouvé, 'was born to be a mind. The body was there as an appendage which he dragged behind that mind all his life. Consequently everything that was a concern of the body, a pleasure of the body, seemed alien to him . . . Such violence as he depicted on the screen always seemed to me to be an attack by him on that enemy of his, the body, to prevent it taking possession of the mind and destroying the mind.'

Was Anthony Asquith the man in the rubber mask strapped between the wooden pillars at Hyde Park Square in December 1961, gratefully accepting the lash from guests, grovelling under the table as those above scoffed peacock? Ward's friend Warwick Charlton said Asquith did attend Novotny's parties. Hod Dibben acknowledged that he had been a guest. Asked whether he had been the masked man, he merely smiled secretively. He did not deny it, as he had the names of other possible candidates.

The matter must rest there. The authors believe it very possible that the Honourable Anthony Asquith, son of a prime minister, was indeed the Man in the Mask.

In 1963, Lord Denning succeeded only in dispelling the notion that the Man in the Mask had been a minister in the Conservative government. He could not alter the wholly accurate impression that members of society's elite led private lives that made a mockery of their public role as defenders of respectability and the public good. 'It is a fond illusion,' Labour Member of Parliament Sydney Silverman was to say in the House of Commons in 1963, 'that Lord Denning's Report established the falsity of the rumours. It did nothing of the kind – it established their accuracy . . . He established the truth of every one of them. Do not let us fool ourselves.'

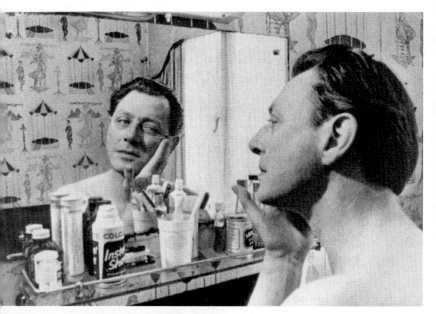

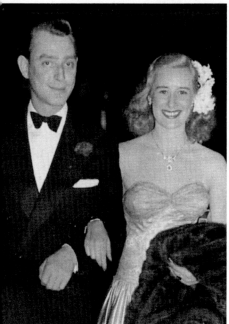

Stephen Ward was a sexual enigma, voyeur as much as participant.

With actress Celia Lipton at a premiere, 1948. He cultivated high society.

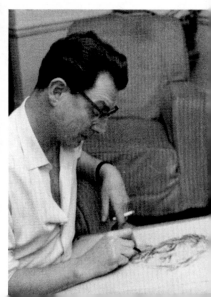

Though an osteopath by profession, Ward was also an accomplished artist.

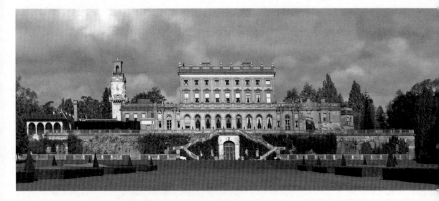

Lord Astor's vast mansion at Cliveden. At a cottage on the estate, Ward entertained many women.

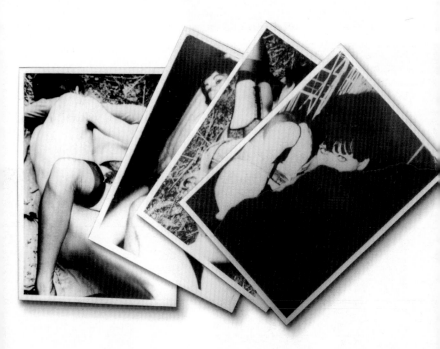

These sex photographs, allegedly taken by Ward, are part of a batch that has surfaced. Some of his female associates are recognisable in uncensored versions of the pictures.

John Profumo was Her Majesty's Secretary of State for War – until his resignation because of his affair with Christine Keeler.

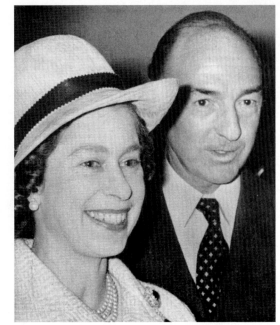

Captain Yevgeny Ivanov, the Soviet agent against whom MI5 ran a 'honeytrap' operation – in uniform and as sketched by Ward.

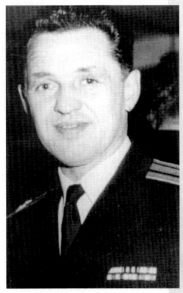

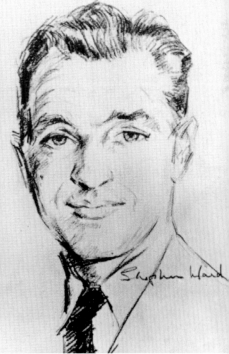

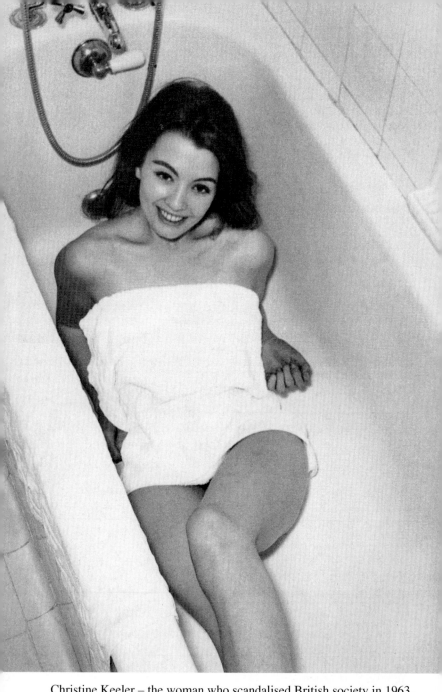

Christine Keeler – the woman who scandalised British society in 1963.

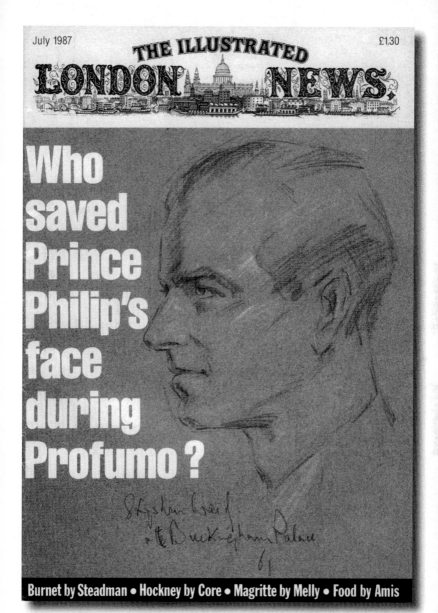

July 1987 £1.30

THE ILLUSTRATED LONDON NEWS

Who saved Prince Philip's face during Profumo ?

Burnet by Steadman • Hockney by Core • Magritte by Melly • Food by Amis

Prince Philip, sketched by Ward in 1961, a day after Ward had been visited by MI5. Ward had met the Prince socially years earlier. Soviet spy Ivanov claimed he sent 'candid' photos of the Prince, obtained from Ward, to Moscow.

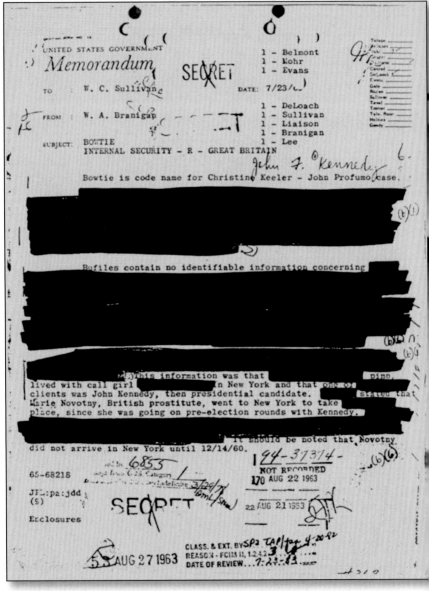

UNITED STATES GOVERNMENT

Memorandum

TO : W. C. Sullivan

FROM : W. A. Branigan

SUBJECT: BOWTIE
INTERNAL SECURITY - R - GREAT BRITAIN

DATE: 7/23/

1 - Belmont
1 - Mohr
1 - Evans

1 - DeLoach
1 - Sullivan
1 - Liaison
1 - Branigan
1 - Lee

John F. Kennedy

Bowtie is code name for Christine Keeler - John Profumo case.

Bufiles contain no identifiable information concerning

This information was that   pimp,
lived with call girl   in New York and that one of
clients was John Kennedy, then presidential candidate.   that
Marie Novotny, British prostitute, went to New York to take
place, since she was going on pre-election rounds with Kennedy.

It should be noted that Novotny
did not arrive in New York until 12/14/60.

65-68218

JFL:pa:jdd
(5)

Enclosures

94-37374-
NOT RECORDED
170 AUG 22 1963

22 AUG 21 1963

AUG 27 1963

CLASS. & EXT. BY SP2
REASON - FCIM II, 1-2-4-2
DATE OF REVIEW... 7-27-83

The American connection – from the FBI's BOWTIE dossier on
the Profumo case. It informs the Assistant Director in charge of
Counterintelligence of allegations that – before he became President
– John F. Kennedy slept with two women linked to Stephen Ward.

Dear Noel
I'm sorry I
has to do this here...
It's really more than I
can stand - the horror
day after day at the court
and in the streets - it's not
only fear - it's a wish not
to let them get me. I'd
rather get myself. -

2 I do hope I haven't let
people down too much.
I (tried) to do my stuff, but
after Marshall's summing up
I've given up all hope
The car made out in the
gene box. By the way, he
happy in it.
Evidently it was surprising
easy - required no guts.
I'm going to addapent the

3 vathier - Poral Hope
This has done the rest.
delay resuscitation nothing
no possible.

There was strong evidence that Ward committed suicide by swallowing barbiturates – this letter was addressed to his host, Noel Howard-Jones. Former MI6 operative Lee Tracey, however, (inset) has now said – on the record – that Ward was killed.

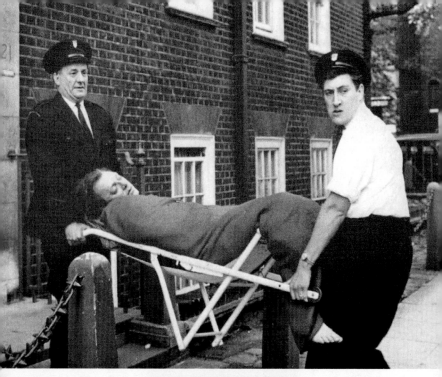

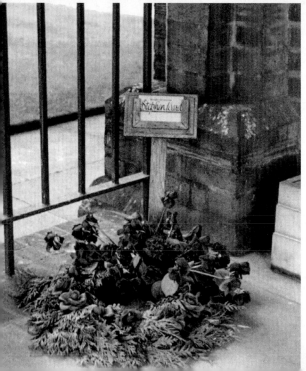

Ward died abandoned
by his wealthy friends.
There was only one
wreath at his funeral.

CHAPTER 17

Things Fall Apart

During 1961, Stephen Ward became somehow shabbier. 'He started to look scruffier and more down at heel,' the 4th Lord Dudley told us. 'There was a deterioration in his lifestyle. I think that's when he was getting involved with sort of, rather sleazy people . . .' Lord Dudley had a point. The best and most beautiful girls were behind Ward now. As he continued to strive to keep wealthy friends happy, he lowered his standards somewhat.

One night in 1961, a prostitute using the name Adrienne left her flat in Curzon Street, Mayfair. Adrienne was a drug addict, on her way to the pharmacy round the corner. A white Jaguar pulled alongside as she walked, and the driver struck up a conversation – Ward, offering to find her clients.

Adrienne – that was not her real name – had retired from the prostitution game by the time she spoke with the authors. Nudging sixty, though still showing traces of the looks that attracted Ward, she lived now in a basement flat in West London. Ironically, Adrienne was never called as a witness at the Ward trial. Because she had thought Ward 'kind and honourable', she had denied knowing him when approached by the police. Had she not done so, the prosecution's case against Ward would have been stronger.

Adrienne still remembered the clients Ward sent her – 'some peers and MPs, and plenty of Americans.' She had given Ward a handful of her business cards, and the men he sent all brought one with them. One, she said, was the 10th Duke of Marlborough, whose wife died in the summer of 1961. Though he initially annoyed her by sending his chauffeur round to take an advance look at her, the Duke became a regular customer. Another aristocratic client, and a close friend of Ward, whom Adrienne remembered as 'a rather sinister bisexual' would insist that she sign a written agreement before each sex act.

Adrienne was still a heroin addict when interviewed for this book – a survivor of a forty-year habit that included being provided with the drug by society doctor Lady Isabella Frankau. Frankau, who prescribed it in the mistaken belief that she thus spared junkies the black market, had operated from a surgery in Wimpole Street just around the corner from Stephen Ward's flat.

The drugs disaster was just starting in England at the time of the Profumo Affair. For most people using drugs meant only 'reefer parties', and marijuana supplied by West Indian immigrants, but the greater evil was gaining ground – and affected some of those around Stephen Ward. Though Ward was to insist in 1963 that he had done all he could to protect his girls from drugs, he was tolerant when Christine Keeler first got interested in marijuana. That was a mistaken indulgence, for the drug connection played a key role in the way the Profumo Affair broke.

Later on the night of the Man in the Mask Party in December 1961, Mandy Rice-Davies aroused the wrath of her lover Peter Rachman by arriving at his place smelling of marijuana. She had inadvertently picked up the smell on her clothes, she told the authors, by sitting next to Keeler in Ward's Jaguar. Keeler had been drawn to marijuana in recent months, certainly since a night in October when she, the portrait artist Vasco Lazzolo and Ward had visited the El Rio Café in Notting Hill. Ward and Lazzolo liked the raffish atmosphere – the café was a hang-out for young

West Indian immigrants, and a place where drug deals were made.

Lazzolo was leery of buying any marijuana, but wanted some. Keeler, who thought he and Ward came over like plain-clothes policemen, told them to wait outside while she tried to buy some. At the back of the premises, where the toilets were, she came across a West Indian man who sold her ten shillings' worth of dope – a price that, though in literal terms equal to fifty pence in modern currency, was in real terms much more at that time. Then, believing Keeler to be a prostitute, he kept her talking. Keeler, who knew Ward had a penchant for black girls, told the man they might be able to get together again – if he could supply 'a sister for my brother'. The man had plenty of sisters, he said, and Keeler gave him the telephone number of Ward's Wimpole Mews flat.

This had been a fateful encounter, one that would prove very unlucky for a number of people. The West Indian was Aloysius 'Lucky' Gordon, a thirty-one-year-old who had arrived in Britain more than a decade earlier. While doing his then obligatory National Service in the Army, he had been discharged for threatening an officer. Later, he had been deported from Denmark for another assault. Another offence on his record, according to Keeler, had been 'sticking a knife up a girl's vagina'.

Gordon phoned two days after the episode at El Rio to invite Keeler and Ward to a party. A combination of drink and drugs made Keeler ill, and Ward had to take her home. The persistent Gordon kept calling, however, saying he wanted help in fencing some jewellery. Keeler thought she could help, for she and Ward had been to a club frequented by criminals. So it was that she went with Gordon to a house, ostensibly to take a look at the jewellery he had mentioned. There, by her account, he held her at knifepoint and repeatedly raped her. She only got away from him, she said, when she promised to see him again.

Gordon turned up soon after, accompanied by a drug dealer, at the Wimpole Mews flat. He wanted to see Keeler in private, he said, to apologise. Once in her bedroom, he again became violent. Ward called the police, but – as Keeler had no visible injury – no charges were brought. According to Ward, he thereafter did what he could to get Keeler back on the straight and narrow, taking her to see a senior Drugs Squad officer at Scotland Yard. Keeler denied this. Ward's psychiatrist friend Dr Ellis Stungo, however, recalled the osteopath sending Keeler to him because she was smoking marijuana and seeing black men.

By early 1962, Christine Keeler was staying with a friend in Dolphin Square, not far from the House of Commons. She and Mandy Rice-Davies rarely lived in one place for more than a few months – sometimes just weeks in Keeler's case – during that period. By Keeler's account, she was now regularly using marijuana. Her playground, now more than ever, was the bars and nightspots of what would soon be known as 'Swinging London'. At home, she said, she and friends 'thought nothing of wandering around or answering the door entirely in the nude'. One of the people who appeared on the doorstep was Lucky Gordon.

He rampaged through the flat, according to Keeler, for some forty-eight hours, threatening her and her friend with an axe. The police were eventually called, and this time they did charge Gordon – only for the charges to be dropped after Gordon's brother assured Keeler that she would never be bothered again. Gordon did persist in making contact, however, and she went on seeing him in spite of everything. By summer 1962, he was sleeping on the fire escape of the flat at Dolphin Square. Keeler briefly shared a room with him at his brother's place. Then she went back to an old lover, Michael Lambton, before boarding a liner with Mandy Rice-Davies – tickets paid for by Lambton and Peter Rachman – bound for the United States.

During the crossing, according to Rice-Davies, 'Christine took a fifteen-year-old's virginity in a ship's lifeboat, slept with the first officer and the captain, all in five days.' The visit to America proved disastrous. Following an excursion to Fire Island, famed as a homosexual community, both young women suffered severe sunburn. They sent home for extra money, then – only a week after arriving – flew back to London.

Lucky Gordon was waiting – and Keeler turned for help to another West Indian, John Edgecombe. 'I was going about my business one day,' fifty-five-year-old Edgecombe told the authors in his first interview since 1963, when 'Christine, whom I didn't know, and Paula Hamilton-Marshall were in a taxi going the other way. They stopped it and called me . . . And Paula opened the taxi door . . .'

Edgecombe knew Hamilton-Marshall, who had a police record as a prostitute. She had a flat in Devonshire Street, near Ward's consulting room, and used to go round to Wimpole Mews to indulge in sexual activity, and that was where the trio headed. At the time in question, she was pregnant by a black US Air Force officer who had gone home to the States.

When Hamilton-Marshall, Keeler and Edgecombe got to Wimpole Mews, Edgecombe said, 'there was a guy in the doorway with his hat down, and Christine fell on the floor of the taxi and started saying "That's him [Gordon]!" Eventually we went upstairs, and every time the doorbell went, Christine hid in case it was Lucky . . .'

Edgecombe, who also went to bed with Keeler, concluded that he had been recruited to protect her from Gordon. Keeler, however, seemed unable to stay away from her persecutor – even when, according to her, he beat her up in the street. Keeler was mesmerised by Gordon, by black men in general, and by the drugs scene. Her involvements with the West Indian men brought a different sort of danger. For both men in due course learned of Keeler's affair with the Minister for War – an affair that, according to the Denning Report, had supposedly ended in late 1961.

During the summer of 1962, Gordon was to tell a detective a year later, Keeler tried to get rid of him by mentioning that 'she had friends in high places, including a Cabinet Minister, and that – if he didn't stop pestering her – she would have him dealt with by the Minister'. One evening, Gordon said, he saw a man enter Christine's flat, stay for about an hour, then leave. The visitor, Keeler told him afterwards, had been John Profumo. A few days later, when Gordon saw Profumo's photograph in the newspaper, he thought he recognised him as the mysterious visitor.

Edgecombe also heard about Profumo. 'This chick,' he told the authors, 'looked as if she had some class, and I asked her what she was doing running round with a cat like Gordon . . . To turn it around she told me about Profumo. I took it all with a pinch of salt – I mean, I didn't know who the fuck Profumo was anyway . . .'

Edgecombe soon learned more about the Minister. 'If she needed some bread,' he said, 'she could always ring up and arrange to see Jack. She would go off and see him, and he'd give her some money. I don't think it was a lot, fifteen or twenty pounds, maybe. Yes, she was sleeping with him – she wouldn't see the guy for anything else. I don't know how many times she rung him . . .'

Keeler's rackety life had begun to threaten John Profumo. Stephen Ward, for his part, was walking a social tightrope, with Keeler in a West Indian dive one day, hobnobbing with aristocracy the next. The mix was ever more dangerous, for he was also still cultivating Yevgeny Ivanov.

In the third week of June 1962, Ward took the Soviet diplomat to an Ascot Week house party thrown by Lord Harrington. 'There were so many guests,' Ward wrote, 'that a large marquee had been put up in the garden, and was known as the House of Lords . . . until we came, the inhabitants were all peers of the realm.' Also in Ascot Week, Ward took Ivanov to the home of the millionaire Paul Getty in Guildford, Surrey.

Ward knew the oil baron's executive assistant Claus von Bülow – real name Claus Borberg – a Danish aristocrat whose functions for Getty reportedly included obtaining a supply of 'rejuvenation' drugs and organising parties. Getty, a relentless womaniser, once boasted of having had sex with five women in a single day.

Ward had been at the Getty spread before – once for dinner, when he brought a woman with him, and once when he arrived dramatically by air in a plane piloted by his cousin, an RAF wing commander. The company on the occasion he brought along Ivanov included Getty's son, a Russian lady aristocrat and a Czech-born girlfriend of Ward – not Mariella Novotny but Ilya Suschenek, who knew Ward through Ivanov and, like so many others in the story, had also visited Lord Astor's estate at Cliveden.

The visit to the Getty residence ended in chaos for everyone involved. 'There was,' Ward wrote in his memoir:

. . . vodka and more vodka, toasts to this and that, and then song, it went on the whole afternoon. When we left most of us were in a sorry state. We loaded Paul's guests into a car and sent them home and set off back to Lord Harrington's. Ivanov, when asked whether he could drive, said, 'I am a captain in the Russian Navy, and I can navigate anywhere.' So he did, and we found ourselves in the middle of the rifle ranges, hopelessly lost. At that moment a head popped over the back seat, and there was one of Paul's guests who had stowed away without our knowledge, very much under the weather . . . We decided to send her back the thirty miles to Paul Getty, C.O.D. From then on we had a series of horrifying bulletins of her progress across the countryside. As each one was brought in by the butler we laughed louder and louder – and eventually, to cap it all, a message from Mr Getty that he would not pay the taxi, and that it was all the fault of the Russian captain . . .

In April 1962, MI5 received a report from the police Special Branch, which had been running surveillance on Ward and Ivanov as they cavorted in high society and attended diplomatic functions. Special Branch also passed on reports of Ward's alleged communist sympathies. As he was to insist, however, Ward himself kept MI5 briefed on his contacts with Russians. An MI5 report, written following a further meeting between the osteopath and Wagstaffe, expressed alarm that 'without knowledge Ward was used by the Foreign Office . . . to pass off-the-record information to the Russian Embassy'. MI5 subsequently confirmed that 'suitably tailored material' had been channelled to Ivanov through Ward. The Foreign Office, told that Ward was 'both naïve and indiscreet', chose to ignore the warning.

As Ward made the social round with Ivanov, Christine Keeler's dark odyssey continued. By now really afraid of Lucky Gordon, she resolved, as 1962 dwindled, to shake him off once and for all. She would, she decided, purchase a gun. She gave 'a very respectable bloke' – Ward would later say he was a 'criminal negro' and that the gun had previously been used in a hold-up – £25 for a German gun and ammunition. Then – in the countryside near her parents' home – she practised firing the weapon. 'It worked,' Keeler said later. 'If Lucky Gordon came at me again, I was going to kill him . . .'

Christine Keeler was never to get the opportunity to use her gun on Lucky Gordon, for John Edgecombe took it away from her. Shots Edgecombe himself would loose off, however, were to ruin the career of the British Minister for War and destroy Stephen Ward. Before those shots were fired, though, the world would come close to a nuclear holocaust.

CHAPTER 18

The Missiles and the Messenger

On a bitterly cold evening in the autumn of 1962, a man stood on the runway of the American airbase at Greenham Common in Berkshire. He was US Ambassador to London David Bruce, and he had no idea – thus far – why he had been summoned to the base after normal hours, with advice that he come armed with a service revolver. At the same time, another man – Stephen Ward – sat hunched in his Jaguar, heading back to London after a damp weekend at Cliveden. Bruce was already caught up in the most serious international crisis of all time, and Ward soon would be.

Sunday, 21 October marked the start of the Cuban Missile Crisis, a drama so far hidden from all but a trusted few. Aboard a US Air Force Boeing, high above Ambassador Bruce, was the elderly man who would shortly explain all to him, former Secretary of State Dean Acheson. With him were three CIA agents, three armed guards and a briefcase. This was a very secret mission.

For a moment, when the ambassador welcomed the statesman on the tarmac, there was laughter. Bruce proffered a bottle of whisky and told Acheson to feel the gun that nestled in his pocket. 'I was told by the Department of State to carry this when I met you,' Bruce said. 'There was nothing said about shooting me, was there?' responded Acheson. With no further delay, the men then got down to business.

Acheson had flown to England on the orders of President Kennedy, with aerial surveillance photographs of Soviet missile sites under construction in Cuba. Through an extraordinary series of contacts between a senior GRU agent and the President's brother Robert, Nikita Khrushchev had for weeks been sending assurances that Soviet aid to Cuba would include no offensive missiles. This was a lie. At breakfast on 16 October, still in his dressing gown, Kennedy had been shown photographs proving that missile launch sites were under construction, that missile erectors had been deployed and that a storage site for nuclear warheads was in position. Missiles might already be on the island, and more Soviet freighters with suspect cargo were on the way.

The launch sites were for medium-range ballistic missiles, capable of hitting American cities. Once operational, they would irrevocably alter the nuclear status quo. The Cuban Missile Crisis had begun.

Britain's government and its intelligence services were factors in the crisis from the start. GRU traitor Oleg Penkovsky, who was being handled by MI6, had provided information that, according to defence expert Anthony Verrier, 'allowed the CIA to follow the progress of Soviet missile emplacement in Cuba by the hour'. As important was Penkovsky's demolition of the myth Khrushchev had propagated that the Soviets had more intercontinental ballistic missiles, capable of precision attacks, than the United States. According to Penkovsky, the Soviet ICBMs 'couldn't hit a bull in the backside with a balalaika'. His assessment, moreover, was that the Soviet Union had no real intention of going to war. Installing missiles in Cuba was part of a gamble, designed to give Khrushchev greater leverage over the United States and to test Kennedy's resolve.

The MI6 Station Chief in Washington, Maurice Oldfield – later to be head of MI6 – had laboured in the weeks before the crisis to convince the President and other key Americans that Penkovsky was a genuine source rather than a Soviet plant. Kennedy's people had finally been persuaded of this on the eve of the crisis, when surveillance pictures were compared with a missile manual Penkovsky had provided. The match was exact. Armed with this and other intelligence, the President was ready to call Khrushchev's bluff.

By the Sunday Bruce met with Acheson at Greenham Common, American officials were working day and night. Many would soon move camp beds into their offices. The President made time that day, nevertheless, to have British ambassador David Ormsby-Gore to lunch at the White House. Ormsby-Gore, later Lord Harlech, had been a personal friend of Kennedy's since his days in London at the start of World War II. Now, with nuclear war threatening, Ormsby-Gore was the one foreign diplomat promised a place in the presidential fallout shelter. He was a trusted confidant of both Kennedy and British Prime Minister Macmillan – and the families of all three were linked by marriage.

The President was concerned to know how Macmillan would react as the Crisis progressed. During the tension over Berlin, Macmillan had counselled prudence in dealing with Khrushchev. Now, as Kennedy prepared to face down the Soviet leader, it seemed possible that the older man's caution would look like vacillation. Would Macmillan try to play the statesman, to mediate in some way, a move the Soviets might interpret as a sign that the Western alliance was shaky?

In Washington, Ormsby-Gore quietly supported the President's plan to take a tough stance. To convince Macmillan of the urgency of the new situation, he suggested Kennedy send him the telltale missile photographs. So it was that Dean Acheson flew into

Greenham Common with copies, and that the following morning, a Monday, the British Prime Minister sat examining them at Number 10 Downing Street. Late that night London time, as England slept, President Kennedy made a nationwide television appearance. He announced a US naval blockade of Cuba and warned that, if attacked, America would retaliate in kind.

The next day, Tuesday, was a crucial moment in the crisis. Behind the scenes, MI6 learned that Colonel Penkovsky's luck had run out. He had been arrested in Moscow, and would in due course be tried and executed. Given a damage assessment, including a briefing by Soviet embassy officials in London, Khrushchev rapidly learned how serious the leak had been. The Soviet leader had to assume now that Kennedy knew enough of Soviet intentions to call his bluff. How could he climb down without publicly losing face? Until a way could be found, Khrushchev remained very dangerous, unpredictable.

The next day, Wednesday, 24 October, the Cuban Missile Crisis came to Wimpole Mews when Captain Yevgeny Ivanov placed a call to Stephen Ward. 'Ivanov wanted,' Ward wrote later, 'to get a message behind the scenes to the Government. He came armed with full authority, he said, to speak for the Soviet government in this matter, and replies could be obtained from Moscow in a matter of hours direct from the Kremlin. There is no doubt at all that this was so. No one from the Soviet Embassy would dare to speak in this way were it not so.'

According to an MI5 source, the phone call was not the only Soviet approach made through Ward. Ivanov subsequently came around to the Mews accompanied by another Soviet diplomat, chargé d'affaires Vitalij Loginov. There was, as Ward put it, 'practically a Cabinet meeting'.

The Ivanov call triggered days of contacts with the British government, with Ward acting as go-between. Ivanov came to

Ward's Devonshire Street consulting rooms for a meeting with him and Sir Godfrey Nicholson, the Conservative MP who a year earlier, during the crisis over Berlin, had liaised with the Foreign Office on Ivanov's behalf.

'We listened to Ivanov with growing amazement,' Ward wrote, 'as he unfolded his suggestion, no less than the calling of a Summit Conference in London . . . On this offer being accepted the Russians could agree to reverse the course of their ships, at that moment sailing on a collision course with the American Navy . . . On the subject of rockets in Cuba he told me that discussions on a quid pro quo basis would be started at once.'

British officials would later play down the role Ivanov and Ward played during the Cuban Missile Crisis. The Denning Report would call Ward's activities 'misconceived and ill-directed'. Ward, for his part, appeared to think naively that the fate of humanity hinged on him. One day that week, Mandy Rice-Davies was to remember, he said solemnly, 'Pray for me, Mandy. If I fail to bring about the meeting I've planned, it could mean the end of the world.'

While it was characteristic of Ward to inflate his role, anyone alive at the time of the Cuban Missile Crisis would recall that everything was out of proportion that week. It did indeed seem that humanity was about to destroy itself. Ward, moreover, had reason to think the Ivanov approach was serious and that the British government would treat it seriously. The previous year, the Foreign Office had approved Nicholson's communications with Ivanov and, by extension, their delivery to the Soviet embassy by Ward. There is nothing implausible about using lowly intermediaries to carry momentous messages. In Washington, the use of such a messenger was to play a major role in the resolution of the Cuban Missile Crisis. In London, Stephen Ward again acted as messenger.

The Soviets were snatching at any straw of hope that Britain might offer to mediate between Moscow and Washington. It was a move that could delay matters, perhaps help Khrushchev save face. 'The Prime Minister and myself,' British Foreign Secretary Home had said, 'will, once we have checked the present fever, play our full part in an attempt to end the Cold War.' Saying this as he did the day before Ivanov's call to Ward, Home may have given the impression that Britain might intervene in the crisis as 'an honest broker'.

At the same time, British intelligence, drawing either on phone taps or on information from an agent inside the Soviet embassy, learned of an embassy message to Moscow that reported, in essence, that 'the British government is not happy about developments'. The message that Ivanov delivered, through Ward and Nicholson, was that the Soviets thought Britain did offer hope of mediation in the crisis over Cuba.

Ward and Nicholson both followed up on their meeting with Ivanov within hours. Ward phoned the Foreign Office to leave a message for the Permanent Under-Secretary of State, Sir Harold – later Lord – Caccia. Lord Astor, according to Ward, had suggested that the osteopath call to put himself forward as an intermediary. Ward and Caccia knew each other – they had lunched, together with Sir Godfrey Nicholson, following Ivanov's earlier attempt at back-door diplomacy.

Nicholson, who went to the Foreign Office in person, told Ward he had personally delivered the Soviet proposal for a summit to Caccia. Caccia, who had previously thought Ward's activity merely meddlesome, now forwarded Ivanov's message of conciliation to the British ambassador in Moscow. The ambassador was 'sceptical about both the information and the initiative'. Caccia, meanwhile, also briefed the chair of the Joint Intelligence Committee, Sir Hugh Stephenson.

Ivanov, meanwhile, was nervy. Although the message he had delivered had been about peace talks, he was aggressive about the alternatives. The same day, at a coffee bar near Ward's consulting rooms, solicitor Michael Eddowes found Ivanov and the osteopath deep in conversation. Eddowes, who had known Ward for years and been treated by him, joined them at their table and asked Ivanov what he thought would happen if the US Navy prevented Soviet ships from reaching Cuba. 'We will blockade Norway [where American missiles were sited],' the Russian blustered, according to Eddowes. 'Or we will drop a bomb in the sea a mile off New York, creating a tidal wave, or we will destroy England [also the site of US missiles] in seven minutes.'

Seated at the next table, quietly eavesdropping on this conversation, was Conservative MP William Shepherd, and he reported the exchange to MI5.

Events the next morning, Thursday, 25 October, seemed at first to augur well for the Soviet approaches in London, with the news that Soviet chargé d'affaires Vitalij Loginov had called on the Foreign Secretary. Ivanov soon learned, however, that the meeting had been unproductive. It had been a sticky session, he told Ward. Home had told Loginov, it later emerged, that Britain 'had no intention of seeking to mediate'.

Macmillan was to remember the Soviet overtures as an attempt 'to drive a wedge between ourselves and the United States . . . a natural part of the Soviet attempt to weaken our resolution'. At the time, Ivanov justified the need for Britain to mediate with a burst of rhetoric. 'It's like a motor accident,' he told Ward, 'where two drivers are arguing while a victim, which in this case is humanity, bleeds to death.'

In Britain, as in other European capitals, Soviet officials continued to work behind the scenes. Mandy Rice-Davies, who was staying at Wimpole Mews at the time, recalled returning one afternoon – almost certainly that Thursday – to find Ivanov and Ward in a huddle with a new arrival, Lord Astor. 'There was much talk about offensive and defensive missiles,' Rice-Davies remembered. 'But I was very young, and it didn't make much sense to me.'

Ward drove Rice-Davies to Whitehall one day that week and gave her some pro-Soviet leaflets to distribute. She giggled at the memory. 'I just walked into the Foreign Office. Nobody stopped me, and left them all over the place. Stephen waited for me round the corner in the car.' Ward's purpose, perhaps, was to reinforce in Ivanov the impression that Ward was on his side, a man he could trust.

Ivanov told Ward and Lord Astor that he was working on direct orders from Moscow, without the knowledge of the Soviet ambassador. He favoured, he said, the notion of an informal gathering of interested parties, Members of Parliament and diplomats, to take place at Cliveden. It seemed that the Soviet attaché remained convinced that the British aristocracy still had real influence. He would have known, to be sure, about the Cliveden set, the group of aristocrats, under the patronage of Lord Astor's parents, said to have sought to keep Britain out of World War II.

The mere fact of being styled 'Lord', Ivanov evidently thought, meant a man could influence events in Britain. While that was obviously an exaggeration, the notion was not entirely silly in 1963. The Macmillan years saw great power placed in the hands of some aristocrats. A foreigner could be forgiven for thinking that members of the Devonshire, Stuart, Ormsby-Gore and Salisbury families held some of the levers of power. Prime Minister Macmillan himself, though a commoner, had married into the Devonshire family. Ivanov hoped to bypass Foreign Secretary Lord Home and get his message to the very top.

'This time,' Stephen Ward was to write, 'we aimed at the Prime Minister himself . . . I rang Lord Astor and through him arranged to take the Soviet offer to Lord Arran, and thence to the PM . . .'

CHAPTER 19

Not the End of the World

In the midst of the Cuban Missile Crisis, some in London continued to indulge in their bizarre antics – some. At the latest party at her home, Mariella Novotny later recalled: 'Standing against the fireplace surrounded by discarded clothes was William Rees-Davies, a Conservative MP. He was addressing a small group as if in the House or in a courtroom, while a very pretty girl knelt on the carpet in front of him having sex with him orally. He appeared disinterested in her ardent attention, preferring the sound of his own pompous voice deliberating on the Cuban crisis. His orgasm caused him to pause only briefly and call for his glass to be refilled.' Novotny's husband Hod Dibben, who said this episode indeed took place, recalled that Stephen Ward, too, found time to be at the party.

Friday, 26 October found Ward playing messenger boy again. He again contacted the Foreign Office on Ivanov's behalf, and was received by Sir Harold Caccia's private secretary. That same day, in the United States, another Soviet intelligence officer also tried an approach through a private citizen. Late that morning Washington time, the phone rang on the desk of the American Broadcasting Company's diplomatic correspondent, John Scali.

The caller was Aleksander Fomin, officially a counsellor at the Soviet embassy but actually a KGB colonel who headed the KGB office in Washington. Fomin, who knew Scali, asked if they could meet immediately.

The two men lunched together, and Fomin behaved much, it seems, as Ivanov had towards Ward. 'Perhaps,' he said quietly, 'a way can be found to solve this crisis . . .' Should the United States agree not to invade Cuba, he suggested, the Soviet Union would dismantle its Cuban missile bases and pledge never to install offensive weapons on Cuba. Scali had a memorandum of the conversation on the desk of Roger Hilsman, director of intelligence at the State Department, within the hour.

That same afternoon, a rambling but similar message arrived from Khrushchev himself. If the US government would promise never to invade Cuba, said Khrushchev, 'this would immediately change everything . . .' That evening at the White House, President Kennedy told newsman Scali that the proposals Counsellor Fomin had passed on were an acceptable basis for a settlement. He told Scali to see Fomin again, to deliver a message for Moscow. The two sides, it seemed, were edging towards a peaceful solution.

Across the Atlantic, in London, the initiatives Ivanov had started were continuing. Stephen Ward phoned the man Lord Astor had suggested as a conduit to the Prime Minister, the Earl of Arran. Arran, a Conservative Party whip in the House of Lords, was an eccentric known for his peculiar speeches in the Lords and a colourful column in the *Evening News*. He was, nevertheless, a good man to contact. 'Life,' as another peer had put it, was 'one Balliol man after another.' Arran had been to Eton and Balliol College, Oxford, as had Prime Minister Macmillan, and many of his contemporaries were in the upper echelons of the Foreign Office. He was, too, a first cousin to

British Ambassador to Washington Ormsby-Gore, who had the ear of President Kennedy. As the Soviets were aware, moreover, he still retained the ties to British intelligence he had acquired during the war.

Arran responded to the call from Ward by inviting him and Ivanov to drinks the following morning at Pimlico House, his home in Hertfordshire. 'We drove out,' Ward was to write, 'Lord Arran greeted us in the drive, and we sat down to talk – with some excellent rosé for myself and vodka for Ivanov.' Though the best part of a bottle of the hard stuff was consumed during the two hours that followed, Lord Arran would recall that Ivanov remained 'reasonably sober'. The Russian, he thought, 'made himself most agreeable. It became immediately clear that Commander Ivanov's mission was to get a message to the British government by indirect means, asking them to call a Summit meeting in London forthwith. Such an invitation, said the Commander, would be accepted by Mr Khrushchev with alacrity.'

'We went back to London,' Ward continued, 'feeling that it was up to fate from now on. We stopped at the Shack Bar in Swiss Cottage, had lunch and drank to success.' Lord Arran, for his part, not only briefed MI5 on the meeting but saw to it that the Soviet proposals reached the Prime Minister's office within hours. As Macmillan later revealed in his memoirs, he was also briefed by Ward's parliamentary associate Sir Godfrey Nicholson. The Ivanov initiative had gone as far as it could.

Macmillan and Foreign Secretary Home had not closed their minds to intervening in the Missile Crisis. Macmillan had been shaken by the onrush of events. Had deadlock continued, Lord Home was to reveal, the British would have put forward proposals. That Saturday morning, though, even as Ivanov and Ward set off to see Lord Arran, Home had again rebuffed

Soviet chargé d'affaires Loginov. Britain, he declared, would stand by the United States.

In Washington, Saturday proved to be both the worst and best day of a frightening week. Optimism was replaced by alarm and confusion. In the morning came news that a US surveillance aircraft had been shot down in Cuban airspace. Soviet fighters chased another US spy plane, which had strayed into Soviet airspace. A second, much colder, message came in from Khrushchev. In exchange for dismantling Soviet missile sites in Cuba, the Soviet leader now demanded that US missiles in Turkey be withdrawn.

Though the missiles in Turkey were obsolete and already scheduled for removal, President Kennedy could not be seen publicly to bow to such pressure. At the Sheraton Hotel in Washington that afternoon, ABC newsman Scali delivered a grim message. 'If you think the United States is bluffing,' he told KGB agent Fomin, 'you are part of the most colossal mis-judgement of American intentions in history. We are absolutely determined to get those missiles out of there. An invasion of Cuba is only hours away.' Attorney General Robert Kennedy told the Soviet ambassador much the same thing that night – while assuring him privately that the American missiles in Turkey would soon be removed.

On Sunday, at 1 p.m. London time, news arrived that Soviet freighters had turned away from Cuba. 'We had been on the brink, almost over it,' Macmillan remembered later, 'yet the world had been providentially saved at the last moment from the final plunge.'

Stephen Ward had spent that morning at Cliveden, digging his garden. Ivanov was his weekend guest, and they went up to the mansion for lunch. With Lord Astor, Lord Arran and Lord

Pakenham – the future Lord Longford – they gathered in the long drawing room to watch the television news. 'Only vision came, no sound,' Ward recalled. 'To our bafflement and dismay we only saw Khrushchev's face and Kennedy's, and until we got the news a bit later we did not know an epic settlement had been reached. Ivanov looked stunned. "A mistake," he said.'

The Soviet attaché 'kept on saying he couldn't believe it,' Lord Arran wrote later. 'He was sure Mr Khrushchev had some counter-demand to make of the Americans. We all felt almost embarrassed by the man's humiliation.' In a sense, though, Ivanov had got it right. The United States removed its missiles from Turkey within three months. And American covert operations against Castro's Cuba were dramatically scaled down.

In the intermediate aftermath of the crisis, however, Ivanov continue to seethe. Conservative MP William Shepherd had to listen to a stream of polemic from the Russian when, at Ward's suggestion, he met with him at Wimpole Mews. As the meeting broke up, Ward announced that he and Ivanov were heading off to see Conservative Party Chairman Iain Macleod.

Shepherd, who had close links to MI5, for his part warned Macleod to 'be careful, dining with a man I assume to be a Soviet spy.' Macleod denied knowing Ward and claimed Ward and Ivanov had merely dropped in on his daughter's birthday party – while he was out – and subsequently went to great lengths to put this on the record. Shepherd thought Macleod's reaction a little odd. 'It seemed to be taking a lot of immediate precaution,' he told the authors. 'But apparently he was concerned about this, and might have known more about Ward than I thought he knew.'

Macleod, a former member of the Thursday Club, may indeed have known Ward better than he allowed. Mandy Rice-Davies was to recall the strange behaviour of a friend of Macleod named David Davis, whom Ward met at the birthday party. He had later 'hung around', apparently wanting to learn all he could about Ward's movements. Ward, for his part, gave Ivanov a book called *Bridge Made Easy*, by Macleod. The following year, 1963, Macleod would be a prominent defender of John Profumo.

Stephen Ward did not hide the role he had played during the Missile Crisis. He wrote to Harold Wilson, Leader of the Opposition, describing his activity as intermediary and relating how the Soviets had wanted to set up a summit conference. On 5 November, when the crisis was still reverberating, he discussed it at a dinner attended by Alfred Wells, executive assistant to the American ambassador in London. Contacted by the authors in retirement, Wells said the events surrounding the Profumo Affair were 'just a foggy memory'. At the time, FBI files show, he hastened to report the 5 November dinner conversation direct to the ambassador himself.

Wells noted in a memorandum that Ward had 'made loud statements that he had been the principal liaison between the Soviets and the British Government during the Cuban crisis'. He reported, too, that another dinner guest had described Ward not just as an osteopath but as a person who 'procured girls for wealthy clients'.

The Profumo Affair was starting to blow. As early as October, long before government officials in Britain learned what had been going on, security officers at the US State Department had apparently learned the basic facts. According to the veteran Washington writer on intelligence affairs Andrew Tully, the information came from the jilted American mistress of a second secretary at the Soviet embassy in Washington. The diplomat, said the woman, had openly boasted that British Minister for War Profumo had been sharing a girlfriend with one of the Russian's colleagues in London. The CIA confirmed that the story had substance, according to Tully, and informed its counterparts in British intelligence.

American officials received no response from London, Tully said, and that should not surprise readers of this book. It may be that MI6 did not pass on the information to its rivals in the Security Service. MI5 had been playing Ivanov for the best part of a year, and Profumo's amours had vastly complicated a sensitive case.

The fact, though, that word that Profumo was compromised had reached a Soviet diplomat, and thus to a virtual certainty Soviet intelligence, would in the months to come – as this book will show – have explosive consequences for Anglo-American relations.

For Profumo and everyone else involved, time was running out.

At the height of the Missile Crisis, on the night of 27 October, Christine Keeler had been involved in a fracas at the All-Nighters Club in Soho. John Edgecombe, her West Indian protector, had chased the troublesome Lucky Gordon into a corner. A knife had flashed and blood had flowed. Gordon suffered a wound to the face that required seventeen stitches. While Edgecombe called a taxi, Keeler had called Stephen Ward to say that – afraid of retaliation by Gordon – she was going into hiding. She would phone again, she told Ward, 'when it's safe'.

Soon, though, there would be no safety, and nowhere to hide, for Christine Keeler, or Stephen Ward – or for the Minister for War. The partying was over. By now, too many people could hear the rattle of the skeleton in Profumo's cupboard.

CHAPTER 20

Disaster Looms

Suitably enough, it had been the smart set who got the first public whiff of scandal. As early as the summer of 1962, *Queen* magazine – required reading in those days for those with an antique coffee table on which to display it – had offered its readers a tantalising snippit of information. On 31 July, in the gossip section, there appeared one sly sentence. Or, rather, part of a sentence. It read:

> . . . *called in MI5 because every time the chauffeur-driven Zis drew up at her front door, out of the back door into a chauffeur-driven Humber slipped* . . .

Things had, of course, happened that way, give or take a couple of details. Yevgeny Ivanov was not usually chauffeur-driven, and John Profumo usually arrived alone in a Mini, not in a ministerial Humber. As Lord Denning would note dryly in his Report, however, there were indeed occasions when the departure of the Soviet spy from and the arrival of the War Minister at Wimpole Mews had been separated only by moments.

Who had fed this juicy item to *Queen*? Its author was the magazine's associate editor, Robin Douglas-Home, a nephew of the Foreign Secretary and a socialite whose relationship with Princess Margaret was the subject of a KGB file. He was a member of the Chelsea Set, one of the labels the London press applied to the fashionable nightclub crowd.

The authors could not ask Douglas-Home who passed him perhaps the most devastatingly accurate titbit in the history of gossip columns. He committed suicide in the mid-1960s. Some have guessed that the columnist got his information from Stephen Ward himself. If he did, then it was surely because Ward was loose-lipped, not because he wanted to see the dangerous tease in print. Ward was to be appalled when the newspapers finally got hold of the story, would strive to protect Profumo from exposure in the press. The fact was that, with Wimpole Mews a crossroads for promiscuous chatterboxes, the story was bound to reach a journalist in the end, especially one like Douglas-Home, with his pedigree ears pressed to the rich ground of the cocktail circuit.

On the very day the *Queen* article appeared, John Profumo had been considering resignation over something quite different. His superior, the Minister of Defence, wanted to scrap a missile project – a weapon named Blue Water – and Profumo strongly disagreed. The cancellation went ahead anyway, in spite of Profumo's protests to Prime Minister Macmillan. 'The poor boy,' Macmillan later told his press secretary, 'was nearly in tears.'

Though he decided not to resign, he may that week have had a premonition of the personal disaster around the corner. If *Queen* landed on the Belgravia coffee table of Mr and Mrs Profumo, and if he read the Douglas-Home piece, the Minister must have shaken in his shoes. It was a year now since the Cabinet Secretary had warned him, because of the osteopath's friendship with Ivanov, not to associate with Stephen Ward.

Profumo must nevertheless have felt safe enough. If what Lucky Gordon and John Edgecombe said they learned from Christine Keeler can be believed, he still occasionally risked seeing Keeler away from Wimpole Mews. Whether he did or not, Profumo's folly had leaked. Now it was congealing, slowly but surely, in ways that would spell catastrophe.

In early November, as people breathed easier in the realisation that the Missile Crisis had not brought the world to an end, two men went to an Armistice Day service in Worcestershire. George Wigg, a Labour Party MP, was spending the day with Tommy Friend, his local political agent. When he got back from church, Wigg learned that someone had phoned while he was out. He was puzzled, for he had thought only his wife knew where he was. He became even more perplexed when, on asking Mrs Wigg, she said no one had called her. Then the phone rang again. The caller did not identify himself, and his message was brief. 'Forget about the Vassall case,' he told Wigg. 'You want to look at Profumo . . .'

Three weeks earlier, following a trial at the Old Bailey, an Admiralty clerk named William Vassall had been jailed for eighteen years for having given away secrets to the Russians. A homosexual, he had fallen for a Soviet honeytrap. The press suspected a cover-up, and the Prime Minister was shortly to order an inquiry. Wigg, who was considered the Labour Party's expert on intelligence matters, was preoccupied with the case. All the same, the odd phone call urging him to 'look at Profumo' intrigued him.

'Driving back to London,' he said later, 'the nagging question kept recurring: how did the unknown caller know where I was, and how did he get my number?' And what did the message mean, and why had the call been directed at him, George Wigg, with his special interest in military affairs and espionage, and his reputation for tireless investigation? Wigg wondered about this for days. It was therefore all the more unfortunate – for the War Minister – that within two weeks of the mysterious telephone call, Profumo crossed Wigg in Parliament.

Wigg, who came from a soldiering family and had served in the Army for eighteen years – he emerged with the rank of colonel – had been Parliamentary Private Secretary to the Minister for War in an earlier Labour government. He was known as the Army's watchdog in Parliament. For a year now he had been collating information suggesting that – in recent operations in Kuwait – British troops had been ill-prepared for desert warfare and would have suffered heavy casualties in any real combat. He had then struck a deal with Minister for War Profumo, however, one that would avoid political point-scoring and work to the benefit of the Army in future operations. In the event, however – and shortly after the anonymous call that had mentioned his name – Profumo manoeuvred in a way that Wigg thought deceitful and dishonourable.

Until then, the experienced George Wigg had been quite impressed with Profumo. Now, following this personal humiliation, he changed his mind. In the months to come, the beleaguered Minister for War could expect no mercy from Wigg.

Meanwhile, away from the parliamentary chamber that would soon be ringing with their names, drama and disaster continued to dog the men and women around Stephen Ward. Mandy Rice-Davies' lover, slum landlord Peter Rachman, died abruptly of an apparent heart attack, wearing a gold bracelet engraved with the serial numbers of his foreign bank accounts. Months later, before his trial, Stephen Ward would ask a friend, Pelham Pound, to retrieve pornographic material he had left at a flat that had belonged to Rachman.

Distraught over Rachman's death, Mandy Rice-Davies moved to the Wimpole Mews flat for a while. There, one night when Ward was out, she took an overdose of barbiturates and settled down to read *Gone With the Wind*. It was a shame, she thought, that she would never know how the book ended. She survived thanks to Christine Keeler, who found her comatose and called an ambulance.

Keeler had her own problems. A few days before Rice-Davies' suicide attempt, the persistent, ever-violent Lucky Gordon had turned up at the flat asking for her. Rice-Davies told him Keeler was out. 'Give her these, with my love,' the West Indian growled, and thrust a bunch of knotted thread into Rice-Davies' hand – the seventeen stitches with which doctors had repaired his face following the recent knifing at the All-Nighters Club.

John Edgecombe, meanwhile, had gone to ground in an attempt to avoid arrest in connection with the knife attack. Then, tiring of life in hiding, he asked Keeler to help him find a solicitor, one who would arrange his surrender to the police. Keeler, jealous now because of Edgecombe's relationship with another woman, refused. She even told her sometime protector that, when his case came to trial, she planned to testify against him. Her stance had results that no one could have foreseen.

Shortly before Christmas 1962, on 14 December, Edgecombe phoned the Wimpole Mews flat and spoke briefly with Keeler. 'Look, Johnny,' she told him, 'you know how difficult everything is. I told you not to phone . . .' When Edgecombe persisted, Keeler slammed down the receiver. Edgecombe, frantic, slipped into his pocket the gun he had taken away from Keeler – the one she had acquired to protect herself from Lucky Gordon. It was loaded. He phoned for a cab, then headed for Wimpole Mews.

It was about 1 p.m. and Stephen Ward was at his consulting rooms in Devonshire Street, treating a patient. 'The telephone rang,' he wrote, 'and I heard a girl saying someone was shooting at the door. I immediately rang Scotland Yard, and went on treating my rather surprised patient. Little did I know at the time that this was the start of a series of shattering events that would become known all over the world . . .'

The woman on the phone had been Mandy Rice-Davies, informing him of mayhem at Wimpole Mews. Having arrived in his cab, Edgecombe had started banging on the door of Ward's flat. 'Mandy came to the window,' Edgecombe remembered, 'and said, "Christine's not here." I said, "Don't give me that bullshit!" and then Christine came to the window. I said, "I'm no fucking salesman, standing here shouting in the street. Come down to the door!" I said, "Man, this taxi's costing money." So at that she threw a pound out of the window, and that really did it. It really grated. I tried to break the door down, and I kept bouncing off. So I started blazing away at the lock, but that didn't work either. That's when she came to the window, and the gun went off again. I didn't mean to shoot her . . .'

The bullet Edgecombe fired had not in fact hit Keeler, but he knew it had been stupid to shoot at all. 'I had to get rid of the gun, so I ran round the back of the house and stashed it. Then I got in the taxi, because I had another clip of ammunition in Brentford and I wanted to get rid of it before the police came.' The taxi driver was a helpful fellow. 'Hey, man,' Edgecombe asked him, 'do you think I made too much noise?' 'No,' replied the driver. 'I've been revving the engine . . .'

The shooting set off an explosive series of events. Alerted by Ward, Rice-Davies and a neighbour, the police arrested Edgecombe at his home following a short siege. He would be charged with shooting with intent to kill, possession of a gun, and with the earlier wounding of Lucky Gordon at the All-Nighters Club. Keeler and Rice-Davies, as witnesses to the shooting, were asked to come to the police station for questioning.

Reporters, meanwhile, had arrived at Wimpole Mews even before the police – perhaps tipped off by the patient Ward had been treating when Rice-Davies called, the wife of a deputy editor of the *Daily Mirror*. The *Mirror*'s headline next day shouted, 'GIRL

IN SHOTS DRAMA'. This was a story with all the ingredients: two young women attacked at the home of a respected osteopath, a West Indian on the rampage, and the use of a gun – a rare event in the London of those days. Stephen Ward asked Keeler and Rice-Davies to stay away until things quietened down. They went off to a flat in Great Cumberland Place, near Marble Arch, which Keeler had been using for some time as a place to hide from Lucky Gordon. From there she made a phone call – one that lit a hydra-headed fuse.

She was later to say she had needed someone to talk to, someone responsible, and the man she picked was Ward's acquaintance and former patient, Michael Eddowes. Eddowes, who was fifty-nine in 1962, was a larger-than-life figure, a lawyer turned businessman. He ran a property company, a copying-machine company and a chain of restaurants named Bistro Vino. He became publicly known for an investigation of the 10 Rillington Place murder case, which showed convincingly that the wrong man had been hanged for a murder at that address. That case aside, though, the man was something of an oddball – he would later go on to pursue the baseless notion that President Kennedy's alleged assassin Lee Harvey Oswald was in reality a Soviet impostor. Fiercely anti-communist – and very rich – Eddowes' characteristics made him a dangerous new player in the Profumo Affair. For his relationship with Christine Keeler obscured his real motives.

Keeler was to say she met Eddowes at Ward's flat 'when he came round for coffee. He was interested in me. Soon after that first meeting he took me out to supper a couple of times . . .' Eddowes denied having had any sexual or emotional interest in Keeler, but she claimed otherwise. 'He says that he only met me three times altogether,' she said. 'It was many more, and I went with him to his home in Kensington. And then, after I had left Wimpole Mews to live with Johnny Edgecombe, he invited me repeatedly – practically every day for weeks. He tried to persuade me to come and live in the West End . . .'

Edgecombe corroborated what Keeler said. 'She came back one day,' he told the authors, 'to say that a Michael Eddowes had offered to provide her with a flat near Regent's Park, provided she got rid of me – she would go and live at Regent's Park and I would visit her secretly twice a week . . .'

Peter Earle, the crack *News of the World* reporter who got close to Keeler – he was to secure her story for his newspaper – had a different take on what frustrated Eddowes' sallies towards Keeler. 'He was involved with Keeler,' Earle said, 'but she wouldn't leave Ward for him. And that was half the reason he began to dabble in the [Profumo] Affair. Ward had spoiled his chances with the girl.'

When Keeler phoned him following the shooting at Ward's flat, Eddowes responded. As reported earlier, he had himself observed Ward meeting with Yevgeny Ivanov in a coffee bar at the height of the Cuban Missile Crisis. Had that not been enough to pique his interest, something he claimed Ward told him later certainly did. Ward confided, according to Eddowes, 'that both War Minister John Profumo and a Soviet naval attaché, Captain Ivanov, were Christine's lovers'.

Late on the day of the shooting, sitting in the third-floor flat at Great Cumberland Place, Eddowes and Keeler watched television news coverage of the incident. 'I thought it was a good opportunity,' Eddowes recalled, 'to put my questions to her about the possibility of espionage. I asked her if Ivanov and Profumo were friends of hers. She said they were, and that one used to go out of one door, and the other come in the other. I judged the moment propitious to ask her if Ivanov tried to get her to get information out of Profumo. She said, "Yes." I said, "Anything in particular?" She said, "The date of the nuclear warheads to Germany." I cannot discuss whether she tried to get the information.* I was very shocked. I am convinced that Miss Keeler was telling the truth.'

Having heard Keeler's sensational story, Eddowes hired a private detective, told him to make further inquiries, but took no immediate further action. He did nothing else, he was to say, 'because I had good reason to believe the authorities were aware of what was going on . . . I had been informed by Dr Ward that the three people were being watched by the security people, and "It was none of my business."' Ward, who had duly reported to MI5 months earlier, when the Keeler-Profumo affair started, may indeed have told Eddowes this. It may have been no co-incidence that, right after the shooting, MI5 asked the police Special Branch for a report. Its contents have never been revealed.

Meanwhile, another fuse had been lit.

'As we left the police station after making our statements after the shooting,' Mandy Rice-Davies recalled, 'a reporter came up to Christine. He was from the *Sunday Pictorial*. He told her his paper knew "the lot". They were interested in buying the letters Profumo had written her. He offered £2,000. We were both horrified . . . this seemed like very deep water.'

It was indeed deep water. How, though, did a major newspaper know such details at that time? There had been a spy in the camp, one of the immediate circle of friends whom Keeler had allowed into the flat at Great Cumberland Place. This was one Nina Gadd, née Gorchekov, a woman who had met Keeler at least a year earlier and had herself stayed at Wimpole Mews for a couple of weeks in 1962. Unknown to Keeler, Gadd was supplying information to the *Sunday Pictorial*.

---

* By all other accounts, it had been Ward – not Ivanov – who asked Keeler to try to get that information. Eddowes said Keeler 'got it mixed up'.

'I met Keeler and Mandy through a hairdresser,' Gadd told the authors. 'Mandy was more intelligent and knew what was going on. She realised what my game was, whereas Keeler never really cottoned on. I had Keeler marked down as someone to watch. She was talking to everyone . . .'

Gadd was employed by the *Pictorial*, then one of the most powerful of the popular Sunday newspapers, to milk Keeler for information. She infiltrated a reporter into the flat at Great Cumberland Place, posing as her boyfriend, and the *Pictorial* would in the weeks that followed become the first newspaper to get Keeler's account of her relations with Profumo and Ivanov. Unnerved by the possibility of libel action, the paper's editors would be too nervous to publish and would eventually lose the story to the *News of the World*. From now on, the reporters were on the trail.

On Christmas Eve, Keeler went to a party – and met a man who had been waiting more than ten years for an opportunity to destroy Stephen Ward. Now he had that opportunity, and it would not matter who else got hurt in the attempt.

And all the time, British intelligence was watching.

CHAPTER 21

The Man With a Grudge

Fifty-year-old John Lewis, who had made a fortune from the industrial use of rubber, had been elected Labour MP for Bolton after the war, done well for a while, then lost his seat. A document in party files noted that colleagues refused to endorse him for future office, resulting in 'a spate of rumours that John Lewis is not a fit and proper person to represent the Party in Parliament, because of some lack of personal or business honesty or integrity on his part'.

Publicly and privately, he had been an embarrassment. The party got unwelcome publicity when he ended up in court accused of bumping into a police car on the way to a parliamentary debate – three times. He was thought to have used corruption to gain his fairly senior political post. Veteran analyst Roger Whipp recalled Lewis as having been 'a nasty piece of work . . . I remember him making optimistic reports about his own companies, when in fact they were losing money.' The MP William Shepherd thought Lewis 'one of the lowest forms of human existence I've ever met – loathsome in every sense'.

To silence those who found him out in business malpractice, Lewis regularly resorted to the law. He had had won enormous sums in damages against major newspapers, sums that in one case an Appeal Court judge deemed 'wholly unreasonable' and ordered a new trial. When Lewis turned out to be playing a role in the Profumo case, the papers would be understandably gun-shy. Had they not been scared of lawsuits, they might have looked harder at the fact that he became one of the principal sources on the scandal – a source capable of implacable hatred and intent on smearing Stephen Ward.

Sex, as so often in this story, was at the heart of the matter. Lewis' marriage – to a model named Joy Fletcher, who knew Ward – had failed within a year because of his philandering and unreasonable behaviour. The family physician had advised her to get out of the marriage, and that a first step in achieving that would be to 'find yourself a man with whom you can commit adultery'.

The man with whom she did so, the judge accepted, was Ward's long-time friend, the journalist Frederic Mullally. Following one row with her husband, moreover, Mrs Lewis had walked out of the family home and taken refuge with Ward himself. In an interview for this book, Mullally recalled that she had been 'in great distress and didn't know what to do, and called Stephen. And he put her up for the night at his place. It was [just] a totally friendly gesture on his part.' Lewis, though, did not believe that.

Ironically, however, it was not his wife's affair with any man that most enraged Lewis. 'He went potty,' Warwick Charlton explained, when he discovered that Ward had introduced his wife to a *woman* with whom she had a relationship. 'He found Stephen had fixed her up with a Swedish beauty queen, a lesbian, with whom she had an affair. This, he thought, was an assault on his manhood . . . I was with him when he got the news. He said, "I will get Ward whatever happens." From then on, the most important thing in John's life was his burning hatred for Ward, which went on year after year.'

Lewis' vendetta against Stephen Ward, however, turns out to

have been more than just another sordid sideshow in the background of the Profumo case. It was noticed in a quarter one might think highly unlikely – by British intelligence.

Ludicrous though it may seem, MI6 – supposedly limited to foreign intelligence-gathering operations – and MI5 – responsible for internal security – often not only failed to cooperate with each other but acted as though they were rivals. (A similarly difficult relationship, it must be said, has existed between the CIA and the FBI in the United States.) MI5 operations have on occasion run head-on into those run by MI6. A case in point was the handling of Stephen Ward.

When on occasion MI6 'played at home' rather than abroad, the game sometimes involved providing women for visiting foreigners. Ward's potential in that area had become obvious by the 1950s, and MI6 'marked' him accordingly – a full decade before MI5 began its contacts with Ward.

This information came to us primarily from a source with a track record of providing reliable information, a former operative named Harold 'Lee' Tracey, who went to MI6 following wartime intelligence work for the RAF. He agreed in 2013 that the authors may quote him in this book on what he described as his 'involvement in the Stephen Ward saga.'

Once recruited, he was ordered to establish long-term cover as a journalist. Having begun as a photographer on Derbyshire's *Evening Telegraph*, Tracey was moved to London in the early 1950s to join the *Daily Mirror*. Only another MI6 'friend' at the paper, managing editor Cyril Morten, knew his true role. For assignments, Tracey reported regularly to MI6 headquarters.

Not surprisingly, since he had other fish to fry, Tracey was disliked at the *Mirror* because of his odd ability to write his own schedule, and his lack of interest in doing much real work.

Colleagues noted, however, that he took a great interest in the 'vice scene'. MI6 had instructed him, he told the authors, to spot people who could be compromised or recruited. One such potential target was Stephen Ward, whom he got to know as early as 1952. Tracey saw Ward as a social climber:

> someone who needed to 'get on' . . . Sex was the entrée. We learned that Ward wasn't that interested in participating in sex. He liked to watch girls being screwed, especially adult women dressed up as underage girls. Ward would obtain girls, and a boost for us came when he met Lord Astor – and capitalised on Astor's perversion . . . For us, here was a thriving little London set-up with all sorts of big names and diplomats and others swimming in and out . . . MI6 has tentacles everywhere, and someone spotted Ward and felt the set-up might become useful, that some interesting people might walk into it. We could get to know them, do little deals, so that they'd be friends of ours . . .

Nobody, Tracey said, told Ward himself of MI6's interest. Instead, a 'bagman' was placed close to Ward, someone who could on occasion supply funds. As reported in these pages, Ward was hopeless at living within his budget. The bagman, according to Tracey, was the publicist and journalist Warwick Charlton, the Ward intimate who has been quoted elsewhere in this book. The money Charlton supplied to Ward was never much, just enough to tide him over and make him feel indebted. This small investment offered MI6 a degree of control and the reward of a trickle of intelligence – including, as time passed, the progress of the obsessively vengeful John Lewis' plans against Ward.

As early as 1953, according to Ward's friend Frederic Mullally, Lewis 'got hold of an *Express* reporter, a young untrained boy, and gave him what purported to be an exclusive story that Stephen

Ward and I were running a call-girl business in Mayfair . . .' That story was scuppered when *Express* editor Arthur Christiansen – a friend of Mullally's – intervened and killed the story. Furious, Lewis then tried to get the police to investigate Ward for procuring women for his wealthy friends. A list of Ward's alleged clients, which had earlier been given to the *Express*, appears to have been the first seed for the police pursuit of Ward years later, at the time of the Profumo scandal.

Exactly what happened next in the saga remains a blur, somewhat illuminated by a series of letters between Ward and Lewis. Ward, it seems, threatened Lewis with a slander suit over the accusation that he had run a call-girl ring. Lewis' view was that Ward was trying to blackmail him. In a letter to Ward years later, Lewis wrote of Ward having launched a 'malicious action' against him and the *Express* 'when there was not the slightest ground for such an action, hoping that in order to avoid publicity you might affect some settlement'. According to the letters, the outcome was that Lewis in due course won damages for attempted 'blackmail' – with the result that Ward for a time faced bankruptcy.

MI6's Tracey was instructed to keep an eye on Lewis. 'The problem,' he told the authors, 'was, "How do we negate Lewis, and stop him spoiling this promising set-up?" My case officer assigned me to get in with Lewis, and I did, by pretending I wanted an interview for the paper or something. Soon I was going nightclubbing with him – we went to a place called Eve's quite a lot. He was quite open about his hatred for Ward. And I got in with him to the extent that I was helping him plan his anti-Ward campaign – but in such a way as to make sure it didn't come off . . .'

MI6 did get back at Lewis. Through its liaison at Scotland Yard, the Service leaked to the press – the *Daily Mail* and the

Telegraph – information that the Fraud Squad was investigating Lewis' company, Rubber Improvements. Lewis instigated a libel suit, but it cost him dear. Though he won the case, his company was fatally damaged – he was eventually forced to call in the receiver.

Meanwhile, MI6 kept Ward on ice as an available asset – until the opportunity to use him came, years later, with the possibility of turning Soviet naval attaché Ivanov. Ward's initial introduction to Ivanov, at a meeting with *Daily Telegraph* editor Colin Coote, smacks more of an MI6 operation than of MI5's recruitment of Ward.

Then, in 1961, to the irritation of MI6, Ward himself approached MI5, offering to cooperate – prior to any of the contacts mentioned in the Denning Report. The consequences, according to Tracey, were 'disastrous'. Both Tracey and a separate source said that MI6 learned of the development at an inter-service meeting in June that year, when an MI5 officer brought up the idea of targeting Ivanov in a honeytrap. MI5's Keith Wagstaffe approached Ward just two days later. In MI6, according to Tracey, word went out to, '"Scatter . . . Drop it." And we did.' Tracey was sent abroad, to a new cover job on a French language newspaper in Canada. MI6, meanwhile, washed its hands of Ward, and was able to look on from a safe distance when – come the Profumo scandal in 1963 – MI5 found itself compromised.

With Tracey gone, there was now no one to restrain or frustrate Ward's sworn enemy John Lewis. In January 1962, Lewis sent Ward a letter demanding that he pay the money awarded against him in damages and costs in the case Lewis had brought years earlier. Ward responded with a letter saying he was unable to pay.

Instead of paying what he owed, Ward suggested, he would give

Lewis the sketches he had done of members of the Royal Family, the Prime Minister and others. Lewis would have none of it and wrote back saying that Ward should declare himself bankrupt. Ward replied saying he realised that what Lewis wanted was not the money but revenge and that Lewis probably had 'the means of destroying me'. Would Lewis to come to dinner, to 'discuss what actually happened'? Lewis, predictably enough, refused.

He continued to wait for his moment, as he had waited so long. Then, months later, he encountered Christine Keeler – which gave him the opportunity to take his final revenge.

It happened when Keeler, by then on the run both from her violent lover Lucky Gordon and the press, had the locks changed at her flat in Great Cumberland Place. Along with Nina Gadd, though, she allowed in an old friend of hers and Ward's named Paul Mann. He had made visits to the Cliveden cottage in 1961 and had met Ivanov – he had even been at Cliveden the weekend Profumo first met Keeler. Now, in late 1962, Mann was making regular visits to Great Cumberland Place.

So it was that on Christmas Eve 1962 Keeler accompanied Mann to a party 'for old friends from the Cabaret Club', met John Lewis, and – the way Mann told it – poured out her story about Ward and the Profumo/Ivanov sex triangle. That, however, may have been a censored version of what happened. The common denominator, yet again, was lust.

'It happened because Christine was broke,' Warwick Charlton said. 'When she went to Profumo all he gave her was £15 and a bottle of scent. A mean person. So she did what she always did when she was broke. She went round the clubs picking people up. John [Lewis] used to go to a Baker Street club that supplied girls to customers. One night he was just sitting at home at his place, and he sent for a woman. The girl they sent was Christine

Keeler. She came along with no idea who he was or what he had against Stephen Ward, and, during the evening, she began spilling the beans about Ward, Profumo, everything . . .'

Just as she had found security in middle-aged Stephen Ward, Keeler apparently felt safe with the middle-aged, at first seemingly kindly Lewis. He, of course, revealed nothing of his vendetta against Ward. Keeler told him that Lord Astor and Michael Eddowes had failed to help her – they were only concerned about what might happen to John Profumo.* Lewis offered to find her a solicitor. 'Everything,' he told her, 'would be all right . . .'

What Lewis saw was a way that would be all right for him, a way both to wreak revenge on Ward at last and to make a political comeback. 'John,' Warwick Charlton told the authors, 'was desperate to get back in. He had two gifts delivered to him by Christine. One, the Russian security thing. And, two, evidence that Stephen was a ponce. He'd have his revenge, and have little presents to give [Labour MP] George Wigg to beat the Tory Party with, and he might get back and re-establish his reputation with Labour . . .'

There have been two theories as to who made the anonymous call to Wigg in November 1962, urging him to 'look at Profumo'. According to one of them, MI5 files contained evidence that the caller was Victor Louis, a Soviet agent fronting as a journalist. If the Soviets did arrange for the call, though, to hurt the Conservative government, why would they have given him only one bland sentence, nothing tangible he could follow up?

To the authors – and Wigg's biographer – it is more plausible

---

* Lord Astor did get in touch, fretting about rumours that Keeler would bring up Profumo's name when the Edgecombe shooting case came to court, and offering to pay Keeler's legal costs.

that John Lewis made the initial anonymous call to Wigg, or arranged for it to be made. Though he may not have got a full account from Keeler until Christmas 1962, it is possible that by November – when the call was made – he already had some part of the story. Certainly, in the weeks to come, it was Lewis who was to feed Wigg ammunition for his coming onslaught on the government over the Profumo case. Their affiliation to the Labour Party aside, they shared an interest in horse racing. Wigg's secretary was to recall that they often discussed the sport – Lewis owned racehorses, and Wigg had long been involved in the supervision of racecourse betting. When Lewis was ready to spread his poison about Stephen Ward, his acquaintance with Wigg gave him an opening.

He went to Wigg for the first time on 2 January 1963, and outlined what Keeler had told him. Mindful of the earlier anonymous phone call, Wigg expressed cautious interest and asked for more information. Keeler provided it. She talked with Lewis not only of Ward's connection to a man from MI5 but also of Ivanov's request that she ask Profumo when nuclear warheads were to be delivered to West Germany. Lewis covertly tape-recorded all this, then called Wigg again.

Wigg's secretary remembered: 'Mr Lewis constantly rang up during the day when Mr Wigg was about his parliamentary business. I frequently got the impression he wasn't completely sober. But he was insistent . . .' Lewis had already been to the police, he said, but 'nothing had happened'. On 7 January, Lewis told Wigg about the disquieting nuclear warheads angle. Still Wigg hesitated – he had begun to think Lewis 'a nuisance'. It all seemed so far-fetched, and though Wigg considered Profumo 'politically untrustworthy', – he did not see him as a security risk. 'It seemed to me,' Wigg said later, 'that the man to keep an eye on was Ivanov.' Lewis agreed that the matter must be handled exclusively on the issue of security. Now, though, Wigg's secretary recalled, he had got journalists chasing the story.

As a 'stream of information' began flowing in, Wigg quietly began building a dossier.

While the battle lines were being drawn, Stephen Ward carried on as though nothing had changed. Over Christmas 1962, he and Ivanov had gone down to the country home of the then Lord Ednam (later the 4th Earl of Dudley). 'We had two extra women staying with us,' Lord Dudley told the authors, 'and we were giving a big dinner party for Boxing Night so we had the idea of asking Stephen, and Stephen had told us that Ivanov was spending Christmas with him, so it solved our problem.'

Lord Dudley thought Ivanov 'a very attractive man, very jolly, drank incredible quantities of vodka without turning a hair, a great *bon viveur*, with a lot of charm, a gold tooth that flashed, quite typically Russian . . . I knew that he was a naval attaché, and I knew that naval attachés have to do a certain amount of intelligence work. I used to make sort of jolly jokes and say, "Have you been to Portsmouth lately?" and that sort of thing. And he would roar with laughter.'

There was a more serious interest in the man with the flashing gold tooth. When Lord Dudley learned Ivanov would be coming, he called a relative, Edward Tomkins, who was a senior official at the Foreign Office. 'Look,' Lord Dudley told Tomkins, 'our mysterious Russian friend is coming to dinner, and I shall quite understand if you don't feel like coming, being in the FO and all that . . .'

Tomkins, who had served in Moscow, spoke Russian and now worked in London in a department with responsibility for Germany, asked for time to think about it, then rang back to say, 'It's all right. I've talked to the FO, and they rather want me to go to dinner, because they are quite anxious to find out what this chap's up to . . .' The dinner, Lord Dudley acknowledged, became 'slightly what you might call an intelligence operation'.

Ivanov, Tomkins recalled in an interview, 'showed great interest in the details of the Polaris missile deal – it was immediately after Macmillan's visit to America in connection with Polaris'. The Soviet agent also brought the conversation around to the very question he had pursued during Profumo's affair with Keeler: West Germany's prospects of acquiring nuclear armaments.

During the visit that Christmas, Lord Dudley recalled, Stephen Ward for his part made some passing remarks 'about having contacts with MI5'. He also 'dropped some hints about Ivanov and Profumo'. Dudley remembered that especially, for Profumo was a friend of the family. Ward was 'fairly cryptic, but hinted that there was something brewing'.

Something was brewing all right. On 16 January, John Edgecombe was committed for trial on the Wimpole Mews shooting charges. The press, sensing now that this was more than a simple case of armed assault, buzzed around Christine Keeler. In secret, Ward's nemesis, John Lewis, was continuing to drip his poison into the ears of George Wigg.

The press activity – and the rent he was paying – was making Stephen Ward uncomfortable. He moved around New Year's into the Bryanston Mews flat previously used by Mandy Rice-Davies' sugar daddy, the late Peter Rachman.

When Ward came down to Cliveden, Lady Astor saw a change in him. 'I noticed a physical deterioration,' she recalled. 'Whether it was too much coffee-drinking I don't know, but when things were getting difficult, you could see his hands were trembling. He looked dreadfully ill sometimes . . .'

Long envied for his magnetic effect on the female sex, Ward had not given up. 'Don't go,' he said one weekend to Jon Pertwee, who had dropped in at the cottage. 'Wait. You must meet my new friend.' 'Oh my God,' said Pertwee. 'Who is it now?' 'The baker's daughter from the village,' Ward responded. 'I can't believe it,' groaned Pertwee. 'Aren't you ever going to stop?'

On 18 January, Ward saw Ivanov again. The Russian was planning to leave within days. MI5 supposedly gleaned these facts from a telephone tap, but they may well have come from Ward himself. Ivanov did leave London on 29 January – just two months short of the end of his three-year posting to Britain – by ferry to the Hook of Holland, to avoid the press. 'His departure,' the diarist in the *Guardian* wrote, 'was much regretted by his many friends . . .'

Ward, who had so long been the soul of everybody's party, was about to find himself short of friends. The first he learned anything was amiss, he wrote, 'was from Lord Astor, who is always well informed about these things. He had heard a story that the police were interested in me, that it was being said that I had seen people as patients and then charged them high fees for introducing them to girls. I just laughed . . . I did not think for one second that anyone would take such an idea seriously . . .'

John Lewis – reviving the libel he had invented against Ward years earlier – was spreading his falsehoods with skill. Ward the great manipulator was being swept to disaster on a current of events he could not control. Very soon now, the British Establishment would be looking for a scapegoat. Take Lewis and his lies, frighten some witnesses into giving phoney evidence, hold a rigged trial – and Ward was a sitting duck.

John Profumo, though, was one of their own. The Establishment would stand by him to the last.

CHAPTER 22

Profumo at Bay

'When there is an almost universal conspiracy to lie and smother the truth,' the American columnist Walter Lippman wrote of another scandal, 'I suppose someone has to violate the decencies.' US Ambassador to London David Bruce would report to President Kennedy that the truth in the Profumo Affair 'trickles, instead of gushing forth'. It trickled – and this long remained only partially known – because of a massive effort to conceal the facts, and because of John Profumo's arrogance in deceiving his high-ranking colleagues.

The panic began, ironically, over a newspaper story that never was. On 22 January 1963, Christine Keeler's contacts with the *Sunday Pictorial*, the newspaper that had infiltrated Keeler's circle through her friend Nina Gadd, proved productive. For a down payment of £200, and the promise of £800 to come, Keeler told the *Pictorial* everything. An accurate draft story was assembled – a better story in that first draft than would emerge when Fleet Street finally broke into print.

This version had Keeler saying of her relations with Profumo and Ivanov:

If that Russian . . . had placed a tape-recorder or cine-camera or both in some hidden place in my bedroom it would have been very embarrassing for the Minister, to say the least. In fact it would have left him open to the worst possible kind of blackmail – the blackmail of a spy . . . This Minister had such knowledge of the military affairs of the Western world that he would be one of the most valuable men in the world for the Russians to have had in their power . . .

The draft story referred to the request that Keeler ask Profumo about nuclear-armed weapons for Germany. Finally, as proof that there really had been an affair, Keeler had given the newspaper Profumo's letter of 9 August 1961 addressing her as 'Darling'. A copy of the letter was placed in the safe at the *Pictorial*'s office. The story was dynamite, but the editors did not rush into print. What with cross-checking, and the need to have Keeler authenticate the final version, almost three weeks slipped by – time for much skulduggery.

Four days after telling all, on Saturday, 26 January, Keeler had a falling-out with Stephen Ward. Speaking on the phone with Keeler's current flatmate about the Edgecombe incident, and unaware that Keeler was overhearing his every word, Ward said, 'I'm absolutely furious with her . . . she's ruining my business. I never know what she'll do next, the silly girl . . .' Angered by this, Keeler proceeded to tell the Profumo story all over again, this time with Ward the villain of the piece as the man who had made the introductions. She told this version of her story to the next interested party – who happened to be a Metropolitan police officer calling to say Keeler and Rice-Davies would have to appear at John Edgecombe's trial. The detective listened, then returned to the office and filed a report.

It included all the story's main elements, along with the statement that 'Dr Ward was a procurer for gentlemen in high places, and was sexually perverted,' and the fact that the *Sunday*

Pictorial already had the story. The report went to the detective's inspector, who passed it on to Special Branch, the police unit that liaises with MI5.

That same Saturday, a reporter told Ward of the impending story in the *Pictorial* – and he demonstrated a loyalty to his friends that none of them were ever to show him. 'I was anxious,' he said in his memoir, 'to save Profumo and Astor from the consequences . . .' The following day, he hurried to the home of Conservative MP William Rees-Davies, who had high connections in government – and is said to have been an habitué of risqué parties. Next morning, Ward phoned and met with Lord Astor. After taking legal advice, Astor personally took the bad news to the Minister for War. It was 5.30 p.m. on Monday, 28 January.

Profumo's first response was to make immediate contact with MI5 chief Sir Roger Hollis. Hollis was in Profumo's office in just over an hour. Both men remembered the occasion in 1961 when MI5, communicating through the Cabinet Secretary, had asked Profumo to try to ensnare Ivanov in a honeytrap operation and get him to defect. Now, in response to a question from Hollis, who wanted an assurance that there had been no leak of classified information, Profumo said he had no connection with Ivanov. His relationship with Keeler, he suggested, was innocuous. It was Hollis' impression that Profumo now hoped for help in getting a government gag – known as a 'D Notice' – slapped on the *Sunday Pictorial*. Hollis did not oblige. Profumo left the meeting, he was to tell his son David, feeling that 'MI5 were pretty lax'.

MI5 had been having a hard time of late. There had been a second Admiralty suspect in the Vassall spy case and, to avoid the public embarrassment of another trial, he had simply been moved to a less sensitive post. An assistant controller at the Central Office of Information had been jailed for passing information to her Yugoslav lover. An Italian atomic scientist working in England, Dr Guiseppe Martelli, was facing trial on espionage charges. It was suspected that a government minister, a friend of the Prime Minister, had left himself open to blackmail by Soviet agents.

Most serious of all for British intelligence, MI5 was hunting for a Soviet mole at a senior level within its own ranks. Deputy Director General Graham Mitchell was under suspicion and surveillance by members of his own staff. Less than a week before Profumo's cry for help, moreover, MI6 traitor Kim Philby had decamped to Moscow.

MI5 had its own selfish reasons, moreover, for running for cover from the Profumo deluge. Not only had it recruited Stephen Ward in its efforts to entrap Ivanov, it had done so in spite of doubts in its ranks as to whether Ward could be trusted. Those who thought Ward untrustworthy because of the left-wing views he aired had been overruled by those who thought those very sentiments made him more likely to gain Ivanov's confidence. Exposure of Ward's MI5 connection could prove highly embarrassing.

From the police's Special Branch, MI5 learned what Christine Keeler had told the Metropolitan Police detective. It was decided that the best thing would be to leave well alone. 'I think it is wise for us to stay out of this business,' the Special Branch commander noted in a written minute, 'and the Security Service agree.' Plans to interview Keeler again were cancelled.

Though one way to put a lid on things had been blocked, there remained the risk that the story would surface in the *Sunday Pictorial*. MI5 could reason, though, that with Ivanov leaving the country, there need no longer be concern about a security leak. Though that was a weak argument – Ivanov's presence or absence did not change the fact that the Minister for War had made himself vulnerable to blackmail – it was one Lord Denning was later to accept.

On 1 February, MI5 Director General Hollis issued the following instruction, as reproduced in the Denning Report:

> Until further notice no approach shall be made to anyone in the Ward galère, or to any other outside contact in respect of it.
> If we are approached, we listen only.

Hollis had cut Ward and Profumo adrift. They might drown in a sea of scandal, but MI5 no longer wanted anything to do with them. These tactics, brutal as they were, succeeded. MI5's honeytrap operation, and its use of Ward, was to remain secret.

Though John Profumo, Stephen Ward and Lord Astor were now out on their own, one of them still held the power of his ministerial office, and Profumo and Astor were both millionaires. Power and money might yet save the day. All three men met for lunch at Astor's London residence, and Profumo and Ward talked at the Dorchester Hotel.* By 1 February, a Friday, they knew the fuses were burning down on twin disasters: the Edgecombe trial, due to start in a few days with Christine Keeler as principal witness; and the *Sunday Pictorial* story, which would be ready for publication within days, once Keeler signed off to its authenticity.

There followed another frantic weekend. Ward's barrister friend William Rees-Davies met with Profumo's solicitor on both Saturday and Sunday. On the Saturday, Profumo's solicitor

---

* Ward referred in his memoir to having met with Profumo not at the Dorchester but at the Grosvenor House Hotel.

visited Keeler to suggest a solicitor through whom she could negotiate a deal – in Denning's words – 'not to publish her story'. Canny for her years – she was still only twenty – Keeler baulked at being represented by a lawyer the Profumo side had picked. She did, however, accept the services of Gerald Black, a solicitor suggested by William Rees-Davies.

That arrangement was made through Paul Mann, Ward and Keeler's mutual friend. 'I think,' Mann told Rees-Davies, 'that Christine should be made to deny everything and talk proposition-wise as to what it is worth for her to be quiet. I think she is open to a higher bid. She is not satisfied with £1,000.* I told her she ought to have obtained a good deal more.' Mann offered to take Keeler away somewhere as soon as the Edgecombe trial was over, to get her away from the press – if someone else would foot the bill.

On Monday, 4 February Gerald Black, representing Keeler, phoned Profumo's solicitor. He suggested that £5,000 might suffice to persuade Keeler to abandon the *Sunday Pictorial* and leave the country.

Was this blackmail, an attempt to extort money from Profumo? According to Mandy Rice-Davies, there were behind-the-scenes discussions. Already, she said, she had called Lord Astor and his friend Douglas Fairbanks Jr, with both of whom she claimed she had slept, to say, 'Something dreadful's brewing. We're all going to be thrown into it.' 'The idea,' Rice-Davies recalled, 'was that Fairbanks should give £1,000, Bill £1,000 and Profumo £2,000. Christine put the figure up to £5,000, because she had Profumo's letters.'

'It was not a matter of blackmail,' Christine Keeler told Lord Denning. 'I would have asked for £50,000 if it was.' Profumo

---

* The sum due to her under her deal with the *Sunday Pictorial*.

could easily afford the £5,000 requested. 'Let no one judge her too harshly,' Lord Denning wrote later. 'If she had been minded to blackmail Mr Profumo, she would have kept the "Darling" letter herself and not handed it over to the *Sunday Pictorial*.'

Lord Denning also discounted the possibility that there had been improper conduct on the part of Christine Keeler's solicitor. Quite what was going on remains unclear. It is possible Keeler was being lured into a trap, to leave herself open to a charge of extortion, and thus ensure her silence. At any rate, the deal fizzled out on 5 February, when Keeler's solicitor went to Ward's lawyer expecting to be handed £5,000. Instead he was handed an envelope containing only £450, for 'expenses'. This Keeler rejected, and went ahead with plans to continue cooperating with the *Sunday Pictorial*.

Profumo was by now engaged in complex discussions with Attorney General Sir John Hobson, the senior government law officer. He lied, telling Hobson that he had not had sex with Keeler, that the 'Darling' in his letter signified nothing – he had got into the habit of calling people 'Darling' because he was married to an actress. Recent events may have given Profumo some grounds for hoping he would be believed. In the Vassall case, former Civil Lord of the Admiralty Thomas Galbraith had resigned partly because he had addressed the traitor, a homosexual, as 'My dear Vassall' in a letter. Though many had assumed an intimacy, there had been none.

At a further meeting with Attorney General Hobson – on this second occasion accompanied by the Solicitor General, Sir Peter Rawlinson – Profumo maintained he was 'totally innocent . . . a victim of malevolent gossip'. Profumo and Hobson had both attended Harrow – Hobson, the older man by about three years, had been Head of School – and both had gone on to Brasenose College, Oxford. Their encounters were very much 'old school', but Hobson was at first suspicious. Profumo, however, won him over with bravado, saying he would sue for libel if Keeler's story was published, and sue Keeler on the grounds that her request for £5,000 was extortion. If Profumo was prepared to declare his innocence on oath, the Attorney General reasoned, it seemed probable he was telling the truth. John Profumo would continue to abuse the trust of his upper-crust colleagues and associates – at the highest level.

On Friday, 1 February, just as Profumo and Ward were hoping to persuade Keeler not to publish her story, a top *News of the World* executive, Mark Chapman-Walker, asked to speak with Prime Minister Macmillan. In Macmillan's absence – he was abroad for a few days – it fell to his private secretary, John Wyndham, to handle the matter. Concerned that there might have been a security risk, Wyndham summoned MI5 Deputy Director General Mitchell – the official currently under suspicion by his own service. Mitchell told him MI5 was aware of the matter, had discussed it with Profumo in the past few days, and that the Minister for War had hoped for MI5's help in gagging the press.

Asked by Wyndham why this was the first the Prime Minister's office had heard of the episode, MI5's deputy head replied tersely that Britain was 'a free country, not a police state'. The inference was that, given the opinion of MI5 that there had been no security leak, ministers' bedroom follies were no concern of British intelligence. MI5 had not kept the Prime Minister or his office in the loop at the outset – during its honeytrap operation of 1961 – and it did not do so now. This failure to keep the Prime Minister informed left him open to savage criticism.

'It would imply,' Opposition leader Harold Wilson would say in Parliament, 'that the sixty million pounds spent on these services have been less productive than the security services of the *News of the World*.' Macmillan's private secretary, too, would say later that he thought the intelligence services a waste of time and money. 'Much better,' he was to reflect, 'if the Russians saw the Cabinet minutes twice a week. Prevent all that fucking dangerous guesswork.'

Less than satisfied by the briefing from MI5, Wyndham decided to see Profumo himself. The top-drawer dialogue continued when the Prime Minister's private secretary – Eton and Cambridge – confronted Profumo – Harrow and Oxford – late that night. 'The Private Secretary,' Profumo suggested hopefully, 'need not bother the Prime Minister with all this at this stage . . .' Wyndham urged him to see the Chief Whip, Martin Redmayne, part of whose duty it was to keep the Prime Minister advised of potentially embarrassing rumours. Profumo did see Redmayne, with Wyndham, on Monday, 4 February – and lied some more. He told a distorted story of his relationship with Keeler. It had supposedly been no more than 'a giggle in the evening' that never involved sex.

'Look,' said Redmayne, 'nobody would believe that you didn't sleep with her.' 'I know they wouldn't believe it,' replied the Minister, 'but it happens to be true . . . I didn't sleep with her.' Profumo even lied to Leader of the House of Commons Iain Macleod, one of his best friends. Macleod did not entirely believe him. Yet Profumo was adamant that there had been no affair. The Chief Whip told him he need not resign and need not inform the Prime Minister.

The Edgecombe trial, which had been due to begin just days later on 8 February, did not go ahead. A key witness, the cab driver who had driven Edgecombe to Wimpole Mews on the day of the shooting incident, had suffered a heart attack.

That same afternoon, Ward went to a police station to report the theft from his flat of two photographs taken at Lord Astor's swimming pool. One, of Ward, Keeler and two other women, had been taken by Profumo. On the back of the other, which showed Profumo with Keeler and another young woman, Profumo had written 'The New Cliveden Set, J.'*

Ward's MI5 case officer, Keith Wagstaffe, concerned about the possible press fallout from the Edgecombe trial, wrote to Director General Hollis urging him to brief the Prime Minister on the full facts about Profumo and Keeler. 'If after subsequent enquiries,' he wrote, 'we were found to be in possession of this information about Profumo and to have taken no action, we would I am sure be subject to much criticism for failing to bring it to light.'

Responding, Hollis told Wagstaffe that 'No enquiries on this subject should be made by us.' A conference attended by Hollis, his deputy, Mitchell, and eight other officers involved in the Ivanov operation had concluded that the service was safe from criticism – so long as it did nothing. With Ivanov now out of the country, MI5 saw no security implications.

The head of Special Branch, Evan Jones, told colleagues that MI5 'believe it to be true that Profumo has told the Prime Minister of the matter, but they do not know that for certain . . .' One of Jones' officers, James Francke, would recall having been advised by MI5 that 'the sex lives of ministers were no business of proles like us. More culpably, the Prime Minister was also kept in the dark, and subsequently made to seem like a gullible fool.'

What Macmillan was – or was not – told, and when, was to be the subject of controversy.

---

* The photographs were described by Ward's friend Paul Mann, who said he had seen them on the mantelpiece at Wimpole Mews.

CHAPTER 23

When Did the Prime Minister Learn the Truth?

The Prime Minister returned to London from Italy on Sunday evening, 3 February. He was briefed on the Profumo matter the following day, according to the Denning Report. Private Secretary John Wyndham and Chief Whip Redmayne told Macmillan of the rumour and what Profumo had said about it. The Prime Minister, for his part, was to tell Lord Denning he did not bring up the matter with Profumo at all. There were two reasons, said Denning:

1. If a Prime Minister sees a Minister and asks a question of this kind, there is no 'follow-up'. The Prime Minister could either believe it or disbelieve it, and if he disbelieved it, he could not do business again as a Prime Minister with him.
2. He thought it better to get friends of his own age, the Attorney-General, the Chief Whip, and others to talk to him: and if there was anything in it, he would say it to them.

The Prime Minister was 'satisfied completely', he told Denning, that Profumo's denials were truthful.

Not everyone believed this account of Macmillan's role. Some came to believe he was told of the Profumo-Keeler-Ivanov triangle at the beginning of 1963, perhaps even earlier, and took no action. Conservative MP William Shepherd, who knew Profumo and Ward and had been a customer at the club where Keeler first appeared as a showgirl, said he wrote to the Prime Minister six *months* before the scandal blew up. Macmillan had asked him to consult the Chief Whip; when he did so, Shepherd had said he believed Profumo had had sex with Keeler. Shepherd, however, did not keep copies of his exchange of letters with Macmillan, and his account of his conversation with the Chief Whip suggests it did not occur until February 1963.

Much more plausible, and more disquieting, is a long series of reports in US Federal Bureau of Investigation files covering late January and early February 1963 – the period during which Profumo and his friends, including Ward, were hastily trying to suppress the truth. It was, too, when Soviet attaché Ivanov left London. If accurate, the reports suggest the Prime Minister was briefed on the Profumo matter – by an American source – on 28 January. If that was the case, he should have realised on 4 February – when the Chief Whip briefed him – that Profumo's denial was a lie. Yet Macmillan did nothing. Profumo, moreover, was soon to repeat the lie in the House of Commons. Can it be that the Prime Minister was a silent accomplice to that lie?

The information indicating that Macmillan was told of the affair earlier than ever publicly admitted comes from a mass of FBI documents – some declassified since the previous edition of this book – that focus on a US citizen then living in London, Thomas Corbally. Corbally was a forty-one-year-old businessman with a major holding in a company linked to Pearl and Dean, the cinema publicists, and a reputation for having been a playboy in New

York. He divided women into two groups: 'Girls you slept with and took to the Copacabana, and girls you bought a black dress for and took to the Stork.' His marriage, to the tennis star 'Gorgeous Gussie' Moran, had been annulled on the grounds of non-consummation.

There was also a serious side to him. He had worked during the war for the forerunner of the CIA, the OSS, and after the war with US intelligence in Germany. In London, where he was ostensibly involved in advertising, he worked with an American firm of security consultants. According to *Spectator* columnist Taki Theodoracopulos, he had 'great contacts in very high government circles as well as security services'.

Sharing Corbally's London apartment was another American, William 'Billy' Hitchcock IV, grandson of the founder of Gulf Oil and a nephew of the immensely wealthy Mellon family. His monthly income was estimated at $100,000, an extraordinary sum in those days. Some of that money went to financing drug guru Timothy Leary's project to spread the use of LSD worldwide.

Corbally, especially, was a man with an inside track. He was to tell the FBI that as early as 1961, while mixing with 'people of high-standing and prominence', he had heard rumours 'that War Minister Profumo was having an affair with some model'. He knew, he said, that Profumo 'had the reputation of being a ladies' man . . . who stacked his office with pretty girls'.

In early 1963, Corbally and Hitchcock became involved in a bizarre chain of events that may have led to Macmillan learning of the Profumo-Keeler-Ivanov triangle not from his own officials but from the US embassy, and as early as 28 January. When first contacted during the writing of this book, both men still regarded the matter as highly sensitive. Thomas Corbally began talking openly, but then excused himself on the advice of his lawyer, who – he said – happened to arrive while he was talking with the authors on the telephone. He subsequently replied to questions in writing, through his lawyer. From Corbally's lawyer and Hitchcock, and from the files, we learned what follows.

In late 1962, while living in Duke Street, Mayfair, Corbally was suffering from a knee injury so serious that he had been advised only surgery would help. Then, Corbally said, 'I was at a party one night and some bloke I didn't know looked at me and said, "What's wrong with your knee?" It was about as big as my head . . . He put his hand on my knee, and within about thirty seconds I was some place in the flat with my trousers pulled up to my knee. And fifteen minutes later I walked back into the party with nothing, no swelling.'

The miracle worker was Dr Stephen Ward, and a grateful Corbally invited him round to Duke Street. 'He knew a lot of pretty girls,' Corbally said, 'and I like pretty girls. He liked to gossip and talked incessantly about the things he knew . . . I entertained a lot, and Stephen was around my flat a lot . . . I certainly liked him and considered him a friend.'

Corbally was to tell the FBI that 'because of Dr Ward's association with beautiful girls he was always invited to exclusive parties, particularly those attended by high-ranking officials and notables'. Corbally's view, though, was that Ward 'could be characterized as pro-communist' – and he had reason to think this. In late 1962, Ward had brought Ivanov to the Corbally/Hitchcock apartment. The Russian had struck him as 'personable . . . and a man with a keen interest in beautiful girls'.

Corbally also met Mandy Rice-Davies, who knew a woman to whom he had once been engaged. He liked her too – she and he were still in touch when the first edition of this book went to press. He summed up Christine Keeler, whom he also encountered, as a 'pretty face, and dumb'. The solicitor Michael Eddowes recalled having seen Corbally at a party at Duke Street with 'Keeler and Rice-Davies sitting on each side of the armchair'.

Billy Hitchcock, for his part, also knew Rice-Davies. His millionaire relative Center Hitchcock had taken her to a society wedding in Paris. Hitchcock, moreover, had been introduced by a British official to Minister for War Profumo.

On 28 or 29 January 1963, Stephen Ward visited the two Americans again – at the very time that he, Profumo and Lord Astor were trying to silence Christine Keeler and prevent her account of her adventures appearing in the *Sunday Pictorial*. He apparently could not contain himself. 'Stephen,' Hitchcock told the authors, 'proceeded to tell me that Christine had been seeing Ivanov, that he [Stephen] had taken Ivanov to the Astors' place at Cliveden, that she met Profumo and had an affair with him. And so on . . .'

This was an extraordinary story, and Hitchcock decided to do something about it. He placed a call straight to the US ambassador to London, David Bruce. He had no difficulty in getting through for there was a family connection – Bruce's wife, like Hitchcock, was part of the Mellon family. Bruce was familiar, too, with the name Stephen Ward for – as reported earlier in these pages – the osteopath-cum-artist had some time earlier sketched him for the *Illustrated London News*. Lord Astor and his wife, moreover, were personal friends and he had visited their country seat at Cliveden. The Ambassador listened intently to what Hitchcock now told him.

Thomas Corbally also told the authors, through his lawyer, about contact with US Ambassador Bruce. 'Mr Corbally,' the lawyer stated, 'was asked to visit the American Ambassador, and did so on or about the 28th or 29th . . . This at the Ambassador's invitation . . . The Ambassador had been told that Mr Corbally knew Stephen Ward as his patient and friend. When the

Ambassador asked Mr Corbally about Ward's knowledge of the Profumo Affair, Mr Corbally told the Ambassador that Ward spoke about it incessantly . . . Mr Corbally felt that the truth would be served better by the Ambassador talking to Ward direct rather than through him . . .'

Ambassador Bruce was interested all right. He wanted information from Ward, but was about to leave London. 'I can't follow up myself,' he told Billy Hitchcock. 'I'm just about to go to Washington, Wells can handle it.' The FBI dossier shows that Alfred Wells, the Ambassador's assistant, did follow through.

He wrote a memorandum, dated 29 January, which – as reported by the FBI – quoted Corbally as saying that Christine Keeler had sold an article on her amours to the *Sunday Pictorial*. The summary further informed the FBI Assistant Director in charge of counter-intelligence that 'the impending scandal had been brought to the attention of the Prime Minister on the evening of 28 January, and a letter had been written to the [*Sunday Pictorial*], putting the paper on notice that the Government is aware of the story, and that under British law the story could not be published until after the trial of the Jamaican [John Edgecombe] . . .'

Another FBI memorandum from London, one that would be sent in June, at the height of the scandal, repeated that the Prime Minister had been advised of the Profumo-Keeler-Ivanov matter by the Americans on 28 January – a week before, according to the official British account, he was briefed on it by the Chief Whip.

Corbally denied that this information came from him. 'Mr Corbally,' his lawyer told the authors, 'did not know the Prime Minister. He had no contact with him or others in his government . . . He would deeply resent his name being used to besmirch the reputation of a distinguished prime minister who is now dead and unable to answer for himself.' Corbally pointed out, however, that he was 'not aware of what Ambassador Bruce or anyone else told the Prime Minister'. Is it not reasonable, then, to speculate that the information on Profumo's folly was at some stage passed on to 10 Downing Street by the office of US Ambassador Bruce?

Two weeks after the January contacts with the embassy, on 13 February, Bruce's assistant Alfred Wells sat down to lunch with Stephen Ward. The meeting, which not only Corbally but Hitchcock and an unnamed woman said occurred, took place at Simpson's in the Strand. 'Mr Wells,' Corbally said, 'obtained answers to all the questions he put to Mr Ward.' 'Stephen,' according to Hitchcock, 'went into everything about Mr Profumo, absolutely A to Z. You couldn't shut him up.' Wells, he said, subsequently told them that, following the lunch at Simpson's, he passed the further information obtained from Ward to the Prime Minister's office. A senior official had later called back to say that, though briefed accordingly, Macmillan still dismissed the whole story as 'absolutely ridiculous'.

Wells himself, contacted by the authors in retirement, said he could remember nothing at all – either about the 29 January memorandum or his subsequent meeting with Stephen Ward.

The FBI dossier shows that Thomas Corbally left London for the United States at some point and visited the head of the FBI's New York office, John Malone. Also that once the scandal finally broke, it was discussed at a meeting on 20 June attended by the Defense Secretary, the Director of the CIA, the head of the Defense Intelligence Agency and an Assistant Director of the FBI. Though heavily censored, some documents appear to indicate that the London embassy had failed to react to the information it had received in January. One, however, dated the day after the high-level meeting, shows that Secretary of State Dean Rusk sent an emissary to London to sort out what had really happened, and to speak with Ambassador Bruce. The emissary, Deputy Assistant Secretary of State William Burdett, proved unhelpful when contacted by the authors. He 'could not recall' any details of the London visit. No memory at all – just like Wells.

What then of Ambassador Bruce himself? Did he or his office brief Prime Minister Macmillan in late January, as indicated by the FBI's dossier? A State Department document, an 'Eyes Only' report from Ambassador Bruce to President Kennedy sent in June 1963, offers more food for thought. It reads: 'Few people believe that Macmillan, whose private integrity has never been questioned, would have connived at a clumsy attempt to avoid an almost inevitable disclosure if he had known that Profumo had lied. Nor would it consort with the character of the PM to have done so.'

How to explain this message, if Bruce had been given information on the Profumo case as early as January? How to explain it if, as memories of others and the file indicates, he had ordered his assistant Wells to investigate, and if Wells had informed the Prime Minister's office of what Corbally and his friend had learned from Ward, and then what Wells learned directly from Ward – weeks before Profumo repeated his lie to Parliament?

We examined not only Bruce's papers as released by the State Department, but also his journals, preserved since his death by the Virginia Historical Society. Bruce kept a meticulous record of each day's activity, down to comments on people he spoke with or met – even details of food served at dinner. The journal is almost pedantically detailed, and the entries for 28 and 29 January – when the Ambassador or his office supposedly told the Prime Minister's office what it had just learned – contain no mention of Profumo. Oddly, though, an entire page is missing from the journal at the relevant point. There is no way of knowing whether it once contained material on a tip-off to Prime Minister Macmillan.

It may be no coincidence that, in the FBI dossier as released, Ambassador Bruce's response to a report of the FBI's interview with Corbally also turns out to be missing. So is a letter on the subject to Secretary of State Dean Rusk. The FBI files indicate, moreover, that the original information given to Ambassador Bruce was not even passed to the State Department in Washington. It seems possible, therefore, that – until the case became public – Bruce simply decided to sit on it.

The Corbally/Hitchcock episode was held tightly by the FBI. Relevant cables to headquarters were flagged 'extremely sensitive and for Director only'. A 19 June memorandum stated that it had been agreed to 'delete the references to the US Ambassador and his relatives in London'.

Ambassador Bruce and Prime Minister Macmillan were close, and dined together regularly at Buck's Club. Macmillan's diaries make no reference to having discussed the Profumo matter with Bruce until 4 March, when they had a two-hour discussion. On that date, Macmillan wrote only that Bruce 'has been in Washington, from where he had little to report except talk, more talk, and still more talk'.

Whatever Bruce or his office did or did not tell Macmillan or his office, the FBI file indicates that the Ambassador's assistant Alfred Wells and Thomas Corbally briefed another British government official, Clive Bossom, Parliamentary Private Secretary to the Secretary of State for Air, at a meeting on 5 February. Corbally, however, told the authors he never met Bossom. Wells, consistent with his responses on the whole affair, said he remembered nothing of the meeting.

Bossom, however, did a little better. He said he recalled someone at the US embassy telling him, 'in a stupid way, at the end of a dinner, that there was a case pending against a minister of the Forces'. The essence of the story, he went on, was that it involved a minister and Cliveden, but the 'someone' had not told him which minister. According to Bossom, he reported the matter at once to his own minister, Secretary of State for Air Hugh Fraser. 'I knew my minister had a cottage at Cliveden,' says Bossom. 'I asked him, "Are you involved?" and he said, "No, not at all."'

Fraser was indeed friendly with Lord Astor, had like Ward been given the use of a cottage on the Cliveden estate, and had met the osteopath. Soon, realising that the coincidence might prove embarrassing, he stopped using the cottage. Sir Philip Zulueta, who was on Prime Minister Macmillan's staff and had also used a cottage on the estate, was to do the same.

There is no suggestion that either of these officials used the cottages in any improper way. Secretary of State for Air Fraser, however, was a close friend of his opposite number at the Ministry for War, John Profumo. So it was that the information now went full circle – Fraser's secretary passed on what his aide Bossom had learned from the US ambassador's office to John Profumo himself. 'There are always rumours,' was Profumo's lofty response, 'about men in the limelight.'

In the weeks following the initial flap, the rumours – which were of course true – continued to reach the Prime Minister's office. Macmillan was informed, but – according to the Denning Report – continued to believe that his friend and protégé Profumo was telling the truth. 'His lie,' the Prime Minister's private secretary John Wyndham wrote later, was believed 'because his story was so incredible that it must be true. It was as simple as that . . .'

Was it? Macmillan had received a warning about Profumo from his Private Secretary and the Chief Whip. He had also at some stage been tipped off by the US embassy to the fact that Stephen Ward, a man better qualified on the subject than anyone except the participants themselves, had described a sex triangle involving Profumo, Keeler and a Soviet diplomat. Why then would he have simply snorted, 'Ridiculous!' and passed on to other things?

The Prime Minister knew Profumo well, and those who knew him were aware he had a reputation as a ladies' man. It may be that Macmillan preferred to play the ostrich, to 'Hear No Evil, See No Evil' – hoping that this was a problem that would go away. On the evidence, that is the only rational explanation. The truth was staring him in the face. His young friend, himself thought by some to be a potential prime minister, was lying. Ignoring that truth would in the end cost Macmillan his career.

The public so far knew nothing about John Profumo's guilty secret. Happily for him, two potentially damaging events had failed to occur in early February. As reported in the previous chapter, the Edgecombe trial had been postponed.

Deft manoeuvring by Stephen Ward, meanwhile, brought Profumo a temporary reprieve from publication of Christine Keeler's story in the newspapers. First, he managed to persuade an assistant editor at the *Sunday Pictorial*, Fred Redman, that the story provided by Keeler contained major inaccuracies. Redman decided to drop the Keeler story and instead run a relatively harmless story about Ward and young women. Ward also somehow prevailed on the *News of the World* to hold off. The twin miracle was not entirely due to Ward's diplomacy – Fleet Street was scared stiff of costly libel actions.

The first damaging headline came as a sneak attack. On 8 March, a mimeographed newsletter called *Westminster Confidential* ran a thinly veiled story on the Profumo case under the headline, 'That was the Government That Was!' So transparent was the veil that Profumo was called 'Jack ------- the Secretary for W-r'. *Westminster Confidential* was a political broadsheet that went to 200 subscribers, a small but influential group made up of politicians, diplomats and reporters. The man with the guts to publish was an expatriate American called Andrew Roth, and he had based the story on information supplied by – of all people – a right-wing Conservative Member of Parliament.

Roth's source was Henry Kerby, a veteran of wartime service with MI6 who had maintained the intelligence connection. He detested the foreign service elite, the mandarins he dismissed as 'those Foreign Office boys rogering their own rectums'. While intensely patriotic, he scorned what he saw as the self-serving core of the British Establishment in general. These were characteristics that made him very dangerous to John Profumo. 'He was scandalised,' *Westminister Confidential* editor Roth recalled, 'that a millionaire War Secretary from the Establishment "kissing ring" should have made himself so vulnerable through a "tart."'

In a nice irony, the stick first used to beat Profumo in public was coloured both pink and blue. Roth, the journalist, had left the United States during the McCarthy witch-hunt against the Left. His source, Kerby, was a right-winger, and the damning article was eagerly distributed by the Conservative right. Kerby himself, moreover, produced a stream of political intelligence eagerly snatched up by his party's political opposition – in the shape of the Labour bloodhound George Wigg, a man currently consolidating his own information on the Profumo case.

It was later to emerge that Kerby was regularly used by MI5 to leak information. More than twenty years later, in 1987, the public would learn of MI5 plots against a later government – and that prompts a question. Was the Profumo scandal in the end deliberately triggered by forces within British intelligence who saw him as sexually compromised?

In the course of the scandal, Home Secretary Henry Brooke would be told that MI5 had sent Valerie, Profumo's actress wife, anonymous letters about her husband's affair with Christine Keeler. The head of MI5 denied it of course, but Stephen Ward – himself a tool of MI5 – believed that was the case. 'I think,' he wrote in his memoir, 'the matter was ended by MI5 leaking the story of Profumo's affair to Valerie Hobson through some roundabout route'.

'British sources who should know,' wrote *Washington Post* correspondent Flora Lewis, 'are convinced that it was neither accident nor their ingenuity that provided . . . the knowledge gradually used to oust Profumo. Their suggestion is that British intelligence themselves determined that if he could not be removed one way, another way must be found . . .'

CHAPTER 24

Truth in a Tight Corner

To John Profumo, it may have mattered little who was fanning the flames of his destruction. March 1963 was the cruellest month. This time, when a witness failed to show up for the Edgecombe trial – the new date set was 14 March – it worked against the War Minister. For the absent witness was Christine Keeler herself. She had run off to Spain with a girlfriend and Stephen Ward's bridge partner, Paul Mann.

'It would be a question for a jury to decide,' Lord Denning was to say, 'whether they did intend to obstruct the course of justice.' While there was nothing to rumours that either Profumo or MI5 paid for the trip to get Keeler out of the country – the minor sum involved came from insurance money paid to Mann following a car crash – the trio clearly flew the coop deliberately. They holed up for a while in a villa in Altea, in those days a quiet fishing port.

Mann said the purpose in going abroad had been to avoid the press. If it was intended thus to shield Profumo from exposure, the plan misfired. A *Daily Express* reporter tracked them down in Spain. Keeler, for her part, came to believe the trip was conceived by those determined not to protect but to expose the War Minister. That, certainly, was its effect.

Keeler's absence did not help John Edgecombe. Though found not guilty on the slashing and shooting charges, he was convicted of possession of a firearm with intent to endanger life. For this he was sentenced to seven years in jail, of which he was to serve more than five. The police did not pursue Keeler, from whom he had obtained the gun in the first place. Nor did they further investigate the source of the weapon, a 'hot' one that had been used in two hold-ups.

To Edgecombe, the prison sentence seemed racially inspired. 'The Englishmen didn't mind having a black guy for a brother, but they didn't want him as a brother-in-law,' he said, 'The British people wouldn't wear a situation where a government minister was sleeping with the same chick as a black guy. I was an embarrassment to the Government, and they had to put me away and shut me up. If I had been a white guy, it would have blown over.'

Christine Keeler's disappearance, meanwhile, spelled disaster for Profumo. For it provided the press with an opportunity to link the Edgecombe-Keeler case to the War Minister's name. Lord Beaverbrook had long since been keen to get back at the Astor family – he had told his minions he wanted Lord Astor exposed as a 'callous libertine' – and his *Daily Express* fired the first broadside the very day after the trial, 15 March. It did so by the device of placing two articles adjacent to each other on a page. A column away from a photograph of Keeler, captioned 'VANISHED', the *Express* ran one of Profumo and his wife beneath the headline: 'WAR MINISTER SHOCK – Profumo, He Asks to Resign for Personal Reasons and Macmillan Asks Him to Stay On'.

The story was not accurate. Profumo had discussed resignation weeks earlier – not with the Prime Minister but the Chief Whip – and had decided against it. Profumo was able to tell reporters who now gathered outside his home, 'There is no truth in this story at all – I have not seen the Prime Minister. I have been working on the Army estimates.' Though skewed, the *Express* story marked a turning point in the case – and it had been noticed.

On the day the story ran, Macmillan referred to the scandal in his diary for the first time. He had been forced to spend much of the day, he wrote, on 'a silly scrape (women this time, thank God, not boys) into which one of the ministers has got himself. It's Jack Profumo . . .' It was not just an affair of morality, he lamented, because among the 'raffish and disreputable set which centre around Lord Astor . . . was the Russian military attache!' Profumo had been warned off by MI5 but 'unfortunately . . . the girl got into a criminal case. A negro tried to murder her on the grounds that she had given him a venereal disease!

'What adds a certain spice of humour to this degrading story,' the Prime Minister concluded, 'is that I think our people (MI5) were hoping to use the lady to get intelligence out of the Russian.'

Macmillan was later informed that Lord Astor had left the country. 'The old Cliveden set,' he wrote, 'was disastrous politically. The new Cliveden set is said to be equally disastrous morally.'

Having chafed at the bit for weeks, Fleet Street was now off and running. The story was to remain front-page news for weeks, fuelled by more curious burglaries – one on 21 March at Ward's cottage on Lord Astor's estate, another at the London home of Lord Astor himself.

The truth about one of the thefts is no longer a mystery. Trevor Kempson, then a twenty-six-year-old freelance journalist, later admitted to having been the culprit in the burglary at the Cliveden cottage. He and a photographer friend had approached Spring Cottage by boat, commando-style. Having broken in and turned the place upside down, they had finally found pictures of Ward and Keeler inside a jar of coffee. Kempson came close to selling the photographs to the *Daily Mirror*, but the paper cried off on realising they had been stolen. The journalist hid the pictures in his loft, inside some Christmas decorations, and eventually destroyed them.

By late March, few in the political world thought the dam could hold. It was at about this time that MP William Shepherd wrote to the Prime Minister demanding action over 'immorality in the Government'. His primary concern was exposure of homosexual activity – illegal until 1967. At Macmillan's request, Shepherd then followed up by submitting what information he had to the Chief Whip, Martin Redmayne. 'I went through a list of men then in the Government,' said Shepherd, 'some of them at a very high level, whose conduct – mostly in the homosexual field – gave rise to anxiety. I said to the Chief Whip, "You really ought to have contact with the people across the road, at Scotland Yard" . . . One of these men was involved with children, you see.'

Then, as he was about to leave Sir Martin's office, Shepherd recalled, he asked: '"What are you going to do about Jack [Profumo]?" and he says, "If anyone says a word about Jack in public, we will sue for damages . . . Iain Macleod [Leader of the House] is very strongly of the view that we must resist this under all circumstances." This was really the culmination of so many things. There had been the Ian Harvey case,* and two or three others at the same time. And another member of the government had been involved in homosexual activity and had been let off by the police . . . so they were nervous – they didn't want any more.'

What the Conservative Party's high-ups wanted would soon be academic. Labour MP George Wigg had shown his bulging dossier to his political boss, Harold Wilson, and Wilson now cleared him to bring the matter into the open. Wigg looked for a way to raise the Profumo case under the protection of parliamentary privilege, and fate delivered an opportunity.

On the evening of 21 March, the House debated the jailing of two reporters who had refused to reveal sources used in the

---

* Harvey, a Foreign Office minister, had resigned in a homosexual scandal.

coverage of the Vassall spy case. It was close to midnight when Wigg rose to deliver his bombshell. Referring to the Vassall case, he announced:

> Here was a set of rumours that gained and gained in strength, consumed men's reputations – might, in fact, have destroyed them – and which here infringed on the security of the state. But are we sure that the same thing is not happening again? There is not an Honourable Member in the House, nor a journalist in the press gallery, who in the past few days has not heard rumour upon rumour involving a member of the government Front Bench. The press has got as near as it could – it has shown itself willing to wound but afraid to strike. That being the case, I rightly use the privilege of the House of Commons – that is what it is given me for – to ask the Home Secretary . . . to go to the Dispatch Box. He knows that the rumour to which I refer relates to Miss Christine Keeler, and Miss Davies, and a shooting by a West Indian – and on behalf of the Government categorically deny the truth of these rumours . . .

Home Secretary Henry Brooke responded with 'I do not propose to comment' and a swipe at Labour for using privilege to raise such matters. The debate ended, but there was pandemonium behind the scenes. Chief Whip Redmayne woke the Prime Minister after 1 a.m. to say that only a personal statement by Profumo could contain the damage. It had to be made within hours, he said, before the newspapers splashed Wigg's speech across the front pages. When Profumo's telephone was found to be off the hook, an official car was sent to his home in Regent's Park. The Minister for War, who had taken a sleeping pill, climbed from the marital bed – the bed he had once shared with his mistress Christine Keeler – and drove to the House of Commons.

The five men he met with that night personified the elite of the British Establishment. Sir John Hobson, the Attorney General and a former army lieutenant colonel, and Minister without Portfolio William Deedes were old Harrovians, like Profumo. Also present were: Chief Whip Redmayne, Radley School and an honorary brigadier; Solicitor General Sir Peter Rawlinson, Downside School, Cambridge and a former army major; and Leader of the House Iain Macleod, Fettes School and Cambridge, also a former major. Home Secretary Brooke, who was responsible for police and security matters, was conspicuous by his absence. Profumo was closeted with the school prefects of the Conservative government, but this was not an inquisition. It was a council of war.

'Look, Jack,' Macleod asked. 'The basic question is: did you fuck her?' Profumo's answer was instant: 'No.' He was not, a fellow Conservative was to say later that year, 'a man ever likely to tell the absolute truth in a tight corner . . .' Several of those at the meeting thought it likely Profumo had lied. Three months later, in a letter to the Chief Whip, Rawlinson wrote that Profumo had told 'not only a wicked series of lies' but put on a 'brazen and convincing performance'. Deedes perceived a more serious, shared failure. 'We created circumstances which made the truth extremely hard to tell.' The men gathered together that night were not there to question Profumo's word. They were there to stage-manage his next move.

Profumo's son David came to think his father was 'so enmired in his story that he would by then have owned up to only one person, the Prime Minister himself'. Macmillan, however, never did have a face-to-face meeting with his Minister for War. The person Profumo most feared facing, however, was his wife, Valerie. She would one day tell David that her husband had 'thought he could get away with it. After all, most of his friends did.'

By 4.30 a.m. a statement had been concocted. Everyone went home, Profumo to a house besieged by reporters and a wife who had sat up in the drawing room all night with a cat on her lap. At Downing Street in the early morning, the Prime Minister read the draft statement, made a couple of amendments and gave his approval. Shortly after 11.00 a.m., flanked by Macmillan, R. A. Butler, Iain Macleod and the Attorney General, John Profumo rose in the House to tell the lie that would never be forgiven.

My wife and I [went the key part of the Minister's statement] first met Miss Keeler at a house party in July 1961, at Cliveden. Among a number of people there was Dr Stephen Ward, whom we already knew slightly, and a Mr Ivanov, who was an attaché at the Russian Embassy . . . Between July and December 1961 I met Miss Keeler on about half a dozen occasions at Dr Ward's flat when I called to see him and his friends. Miss Keeler and I were on friendly terms. There was no impropriety whatsoever in my acquaintance with Miss Keeler . . . I shall not hesitate to issue writs for libel and slander if scandalous allegations are made or repeated outside the House.

His lie thus repeated, Profumo left the Chamber to the cheers of the Conservative faithful. The Prime Minister walked alongside him, a hand on the younger man's shoulder. That afternoon, Profumo found time to go to the races at Sandown Park, where he allowed himself to be photographed with the Queen Mother. His face in the pictures is that of a middle-aged schoolboy daring the world to call his bluff. That night, Valerie at his side, he went dancing at Quaglino's.

On 25 March, the elusive Christine Keeler resurfaced in Madrid, where – for £2,000 (£500 of which went to Paul Mann) – she agreed to cooperate with an exclusive story in the *Express*.

The following day, they flew back to London – into the press whirlwind.

Days later, over lunch at the Savoy with defence correspondent Chapman Pincher – and having seen the account Keeler had given the *Express* in Madrid – Profumo tried to limit the damage. 'Look,' he said, 'I love my wife, and she loves me, and that's all that matters. Anyway, who's going to believe the word of this whore against the word of a man who has been in Government for ten years?'

'But what about the letters?' probed Pincher, who knew that at least one letter was in the safe at the *Sunday Pictorial*. 'Letters? There are no letters,' Profumo shot back confidently. In fact, Christine Keeler was to say, she had handed at least two other letters to her friend Michael Lambton. She thought Lambton, a cousin of right-wing Conservative MP Lord Lambton, had passed them back to Profumo.

With the exception of the outright falsehood about his relations with Keeler having been innocent, Profumo's statement to the House had been a masterpiece of ambiguity. Just as he now paraded around with his wife as if to demonstrate their marital bliss, in his speech he had three times used the phrase 'My wife and I'. One could infer from it, indeed, that Mrs Profumo had been on friendly terms with Keeler – there were rumours to that effect. Keeler herself was to say on her return from Spain that 'Certainly both he and his wife were friends of mine. But it was a friendship no one can criticise.'

Attorney General Hobson, former head boy at Profumo's school, had played a leading role in drafting the statement to Parliament. 'His understanding of the complex art of the parliamentary draughtsman,' Hobson's obituary would one day say, 'was the result of years of study . . .' His expertise paid off in the short term, but it was flimsy armour on a battlefield crowded with enemies.

CHAPTER 25

Getting Ward

George Wigg had left the Commons after Profumo made his statement, he remembered, 'with black rage in my heart, because I knew what the facts were. I knew the truth and I knew that, just as over the Kuwait operation, I had been trussed up and done again.' Wigg was not to rest until he had forced the government to confront the truth.

In the background were men with more dubious motives, all of them dedicated to seeing Profumo, or Stephen Ward, or both, exposed: Ward's sworn enemy John Lewis, solicitor Michael Eddowes, intervening for his own complex reasons – and the chiefs of MI5, scheming now to mask their own involvement.

George Wigg returned to the offensive on BBC Television's *Panorama*, speaking of a continuing security issue. Stephen Ward saw the programme and then, stung by the implication that he had endangered national security, went to see Wigg. Working from what Ward told him, Wigg drew up what Labour Party leader Harold Wilson was to describe later as 'a nauseating document, taking the lid off a corner of the London underworld of vice . . . blackmail and counter-blackmail . . . together with references to Mr Profumo and the Soviet attaché . . .'

Though Wigg's papers, held at the London School of Economics, are now open to researchers, many documents are still unavailable.

The document Wigg drew up after seeing Ward betrays the osteopath's anxiety and isolation as he saw events slipping out of his control once and for all. It is clear, too, that he bitterly resented the behaviour of Christine Keeler and Paul Mann.

Wilson, for his part, reportedly donated his documents on the case to the *Sunday Times*. The *Times* searched for the papers at the authors' request, but said they could not be found.

On 25 March, Scotland Yard's Commander Arthur Townsend received an anonymous communication alleging that Ward 'was living on the immoral earnings of girls'. Townsend was the man George Wigg had suggested John Lewis contact, when he had come to see him weeks earlier, and Lewis lapped up the information. A year later, when Lewis faced drink-driving charges, Townsend would be his character witness. The dossier sent to Townsend offered the details of Ward's supposed call-girl ring – activity, and names and addresses. Townsend promptly sent the material on to the Commissioner of Police, Sir Joseph Simpson.

Wigg, meanwhile, received the sordid details of the ancient John Lewis divorce case – almost certainly from Lewis himself, for it had been doctored, Wigg would discover later, to make Ward appear a liar.

On 29 March, Michael Eddowes, the solicitor in whom Keeler had confided after the Edgecombe shooting, phoned Scotland Yard to report that he too had important information. Then, at his Knightsbridge home, he gave a Special Branch officer an aide-memoire alleging that Ivanov – not Ward, as most other accounts have it – had asked Keeler to pump Profumo for information about the delivery of nuclear warheads to Germany. According to Eddowes, the Special Branch man responded, 'This is a hot potato. It will be on the Prime Minister's desk in the morning.'

The Special Branch officer, whom Eddowes later said was named Dickinson, shortly afterwards told both Eddowes and his assistant that they should drop the matter. It was, he said, now out of his hands. Special Branch, which took its lead from MI5 on security matters, was following the line taken by MI5 head Sir Roger Hollis. Deny, drop all contacts, run for cover.

On the day of Eddowes' meeting with Special Branch, Home Secretary Henry Brooke had summoned Hollis. MI5 knew of course that Profumo had lied to Parliament – its agents had been aware of the affair with Keeler at the time it occurred. Hollis, though, did not tell the Home Secretary that. To do so would have revealed that MI5 had used Stephen Ward in the honeytrap scheme designed to ensnare Ivanov. Instead, the head of MI5 threw Ward to the wolves.

Hollis told Brooke that Ward had asked Keeler to get information from Profumo on nuclear warheads. Was there, then, the Home Secretary wanted to know, a case for prosecuting Ward under the Official Secrets Act? As well he might – since Ward had been the tool of MI5 – Hollis told Brooke that the evidence was shaky. He had planted a deadly seed, however. The notion was born in the mind of authority that the buck could be passed, not to the foolish government minister, Profumo, but to the foolish 'provider of popsies', Stephen Ward.

Brooke – Marlborough School and Balliol College, Oxford – now turned the guns of the Establishment on Ward, the man from a minor public school and an obscure American college of osteopathy. Did the police have an interest in Ward, he asked Commissioner Sir Joseph Simpson? Simpson, who had received John Lewis' inflammatory dossier on Ward, said there might be a basis for prosecuting Ward in connection with his young women – though evidence would be hard to get.

Suitably enough, on April Fool's Day, an almost manic police investigation began.

* * *

The police 'Get Stephen Ward' team – and it was just that – consisted of a chief inspector, a detective superintendent and three sergeants. Its investigation was highly unusual in that its purpose was not to look for evidence to prosecute a crime that had been committed but to dig for evidence of a crime Stephen Ward might have committed. The team's daily progress reports would soon be going to a list of ten 'interested parties' – a list headed by the Prime Minister.

The very first statements the police took from Christine Keeler contained details of her relations with Profumo that – as Lord Denning acknowledged in his ponderous prose – 'one would think . . . not likely to have been invented'. The police knew, if they had not known already, that Profumo had lied to Parliament. For them, however, that was not the issue. Their job was to get Ward.

'I became aware that the police had started asking questions,' Ward wrote. 'It only came home to me most gradually that these questions were directed against me. Originally the police had told people they were trying to end the rumours. Of course, this had the opposite effect. The police, people reasoned, could not be investigating like this unless there was substance. Now the full horror of the situation came home to me, and I started to feel hunted.'

As Ward flailed around for help, two friends appeared at the flat. One was Lord Astor, offering £5,000 – a huge sum then – to cover the osteopath's legal expenses, and asking Ward to give up the keys to his cottage on the Astor estate. A double mission, it seems. A financial sop on the one hand, on the other an attempt to sever the obvious connection with Ward. Ward, for his part, appeared mostly concerned about the loss of the beloved cottage at Cliveden.

His old friend Warwick Charlton, one of the two MI6 men

under journalistic cover who had been used over the years to handle Ward for the service, also came to the flat. In what MI6 saw as its own interest, it was at this stage trying to protect Ward.

Charlton apprised Ward of what his foe John Lewis was up to and – using information gleaned from his police contacts – told him how the police investigation was progressing. He too offered Ward £5,000, to 'help with a series of articles for *Today* magazine'. Ward could use the money, Charlton suggested, to go abroad for a while. Ward turned the offer down – he was still loyal to his friends.

His mission completed, it was in the event Charlton who went abroad – his role taken over, according to his MI6 colleague Lee Tracey, by a third man used on occasion by MI6, named Stanley Rytter, who fronted as a press photographer. Rytter will figure in the final chapter of this book, which examines unresolved questions surrounding Ward's death.

Meanwhile, Ward was still trying – as he had during the Missile Crisis – to get to the very top. On 7 May he telephoned the Prime Minister's office and spoke to Principal Private Secretary Timothy Bligh. They met that evening with an MI5 man sitting in – there was no getting away from MI5. 'You see,' Ward said hopefully, 'the facts as presented in Parliament were not strictly speaking just like that . . . I made a considerable sacrifice for Mr Profumo . . . I feel I should tell you the truth of what really happened. You probably know as a matter of fact anyway . . . I don't know whether you have any feelings about this, whether there is anything you can do. I know myself here that there is a great deal of potentially extremely explosive material in what I've told you.'

Lord Denning was to characterise this as an attempt 'to blackmail the Government' into calling off the police. Bligh – Winchester and Balliol – was of no help to Ward. The pursuit went on.

Also on 7 May, MI5 Director General Hollis and MI6 chief Dick White briefed the Prime Minister on another pending intelligence disaster, the trial in Moscow of Greville Wynne, MI6's courier in the Penkovsky case. At the meeting, Hollis admitted for the first time that his service had been aware of Profumo's sexual relationship with Christine Keeler for some five months. Macmillan's already low opinion of Hollis now declined even further.

In May an interim report went to Director of Public Prosecutions Sir Theobald Mathew – Oratory School and Sandhurst. It said, as the Commissioner of Police had rather expected, that there was insufficient evidence to prosecute Ward. Someone never identified, however, insisted that – evidence or no evidence – investigators press on. The FBI's senior man in London, Charles Bates – he would rise to the rank of Assistant Director – was to recall what his counterparts in the British police force told him when, most evenings, they met for a pint in the Red Lion pub opposite Scotland Yard. One of his police friends, a key contact during the Profumo Affair, was Joe Jackson, an assistant commissioner. 'I was told,' Bates recalled in an intervieiew, 'that someone was going to take a fall . . . That someone was Ward.'

On 19 May, as he became more desperate, Ward wrote to Home Secretary Brooke:

The Marylebone police are questioning my patients and friends in a line, however tactful, which is extremely damaging to me both professionally and socially . . . The instruction to do this must have come from the Home Office. Over the past weeks I have done what I could to shield Mr Profumo from his indiscretion about which I complained to the Security Services at the time . . .

Possibly my efforts . . . might make it appear that I had something
to conceal myself. I have not . . . The allegations . . . are malicious
and entirely false . . . That I was against this [Profumo] liaison is a
matter of record in the War Office [MI5] . . . May I ask that the
person who has lodged the false information against me should
be prosecuted?

That person, of course, was Ward's nemesis John Lewis. The
notion that he might be prosecuted was, equally obviously,
a futile hope.

The following day, Ward fired off two further letters, to Sir
Wavell Wakefield, his Member of Parliament, and to Leader of
the Opposition Harold Wilson. His hopes of receiving a positive
response were raised, only to fizzle out. Two questions were
tabled in Parliament, then withdrawn. Ward's revelation that
MI5 had been briefed on Profumo's affair with Keeler – by
him – ran into a brick wall. 'There is no truth,' MI5 director
Hollis had reported to the Prime Minister's office, 'in the story
that the Security Service was informed of . . . anything . . . in
connection with Mr Profumo's alleged visits to Ward or to
Miss Keeler'. That was untrue, of course, as several former MI5
officers would shamefacedly confirm nearly two decades later.*
One characterised Hollis' conduct as 'a grave dereliction of duty
and responsibility'.

Labour's Harold Wilson did do something. He wrote to the
Prime Minister, then saw him at the House of Commons. Profumo's
lie to Parliament, which by now would have been obvious to
anyone, was apparently not discussed. Wilson's focus, as George
Wigg had urged it should be, was national security. Macmillan said
he would ask MI5 to 'look again'. Hollis now revealed another

___

* See Chapter 9.

element of the case he had previously kept hidden. On 29 May, he told the Prime Minister about the attempt to have Keeler get the 'bomb-heads' information out of Profumo.

Still Macmillan felt there had been no security lapse, because he did not think Profumo had had access to atomic secrets. He did not want to order an inquiry, his diaries reveal, because he believed Wilson, 'a blackmailing type', was out to hurt the 'the Establishment'. He did now think, all the same, that MI5 had been incompetent – and ordered the Lord Chancellor, Lord Dilhorne, to review the matter.

Had Macmillan finally decided that a way had to be found to clear the air, that the government could no longer get away with turning a blind eye to Profumo's lie? The bubble was about to burst in the press. *The People* was poised to step into the gap left by the *Sunday Pictorial*'s decision to drop the story – exposing Profumo as a liar on the Sunday following the Whitsun holiday weekend. Sam Campbell, editor of *The People*, told Police Commissioner Simpson what was coming, and Simpson in turn tipped off the government.

The tip-off may explain something the Prime Minister did on 30 May, something Denning was never told about. Macmillan instructed his Private Secretary to ask the Police Commissioner to brief Lord Dilhorne. In his reply, Simpson stated that, while he 'recognised the delicacy' of the request, the police 'could not conduct their actions on instructions from the Government'. The Prime Minister, his biographer Richard Lamb has suggested, was hoping that – if Stephen Ward was to be arrested – the arrest could be delayed until he had received Dilhorne's report on MI5's role in the matter. That way, Lamb wrote, the government might 'cushion themselves against the massive publicity about Profumo which was bound to be aroused by Ward's arrest'.

The following day, 31 May, Lord Dilhorne told Profumo he would interview him in a week's time. The Minister responded by going off to Venice on holiday with his wife. Before the weekend was over, however, a telegram from Dilhorne – whose nickname was 'Reggie Bullying Manner' – blew away any illusion he may have had that his lie would hold up. Lord Dilhorne wanted him to return to London. After a long talk with his wife, Profumo headed quietly home by train and boat. Then he owned up and submitted his resignation.

In the absence of the Prime Minister, who was relaxing in Scotland, Profumo told Macmillan's Principal Private Secretary Bligh that he had indeed slept with Christine Keeler. His resignation letter read in part:

> Dear Prime Minister,
>   I said that there had been no impropriety in this association. To my very deep regret I have to admit that this was not true . . . I have come to realise that, by this deception, I have been guilty of a grave misdemeanour . . . I cannot remain a member of your administration, nor of the House of Commons.
>   Yours sincerely,
>   Jack Profumo

Harold Macmillan wrote back from Scotland:

> Dear Profumo,
>   This is a great tragedy for you, your family and your friends. Nevertheless, I am sure you will understand that in the circumstances, I have no alternative but to advise the Queen to accept your resignation.
>   Yours very sincerely,
>   Harold Macmillan

To the general public, the resignation had the appearance of a gentlemanly affair, handled more in sorrow than in anger. It was all very public school, almost as though Profumo had been bowled out by a googly while playing cricket. He and his wife went into hiding for a few days. The 'folk of the village', Lord Denning would note with evident approval in his Report, knew the couple's location but kept it a secret. Extraordinarily quickly, an observer noted, 'Profumo was far from the stage, heading back fast towards obscurity.'

It would not be long before the former Minister for War was to be forgiven, praised for his good works, spoken of as 'poor Jack Profumo'.

Christine Keeler heard the news while watching television with the man who had become her 'manager', Robin Drury. 'Christine was furious,' Drury recalled. 'She had planned to make an announcement herself, about the relationship.'

On the day of the resignation, the Prime Minister's Private Secretary again approached the Police Commissioner, according to Macmillan's biographer Lamb. The Prime Minister 'was confronted with a certain problem of timing . . . and it would be helpful, although the Prime Minister would not in any way wish to be thought to be involved in what the police were doing, to know what the timetable was likely to be in relation to Dr Ward and the police enquiries'.

Then, apparently, Macmillan's Private Secretary and Commissioner Simpson discussed the case, and whether John Profumo would be called as a witness at a trial of Ward. There was, though, according to the record the secretary made, '*nothing of interest that needs to be recorded* [authors' italics]'. Even that pillar of the Establishment Lord Denning, who in 1963 was never shown this material, told Macmillan's biographer that the documents suggest the government 'was trying to interfere with the course of justice' – this was a blatant attempt to delay Ward's arrest.

* * *

Ward had been at Bryanston Mews when the news of Profumo's resignation came through. He was at his wits' end now, harried by reporters, abandoned by his rich friends. When a former patient, film producer Bill Lang, offered him sanctuary at his home in Watford, Ward gratefully accepted. He emerged blinking into the light and squeezed into his Jaguar, only to find the street blocked by reporters' cars. Frantic, Ward bulldozed himself an escape route by driving straight into one of the vehicles obstructing his way. The man with the unflappable charm was finally snapping. For a couple of days, ensconced with the Langs in Hertfordshire, he had time to think.

Ward had made friends with a few of the newspapermen, those who dealt straight with him. By the end, they would be virtually the only people still talking to him. *News of the World* features editor Pelham Pound, who was hoping to buy Ward's story for his paper, had also promised to help Ward get away somewhere for a rest – to the United States perhaps. On 7 June, on Ward's behalf, Pound went to Scotland Yard to see Commander Townsend, the man running the Ward investigation. 'I asked him,' Pound remembered, 'if it would be all right for Ward to go on a holiday abroad, Ward wanted to know if it would be in order. He said that, apart from a few formalities, there would be no problem.'

Another untruth. The next day, as Pound arrived to tell Ward all was well, two police officers appeared – to arrest Ward. 'It was,' Pound said, 'another example of police deviousness and lying.' To avoid embarrassing his hosts, Ward made a courteous exit. He walked a little distance from the house, dressed in an open-necked shirt, dark glasses and carpet slippers. There they arrested him.

Five hours later, at Marylebone Police Station, it was charged that 'he, being a man, did on diverse dates between January 1961, and 8 June 1963, knowingly live wholly or in part on the earnings of prostitution at 17, Wimpole Mews, London W., contrary to Section 30 of the Sexual Offences Act, 1956'. There would eventually be a total of nine charges.

While John Profumo, the man who had put the nation's security at risk, faded from the limelight, Ward was detained like a felon in Brixton Prison. He would not be granted bail for weeks to come.

'Ward,' the respected commentator Ludovic Kennedy would observe, 'was a whipping boy for the humiliations the Government had suffered as a result of the Profumo affair.' As the public scourging proceeded, the private security panic continued. The exposure of Profumo's sexual peccadilloes now placed the presidency of the United States in jeopardy.

CHAPTER 26

The 'Bowtie' Dossier

On the day Stephen Ward was arrested, 8 June, an FBI official in Washington DC opened a new file. The initial file title, 'Christine Keeler, John Profumo, Internal Security – Russia, Great Britain', was soon to be replaced with a codename, 'Bowtie'. Some code clerk, perhaps, imagined that bowties, like bowler hats, were the hallmark of the English gentleman.

More than a thousand pages of the 'Bowtie' dossier, along with many others from US Air Force, US Immigration, and Central Intelligence Agency files, were obtained under the Freedom of Information Act during the writing of this book. Many pages were largely blacked out by the censor's pen in the name of national security or personal privacy. What survives, however, provides a glimpse of how serious the Profumo Affair really was. One Englishman's folly with a teenager opened up a can of American worms, a scare about Air Force security, and the discovery that President Kennedy himself was implicated.

The day before the 'Bowtie' dossier was opened, the *New York Post* ran a story on 'the notorious British prostitute, Christine Keeler'. 'Information had been forwarded,' said the report, 'on the possibility that American diplomats or politicians may have been compromised.' That worry was kept out of the written record as much as possible, but the Profumo case received prolonged attention at the highest level. There were a series of meetings, attended by Defense Secretary Robert McNamara, CIA Director John McCone, Defense Intelligence Agency boss General Joseph Carroll and, usually, a senior aide to FBI Director J. Edgar Hoover. At the FBI, which is responsible for internal security, the case was handled by two Assistant Directors, William Sullivan of counter-intelligence and John Malone of the New York Field Office. Progress reports, which were almost entirely censored as released to the authors, went to Hoover, Attorney General Robert Kennedy and the office of the President.

Hoover informed Robert Kennedy on 14 June that there was a possibility 'some Air Force enlisted personnel may have had relations with Christine Keeler'. One airman had admitted to air force investigators that he had spent several nights with Keeler, for money. Frantic inquiries in Britain, particularly at the US airbase at Ruislip, established that several airmen had 'closely associated' with Keeler. All of them black, they had met Keeler at London nightspots.

According to a former airman named Albert Hammond, who served at Mildenhall airbase in 1963, the investigation was 'heavy . . . Thirty or forty guys were flown back to the States under tight security'. The Air Force never did admit the extent of the security flap – public statements mentioned the investigation of only three airmen. They were Technical Sergeant George 'Hoppy' Hopkins, aged twenty-nine, Airman Charles Wright, twenty, and a colleague identified only as Hamilton. There are also references to a fourth man, whose name is blanked out in the file for reasons that will become apparent.

Airman Hopkins acknowledged that he had frequented the All-Nighters Club, where Edgecombe and Lucky Gordon had their fight over Christine Keeler, and the Roaring Twenties. 'Many girls go there,' he said, 'and are picked up by the GIs. These girls are usually well-dressed and attractive and have wealthy boyfriends – sugar-daddies – who provide their flats and clothes. Usually these girls come in late at night after going out with their sugar-daddies . . .'

Johnny Edgecombe well remembered the All-Nighters Club. 'Ward used to accompany me and Keeler there,' he said. 'The attraction was drugs. Many of Ward's upper-class friends wanted to try drugs, and the only way to get them was to go down to the shady side of life.'

'Sometime in 1961,' Sergeant Hopkins told investigators, 'I was introduced at the All-Nighters to a girl by the name of Ronna . . . Ronna knew this year that my birthday was coming and arranged a party for me on 6 February 1963, to be held at her flat . . . At the party Ronna introduced me to a girl called Christine, whom I later saw in the newspaper as Christine Keeler . . . Christine came to the party with a girl known to me as Paula.'

'Ronna' was Ronna Riccardo, a prostitute who had known Ward since about 1960. She was to figure prominently at his trial. 'Paula' was Paula Hamilton-Marshall, the convicted prostitute then spending much time with Keeler. In an interview for this book, Riccardo well remembered her times at the All-Nighters. 'We'd start in the Club on Fridays,' she said, 'take some pills, crash out during the day, go to another club on Saturday night, take some more pills, then go to a Sunday afternoon dancing session . . . Stephen didn't like to dance, but he liked to mix.'

According to the records, both Riccardo and one of her friends had babies by American servicemen – though Riccardo denied to the authors that she had borne an airman's child. Keeler had had her American baby as long ago as 1959.*

The other airmen questioned told similar stories, including

---

* See Chapter 8.

references to key characters such as Lucky Gordon and Paul Mann, but satisfied investigators that no classified information had been discussed with Keeler or her friends. A senior Defense Department spokesman early on assured the press there had been no security leak. Further investigation of people who might have known Keeler, or the other young women involved, or Stephen Ward, continued for months. The inquiries into Ward's background reached right back to World War II and included a reference to a 'Miss Kolb' of the OSS, the forerunner of the CIA.

The Defense Department spokesman made no mention of the fourth man questioned. It appears from the FBI record, though, that there was interest in a US Air Force man, rank unknown, named Hawkins. On the day the other three airmen were returned to duty following questioning, Hawkins received an honourable discharge from the service. In a reference at Ward's trial that meant nothing at the time, Riccardo said: 'I never met a man in Stephen Ward's flat except my friend "Silky" Hawkins . . . the only man I have ever had intercourse with in Ward's flat.' One US airman at least, it seems, visited the flat during the year Keeler met War Minister Profumo. Why this area was so sensitive to the US Air Force remains unknown.

The US security inquiry prompted a rash of newspaper stories in June 1963, most notably in New York's *Journal-American*. The paper's editor, Guy Richards, was a right-winger with excellent contacts in intelligence, and some of its stories appear to have been inspired by deliberate high-level leaks. In the wake of the Air Force probe, Richards asked one of the stranger figures in the Profumo case, Michael Eddowes, to fly to the United States.

Eddowes had become angry and suspicious when Special Branch failed to follow up his dramatic information that – according to Keeler – she had been asked to get nuclear information out of Profumo. On 13 June, Eddowes wrote a letter to the Prime

Minister. 'The apparent disregard of my report and suggestions,' he said, 'has been a matter of deep concern to me from the security angle, and in case the whole contents of my report did not reach you, as Head of the security forces, I feel it is now my duty to draw your attention to it.'

Eddowes had no sooner raised the security bogey, however, than he inexplicably clammed up, pulled out of a planned appearance on Granada TV's *World in Action* programme and left for the United States. A subsequent *Journal-American* article, the first in a planned series of six, claimed that 'Anglo-American security and the Anglo-American alliance had been jeopardized by the affair'.

Two days later, FBI Assistant Director John Malone visited Eddowes at his hotel. He was then driven to the FBI office to be questioned at length. The office of the President, the Attorney General, the Secretary of State, the Secretary of Defense and the Director of the CIA all then received briefings on what he had said. According to recent document releases, it seems that Eddowes had passed on what he had learned from Christine Keeler and Stephen Ward. Ward, he said, had revealed that Keeler was having sex with both Profumo and Ivanov, that 'when one of these men would come in one door, the other would go out the back'. Ward, he had added, had thought it 'an amusing thing that [MI5] was covering both doors'.

Most serious, from the point of view of the Americans, was what Eddowes said of Profumo having been pumped as to when 'American warheads were planned to be sent to West Germany'. If he was to be believed, moreover, the question had not only been put to Profumo but 'had succeeded in unearthing such intelligence information'. This was 'political dynamite', Eddowes thought, and some of his American audience agreed. Defense Secretary McNamara, for one, was especially concerned.

Eddowes himself would not discuss with the authors what exactly he had told the FBI, or what he learned from American officials. It is clear, though, that the FBI was keenly interested in hearing from Thomas Corbally, the American citizen who – as reported earlier – had given information on the case to the US embassy in London. Corbally was now back in the United States, and gave information both directly to the FBI and through his attorney Roy Cohn. Much of the information he gave to Roy Cohn is still classified today.

The FBI's man in London, Legal Attaché Charles Bates, was an Anglophile. Affectionately known to friends as the 'Legal Beagle under the Eagle', he liked his posting so much that he stayed on in Britain for eight years. Interviewed in California for this book, Bates remembered the Profumo Affair well. In June 1963, he said, he had been bombarded with requests from headquarters in Washington for more information. Bates had a direct line to Scotland Yard – as noted earlier he had become a personal friend of Assistant Commissioner Joe Jackson – and a scrambler telephone to MI5. Now, though, Bates found his contacts strangely reticent.

'I knew Washington was worried,' Bates told the authors. 'There had been some references to high-level or prominent Americans involved and of course my HQ sent cables saying "Is this true? What can you find out?" I didn't know the extent of it – they weren't transmitting to me all they were picking up in the States. They often didn't. But I began to feel that I was kind of all alone on a desert island someplace. I couldn't raise a thing out of MI5. Some of the time I couldn't get much out of Scotland Yard. But my friends at MI5, they'd just pulled the blankets over their heads.'

The CIA Station Chief in London was Archibald Roosevelt, a relative of the late President. He obviously had a direct line to

British intelligence, but it too was now virtually useless. 'I took it up with Roger Hollis at MI5,' Roosevelt remembered, 'and made myself a nuisance. But they never came up with anything.' Something about the messages from Washington puzzled Roosevelt. 'As far as I was concerned,' he says, 'it was a strictly British scandal. But Washington persisted. They asked me all the time: "Are you sure there isn't any American involvement?" But they never spelled it out to me, so that I could understand what they were on about.'

One of those pushing from Washington was the CIA's Walter Elder, Executive Assistant to Director John McCone, who was attending key meetings on the Profumo case. Elder remembered the case as 'painfully hilarious'. 'There was great excitement,' he said, 'and we kept pushing to find out what the American involvement was . . .' Elder knew the scare about the American airmen had come to nothing. Separate from that, he heard that 'some Americans may have met the ladies in question', but that was all he was told. With no information on the security aspects of the matter, he kept his peace.

The man at the FBI's listening post, Charles Bates, was shown the police interviews in which Christine Keeler and Mandy Rice-Davies claimed they had slept with film star – and friend of royalty and the Astors – Douglas Fairbanks Jr. 'What do you think about this story?' Fairbanks' wife Mary had been asked at a reception. 'My husband,' she replied, 'doesn't have to pay for anything. He can get any woman he wants for free . . .' An FBI document, however, quotes Fairbanks as having acknowledged that he 'met Christine Keeler on two occasions, and – as he "touched wood" – said he was not one of her customers. In passing, Fairbanks stated that half of the House of Lords could be named between the Ward-Keeler combination.'

Fairbanks had told the American naval attaché in London

that he thought Stephen Ward not only a 'left-wing fellow traveler' but also a 'procurer' running a 'sex den'. Profumo, he said, was a 'blackmail victim'. The Navy, for its part, thought Fairbanks might be 'more involved with Ward than he had indicated'. Naval Intelligence told the FBI that it thought Fairbanks 'unstable . . . unfortunate in his associations . . . disposed to converse indiscreetly on matters of naval interest'.

Most of this information was passed by the FBI to Attorney General Robert Kennedy. In London, as the scandal developed, the FBI's Charles Bates was hearing more on the American angle from his Scotland Yard contacts. It was mostly hard information, he told the authors, and some of it referred to 'high-level Americans involved'. None of that, however, would appear in the Denning Report.

On 10 June, in the United States, a crack appeared in the wall of silence. The New York *Daily News*, reporting from London, said US officials were sure the women around Ward were 'only part of a bigger set-up with American ramifications'. It was a reference to the prostitution case, two years earlier, of Harry Towers and Mariella Novotny – the young woman who had claimed, following her return to Britain, that one of the men she had had sex with was the man who was now President, John F. Kennedy.* The *News* now further reported that there was 'an American-based organization' attempting, through vice rings, to blackmail 'influential people'.

The London correspondent who had filed this story, Henry Maule, told Labour MP George Wigg – who was still energetically collecting information – that he had been pursuing the story for many months, and had been looking especially into the activities of the wealthy American Thomas Corbally.

---

* See Chapter 9.

Corbally, according to Maule, had made a practice of finding out the names of men associated with Rice-Davies and Keeler for the purposes of blackmail. Maule also brought up Harry Towers' name, and that of another American who, he said, had left the country. His information, he told Wigg, was coming from reliable sources.

Wigg followed up by referring in a press interview to three people 'actively connected with blackmail on an international scale, who got out of London last weekend as quickly as they could when they knew that Dr Ward had been arrested . . .' While he did not name the 'three people' publicly, he passed the names to the police and, later, to the Denning inquiry. Its Report, however, made no reference to the blackmail angle.

The authors did get a lead as to the identity of one of those involved in the alleged blackmail. Dr Eric Dingwall, the British Museum official who dealt with pornography donations from anxious socialites during the Affair, had regular contacts with Scotland Yard. 'One of the key figures behind the sexual side of the Profumo scandal,' Dingwall said, 'was a woman who called herself "Carmen". She originally ran an expensive sex service in Washington. Elaborate sexual displays were put on, covering every conceivable anomaly and perversion, and elaborate charades were enacted. At some point, Carmen moved her operation to England. She owned a large country house in Berkshire, catering to people with the money to participate. This was in the late 1950s and early 1960s.'

One of Carmen's customers, according to Dingwall, was none other than Minister for War John Profumo. 'Profumo,' Dingwall said, 'used to go down there [to the Berkshire country house] quite a lot . . . I heard that he favoured a "babies and nursemaid" scene, in which he played the nursemaid.'

While the authors did not succeed in tracing 'Carmen', they

did interview a prostitute who brought a measure of corroboration to this extraordinary allegation. The prostitute, who herself catered to people with bizarre sexual tastes, said she knew about Carmen's operation, and believed Profumo had been a customer.

In the United States in 1963, the *Daily News*' pursuit of the sex blackmail of prominent figures continued only briefly. The *News* ran a story mentioning Thomas Corbally. Corbally then threatened a million-dollar lawsuit, and the story died. The *Journal-American* took up the cudgels a week or two later, however, on 20 June 1963, with more on Harry Towers and Mariella Novotny. On the heels of references to Christine Keeler and Soviet attaché Ivanov, the paper referred to the 'espionage' activities of an unnamed Hungarian woman who had reported to a Soviet contact.

The Hungarian, who was identified in FBI files as Ilona Bata, had been named by Novotny as one of the prostitutes she had 'done dates with'. The FBI characterised Bata as having been the madam controlling Novotny.

The Novotny case, it was reported, had been linked to a vice ring that had United Nations diplomats as customers. On 24 June, Congressman Harold Gross, a right-winger often used as a mouthpiece by FBI Director J. Edgar Hoover, called for an inquiry into the UN angle. UN Secretary General U Thant called for further investigation. A woman named Evelyn Davis was arrested on vice charges, and three women linked to the UN case – respectively English, American and Hungarian – were reported to have arrived in Prague. The bottom line, in a complex story, was the theory that Soviet puppets, notably the Czechs, had been using the sexual-compromise ploy in New York – the honeytrap technique.

As the authors have reported, American officials were to suffer memory lapses on the subject of the U.S. side of the Profumo case, lapses remarkable even allowing for the passing of the years. Ambassador Bruce's assistant, Alfred Wells, who dined with Ward more than once, said his mind was a blank. Dean Rusk's troubleshooter, William Burdett, had a similar problem. In California, John McCone, the man President Kennedy chose as CIA Director when Allen Dulles failed him, listened silently to what the authors had to say. Then he said he was sorry, but he had 'no recollection'. McCone's former assistant, Walter Elder, was simply mystified. 'Washington,' he said, 'was terribly interested, but I didn't quite know why. Because I didn't have the background.'

People who did have the background were President John F. Kennedy himself, probably his brother Robert, and some trusted male friends – and at least one of the young women close to Stephen Ward. Humans hide to have sex, a fact that has saved many a potentate. It is clear, though, that the explosion of the British scandal shook the White House.

CHAPTER 27

The White House Trembles

In December 1962, as the Profumo case was about to break, Kennedy had met the British Prime Minister in the Bahamas. The President was no longer intimidated by the older man – he jovially addressed him as 'Mr Prime'. In the heat of a Nassau evening, as he chatted over the whiskey with Macmillan and his deputy, R. A. Butler, reporters eavesdropped on an aside that would become legend. 'You know, it's funny,' Kennedy confided, eyeing a nearby young woman, 'but if I go too long without a woman, I get a headache . . .'

Years later, when the President was long dead, Macmillan would criticise him for having spent 'half his time thinking about adultery, the other half about second-class ideas passed on by his advisers'. Adultery was a sore point with Macmillan, whose wife for years betrayed him with one of his own friends.

Kennedy was an Anglophile who had what a female friend described as the 'aristocratic English attitude' towards women. A favourite book was Lord David Cecil's *Young Melbourne*, a heady celebration of sexual adventure and politics. In spring 1963, as the Profumo case began to break, the President showed an almost obsessive interest. The first anecdote comes from a surprising source: Mandy Rice-Davies.

In the wake of the scandal, Rice-Davies was to meet future Israeli Prime Minister Shimon Peres. Peres, who had been Deputy Defence Minister at the time, told her of having visited President Kennedy at the White House in March 1963, on the same day as British Opposition leader Harold Wilson. 'Everyone was allotted a certain time with the President,' goes the story as related by Rice-Davies. 'Shimon was waiting in the ante-chamber, and Wilson was supposed to be in there for just a little while. But he stayed in there about two hours, and Shimon couldn't believe it. "What the hell have you and Kennedy been talking about?" he asked Wilson when he came out at last. And Wilson said, "I couldn't believe it. The man just talked and talked about the Profumo business. He really grilled me on what I knew . . ."'

In London during the weeks of crisis, Lord Astor had come hurrying to see Stephen Ward – at that point still a free man. 'Astor was just back from Washington,' Ward's friend Warwick Charlton recalled. 'He had been to see President Kennedy for lunch at the White House. Partly JFK was joking, asking Astor about the girls, and saying he was disappointed Astor denied having had them himself. He also wanted to know everything that was coming out . . .'

Kennedy, who also discussed the Profumo case with his London ambassador David Bruce, ordered that all London embassy cable traffic on the subject be routed to him personally. Kennedy 'felt terribly sorry for Profumo', his friend Charles Spalding recalled, 'and he sympathised with the way Profumo was caught. Jack also thought the girls involved were kind of cute.'

The President's advisers had good reason to distance him from stories about sexual high jinks in Britain. They were already struggling to protect Kennedy – the first Catholic president, projected to the public as the good family man incarnate – from his own indiscretions. A year earlier, at an embarrassing luncheon in the White House, FBI Director Hoover had confronted Kennedy with evidence of his affair with starlet Judith Campbell, a woman then also seeing a top Mafia leader. A few months later, when Marilyn Monroe died, he and his brother Robert had only barely prevented exposure of their affairs with the actress. The Kennedys' womanising had their advisers worried.

In June 1963, as the Profumo Affair unwound, the President prepared for an important European tour. 'With the case of the British War Minister and the call girls building up,' said the *Washington News*, 'we can think of no better time for an American president to stay as far as possible away from England.' 'Strong pressure was exerted,' it was later reported, 'to postpone a visit to London, for fear President Kennedy might become in some way involved.'

The State Department, however, was keen that Kennedy should visit London, to show that the 'special relationship' with Britain was as strong as ever in spite of the crisis. London was on the itinerary when the President left Washington on 21 June. First, he made his famous speech in West Berlin. 'Two thousand years ago,' said Kennedy, 'the proudest boast was "*Civis Romanus sum*." Today in the world of freedom, the proudest boast is "*Ich bin ein Berliner*." . . . There are some who say that Communism is the wave of the future. Let them come to Berlin.'

As Kennedy was capturing the hearts of Berliners, an obscure twenty-two-year-old named Mariella Novotny began making dangerous noises. 'Now,' she said, answering a London reporter's questions about the Americans and the Profumo case, 'they are just trying to put up a smokescreen . . . In case they blundered over two years ago . . . I suppose the Americans will want to interview me.' In New York, the *Journal-American* did notice and fired off a telegram asking Novotny for an interview. Before she could respond, however, another troubling story came out of London.

On 28 June, as Kennedy visited the Republic of Ireland, home of his forebears, the *Washington Post* ran a story filed from London by the powerful columnist Dorothy Kilgallen. 'The Novotny story,' Kilgallen wrote, 'may challenge Christine Keeler's saga before the international call girl scandals become history.' Kilgallen suspected, according to her biographer, 'that the British counterpart of the CIA knew a whole lot more than it was telling about the international ramifications of the case . . .'

Next day, as the President arrived in England, the *Washington Post* hinted heavily that there were skeletons yet to be uncovered. 'Britishers who read American criticisms of Profumo,' wrote Drew Pearson, 'throw back the question "What high American official was involved with Marilyn Monroe?"'

Kennedy arrived at Birch Grove, the Prime Minister's country residence, by helicopter. 'I can see him now,' the Macmillan would recall in old age, 'stepping out from the machine, a splendid, young, gay figure . . . The excitement was intense . . . The roads were packed outside the front gates. The crowd included a hundred CND [Campaign for Nuclear Disarmament] marchers, with banners demanding that we should abolish nuclear tests. Since it was the main purpose of our meeting to achieve this, the demonstration seemed hardly necessary.'

The President found the British Prime Minister worn out by the Profumo Affair, 'tired and lacking in ideas. Macmillan could not convey any sense of excitement and optimism for the future, because he did not feel any . . .' Kennedy, for his part, was striving to hide his own exhaustion – his chronic back problem was giving him hell. And that Saturday evening, as he dined with

Macmillan, he learned that the Profumo case was about to touch his presidency.

In the United States that day, the noon edition of the *Journal-American* carried this teaser: 'One of the biggest names in American politics – a man who holds "a very high" elective office – has been injected into Britain's vice-security scandal . . .' The headline read: 'HIGH US AIDE IMPLICATED IN V-GIRL SCANDAL'. In 1963, those in the political know understood that the story referred to the President.

The story remained in the paper for only one edition. In Washington, the President's brother Robert, the Attorney General, took urgent action. The *Journal-American* dropped the item from subsequent editions. FBI Assistant Director Courtney Evans, who acted as liaison between Hoover and Robert Kennedy, told the FBI's weekend supervisor that the Kennedys wanted to know what was going on. A phone call disturbed the President at Macmillan's home in England. Through his brother, he expressed his 'concern'.

In London, FBI representative Charles Bates was told the President wanted to be briefed in person. He drove down to Sussex the following day, Sunday, where he found Kennedy in characteristic pose, feet on the desk, tie askew. 'Charles,' said Kennedy, 'if anything develops on this case, anything at all, we'd like to be advised. Get it to us in Rome.'

The President was on his way to Italy, and the FBI's man watched as a helicopter bore him away to London Airport. So did Macmillan. 'Hatless, with his brisk step, combining that indescribable look of a boy on holiday with the dignity of a President and Commander-in-Chief, he walked across the garden to the machine. We stood and waved . . .'

Back in Washington, Robert Kennedy took swift action over the *Journal-American* story. Within forty-eight hours, on Monday,

31 July, the journalists responsible for it faced the Attorney General – having been hauled from their homes in New York and flown to Washington in the Kennedys' private plane, the *Caroline*. They were the paper's managing editor James Horan, winner of the Pulitzer Prize and numerous other awards, and a younger reporter named Dom Frasca. In the words of a senior colleague, 'Horan was the best investigative reporter they ever had. If he wrote it, it was true.'

Horan and Frasca died before work began on this book, but their ordeal in front of Robert Kennedy survives thanks to FBI liaison man Courtney Evans. According to an Evans memorandum, the President's brother asked the newsmen to name the 'high US aide' who, according to the article, was being linked to the Profumo scandal. Horan replied that the reference was to the President, and that – according to the newspaper's information – he had 'been involved with' a woman – not Novotny – shortly before his election.

The meeting between Kennedy and the reporters was less than cordial. 'It is noted,' Evans wrote afterwards, 'that the Attorney-General treated the newspaper representatives at arm's length ... in fact, there was almost an air of hostility ...' He berated them for, he claimed, having published 'without any further check being made to get to the truth of the matter.'

Nothing was resolved. The reporters refused to reveal their sources other than those already mentioned in print. Kennedy offered them no information, and the meeting ended in frosty deadlock. The Attorney General then did something odd, 'admonishing' the FBI's liaison man Courtney Evans 'not to write a memorandum' on what had occurred. Evans promptly reported orally to Director Hoover. When Kennedy learned that the following day, he said he hoped Evans 'had not misunderstood' his earlier instruction not to write a report.

According to Mark Monsky, a future vice-president of NBC News, Robert Kennedy acted ruthlessly behind the scenes. Monsky, a godson of Randolph Hearst, owner of the *Journal-American*, said he learned how the Attorney General resolved the matter. At a meeting in Manhattan, Kennedy threatened the paper with a government anti-trust suit if it did not cease to pursue the story. The story was dropped. The investigation was called off, managing editor Horan was to tell his sons, because of pressure from Robert Kennedy.

On 2 July, Robert Kennedy asked J. Edgar Hoover to find out what Christine Keeler and Mandy Rice-Davies had been up to during their visit to the States a year earlier. Nothing untoward was discovered. The following day, as John Kennedy met the Pope in the Vatican, his brother learned of yet more trouble. There were now allegations linking 'highly placed Government officials' with a woman of East German origin called Ellen Rometsch.

'Robert Kennedy definitely knew,' Vice-President Johnson's assistant Bobby Baker wrote in his memoir, 'that Ellen Rometsch had been one of the women Jack Kennedy had asked me to introduce him to. I accommodated his request.' Rometsch was packed off back to Germany following an FBI probe. She refused the authors' repeated requests for an interview.

President Kennedy's endless womanising was catching up with him all in a rush. Weeks earlier, in England, Christine Keeler had spent four evenings putting her experiences on tape for Robin Drury, the man now acting as her business manager. The tape was eventually handed over to the police under a court order, and the contents were never made public. 'You know,' Drury later said, 'there were a lot of big American political names involved in this thing. It never came out because it was hushed up by the British Government for political reasons.' What Drury learned was passed on to Washington by the FBI – as an 'allegation against President

Kennedy'. A related document remains entirely blanked out by the censor.

The 'big flap' – as FBI man Charles Bates called it, looking back – was not about Christine Keeler herself. The only John Kennedy she knew was the manager of the pop singer Tommy Steele. Nor was it just about Mariella Novotny, and her claim to have slept with Kennedy. 'One of Novotny's closest girl chums,' columnist Kilgallen had written during Kennedy's European visit, 'was involved with a very big man on the other side of the Atlantic.'

On the evening of 29 June, as Kennedy dined with Macmillan, Bates had sent coded telegraph 861 to FBI headquarters. It was rated 'VERY URGENT', and concerned the President. Of twenty lines, seventeen were obliterated by the censor as released. What remains reads: '... [NAME CENSORED] TALKED ABOUT PRESIDENT KENNEDY AND REPEATED A RUMOUR THAT WAS GOING AROUND NEW YORK...' A second document, though stripped of names, provides further background. A report addressed to the FBI's Assistant Director in charge of counter-intelligence, William Sullivan, offers – between the censored chunks – information that 'ONE OF [NAME BLANKED OUT] CLIENTS WAS JOHN KENNEDY, THEN PRESIDENTIAL CANDIDATE. [NAME] STATED THAT MARIE NOVOTNY, BRITISH PROSTITUTE, WENT TO NEW YORK TO TAKE [NAME]'S PLACE, SINCE SHE WAS GOING ON PRE-ELECTION ROUNDS WITH KENNEDY.'

In his interview, Charles Bates threw some light on the censored cable traffic. His information, he says, came from Assistant Commissioner for Crime Joe Jackson at Scotland Yard. 'They had questioned a woman,' Bates said, 'apparently Mariella Novotny. She had taken the place of another woman, who had looked after Kennedy during the campaign.' Bates could not remember the other woman's name. Who was she?

Gossip columnist Dorothy Kilgallen had suggested that there was a 'girl who could "tell all"... reported to have committed suicide not long ago.' The women around Stephen Ward did have a tendency to die by their own hand. Yvonne Brooks, who knew Lord Astor and was kept by an American businessman in London, tried to kill herself just as the Profumo Affair was breaking. Another Ward protégée, Pat Marlowe, a regular visitor to the United States and friend of another presidential mistress, Marilyn Monroe, had succeeded in killing herself in August 1962 – just days after Monroe.

Research suggests, however, that the mystery woman was neither Brooks nor Marlowe, and that she survived the events of 1963. Before it was silenced, the New York *Journal-American* said she was 'a beautiful Chinese-American girl now in London'. The highest authorities, said the paper, 'identified her as Suzy Chang... who later went to London and operated as a call girl from the fashionable layout of Dr Stephen Ward...'

Who was Suzy Chang?

CHAPTER 28

The World of Suzy Chang

For a long time during the work on this book, Suzy Chang remained a mere name on an old newspaper clipping, a frustrating enigma. Then, gradually, we were able to put a face to the woman alleged to have been a mistress of John Kennedy. We obtained immigration records that covered Chang's comings and goings to and from the United States. Using them, we started to reconstruct a life.

Though Chang used a string of different names – largely for transliteration purposes – her birth name was Su-Yang Chang. She had been born in Tientsin, China, in 1935. Her parents, both doctors, moved to Hong Kong in the wake of the communist revolution. During the 1950s, they settled in Delaware in the United States. Suzy, for reasons unknown, did not follow immediately. At the age of nineteen she was in England, starting adult life as a nurse in Birmingham. Then she headed for the bright lights of London, where she worked first at the Pigalle Club as a cigarette girl, then at the Casanova, near Claridge's hotel.

By 1960 or thereabouts, when she reportedly spent time with President Kennedy, Chang was a strikingly lovely model and aspiring actress. She got a part in the film *Nudes of the World*, and publicity shots show her in the pose one would expect: slinky oriental-style dress cut to the thigh, fitting tightly on a figure to make any man take a deep breath. The movie's producer, Arnold Miller, said Chang knew who was who in the world of London nightclubs. She was, he remembered, 'always elegantly and expensively dressed. And she obviously wasn't doing the film for the money.'

For three months in 1961, Chang acted in the film *The Road to Hong Kong*, made at Shepperton Studios. The lead parts were played by Bob Hope, Bing Crosby and Joan Collins, and a glittering list of guest stars included Frank Sinatra and Dean Martin. For us, here was a first hint of a possible link between Chang and the people in the Profumo case. Bob Hope and his manager Louie 'Doc' Shurr were shortly to become friendly with Mandy Rice-Davies.

In California we traced Chang's second husband Glen Costin, who had first known Chang in London in the early 1960s. He remembered a woman who 'moved in very wealthy circles'. She did indeed, but at the height of the Profumo Affair in 1963 Chang was involved in some strange adventures. In May that year she was in court giving evidence against Alfred Davis, an Olympic Airways official accused of stealing her handbag containing cash and a ring worth £900 – a great deal of money at the time. This unrelated case produced a tenuous connection to Stephen Ward. Alfred Davis was described to us by his friends Tony and Barbara Pistalo – both of whom were patients of Ward's – as having been 'a big gambler who always had money, and hung about in Chelsea. He was more or less living in Nell Gwynne House at the time . . .'

Suzy Chang, moreover, was staying in Nell Gwynne House herself. More than one call girl lived at that address, but there is no evidence that Chang was ever a prostitute. Those who knew her say she was in a much higher league.

Ronna Riccardo, the London prostitute who was close to Stephen Ward, knew Suzy Chang. 'I remember Suzy,' she said, 'from when I was living in Nell Gwynne House. She had long hair down her back. We all stayed there at one time or another, me and Paula and Suzy. Stephen knew Suzy. We were a tight little clique.'

Chang's tangle with Alfred Davis – he was said to have taken the handbag during a car ride from Nell Gwynne House – led to another odd coincidence. Davis' defence counsel was James Burge, the barrister who would shortly defend Stephen Ward. Burge persuaded Chang, in court, to reveal whose flat she had been in that day at Nell Gwynne House. She said it belonged to a 'Mr Slazenger'. 'I had been staying there a few days,' said Chang. 'Slazenger' was in fact John Schlesinger,* a multi-millionaire American-born film producer and businessman. In South Africa, where Schlesinger lived later, a film distributor described him to the authors as 'the best-known womaniser in the history of South Africa'. In 1958, at thirty-five, he had been involved in a particularly messy divorce.

Another curious aspect of the handbag theft case was Suzy Chang's use of another name. 'Film actress Jackie Chang,' one paper reported after the case, 'is determined not to change her name. "Why should I? It's my name, and the one I've always had . . ."' It wasn't, of course – Chang told the court she had been calling herself 'Jackie' only for the past few years. Another woman of oriental extraction, however, took great exception to Chang using the name – with reason.

---

* This is not the celebrated John Schlesinger who made *Far from the Madding Crowd*, *Yanks*, etc.

Jacqui Chan, who played in the film *The World of Suzie Wong*, began a libel action against a newspaper that had mistakenly printed 'Chang' as 'Chan' in connection with the Davis theft case. Why did she bother? The silly little episode throws a little more light on Suzy Chang.

Jacqui Chan had in the 1950s been the girlfriend of Antony Armstrong-Jones, the future Lord Snowdon, before he married Princess Margaret. Armstrong-Jones, then a young photographer, seems to have been fascinated by Chinese women – he produced two portfolios of photographs on the theme. He also knew Suzy Chang. And Chang seems to have begun using the name 'Jackie' at about the time Armstrong-Jones broke up with Jacqui. The authors wrote to both Lord Snowdon and Jacqui Chan asking about Chang, but they did not reply.

Armstrong-Jones had known Stephen Ward from the early 1950s. After leaving Cambridge, he had begun his photographic career as assistant to Ward's good friend, court photographer Baron. Ward did not much like Armstrong-Jones. Not long before the Profumo case broke, when Ward sketched Princess Margaret while doing portraits of members of the Royal Family, he thought hers 'probably the most difficult face to draw' he ever attempted. Armstrong-Jones, now Lord Snowdon, told him he had 'got the nose too long'. The Princess' husband was Ward's next sitter, but he never finished the sketch.

Suzy Chang – friend of Armstrong-Jones and alleged mistress of John F. Kennedy – also knew Stephen Ward. Billy Hitchcock, who knew Ward and first tipped the US ambassador to London to the Keeler/Profumo/Ivanov love triangle, remembered Chang as 'one of Stephen's girls', and said he heard rumours about her and Kennedy at the time. Chang's former husband Glen Costin remembered her telling him at the height of the Profumo

Affair that she was acquainted with the people in the case. 'I know them, I know them,' she told Costin. She said, specifically, that she knew Ward. She did not, however, tell him anything about Kennedy. Was Chang really involved with him?

Those heavily censored FBI and US Immigration Service documents reveal that Chang travelled to New York in 1960 and 1961, and over the Christmas period of 1962. Earlier in 1962, she applied to get on to the Chinese visa quota for the United States. Chang's mother, who was already living in America, filed a petition to the Immigration Service on her daughter's behalf. She did so through the prestigious New York law firm of Donovan Leisure Newton & Irvine. William Donovan, who started the firm, had been the founder of the OSS, the precursor of the CIA, and the law firm had always had strong connections with the government in power.

This was a surprisingly powerful helping hand for a minor actress. 'Someone,' a former FBI official told us, 'was protecting her ass. They wanted someone with real clout to carry the ball, to run interference for her . . .' Suzy Chang got on to the visa quota within a fortnight.

A 19 July 1963 report in the Immigration Service file – soon after the flap over the *Journal-American* article hinting at the President's involvement in the Profumo case – reflects an extensive investigation of Chang. The report lists nine people, most of them British models, who had been linked to Chang. All the names are blanked out. Another document shows that the authorities had combed the file on the Mariella Novotny prostitution case, looking for a connection to Chang. They did not find one.

The most suggestive document is dated well after the Profumo case, in 1965. It notes that Chang 'arrived in US at New York, via Flight 701, on 22/12/63. She was the [blanked-out section in report] . . . she was questioned regarding the "Profumo Affair," and alleged to be a close friend of Stephen Ward.'

As this book went into its first edition, the authors finally traced Suzy Chang, who had taken a new name and lived on the eastern seaboard of the United States. She confirmed that she had known many celebrities, including Antony Armstrong-Jones and key figures associated with the Profumo Affair – notably Thomas Corbally, who played a leading role in alerting the American ambassador in London to the looming scandal, Kennedy, and Stephen Ward.

'Stephen was a good, good, good friend . . . I knew him a long time,' Chang said. 'He used to come to my house to eat . . . I loved Stephen . . . I knew all the people Stephen knew . . . I really cared about him.'

When the authors asked Chang about the reports that linked her to John F. Kennedy, she paused, then cautiously acknowledged it. 'Well, John – John was the President of the United States . . . Well, I used to come and visit my mother [in the USA]. And well, anyway, we'd meet in the 21 Club. You know, everybody saw me eating with him. It wasn't behind anybody's back. I know Stash Radziwill, but I don't know Lee very well, you know what I mean?'

'Stash' was Prince Stanislas Radziwill, married to Lee, sister of the President's wife, Jacqueline. The President did visit New York's 21 Club between his election and his inauguration. Asked whether she had an affair with him, Suzy Chang denied it. She said, 'I think the President was a nice guy, very charming.' Then she laughed. 'What else am I going to say?' she asked.

Interviewed again in 2006, Chang – still lovely in old age – was courteous but still very careful what she said. Now, though, she indicated that although she had spent time with Kennedy at the 21 Club in New York, she had actually met him at the 21 Club in London.

Beyond that, and while happy to talk about many other famous names she had known – and in some cases still knew – she remained tight-lipped about Kennedy. She did say, with a giggle, that she preferred 'men with a lot of hair on their heads'.

But: 'I prefer not publicity. These were friends, and so many of them are dead.'

Two British journalists, Alastair and Sheila Revie, who covered the Profumo case in depth in 1963, went to great pains to interview as many women as they could trace who had been close to Ward. 'The Ward girls,' the Revies said, 'were all talking about Kennedy. And Chang was one of the girls discussed. A coloured girl, a Eurasian, who lived at Nell Gwynne House, was believed to have gone with the President.'

Charles Bates, the FBI man in London during the Affair, remembered being shown Scotland Yard reports on the way Kennedy's name had come up in the Profumo case. 'I saw something about a couple of girls who went over to the US in 1960, during the JFK campaign. They went to New York, they were in a hotel there. One or both later rode the campaign train to furnish her wares to those who wanted it. Also, one of them was given an assignment to meet a man in a certain hotel room. Then the other girl was sent over to take her place. That's vivid in my mind – the business about the hotel in New York, and the report referring to the man by the initials JFK . . .'

On 22 July 1963, nearly a month after the flap had started, the President's brother had a meeting with FBI Assistant Director Courtney Evans, who had sat in on the encounter with the *Journal-American* reporters who had written the Chang story. Now Evans reported to Hoover:

The Attorney-General was contacted last evening and orally advised of the information developed by [name blanked out] that [name blanked out] had lived with [name blanked out], a New York City call girl, and that one of her clients was alleged to be the then presidential candidate John F. Kennedy. He was further informed that Mariella Novotny had allegedly gone to New York to take [name blanked out]'s place, as she was travelling on pre-election rounds with the presidential candidate. As a matter of fact, Novotny did not enter the United States until 14 December 1960, nearly six weeks after the election. The Attorney-General was appreciative of our bringing this matter to his attention personally. He said it did seem preposterous that such a story would be circulated when a presidential candidate during the campaign travels with scores of newspapermen. He added that with the next presidential election now less than eighteen months away, he anticipated there would be similar stories and he would like us to continue to advise him of any such matters coming to our attention on a personal basis, as he could better defend the family if he knew what was being said.

Donald Stewart, an FBI espionage supervisor in Washington at the time, remembers Robert Kennedy's intervention during the Profumo Affair. 'Everything we got,' says Stewart, 'had to go through him. One night I got a call from [Assistant Director] Courtney Evans and he said "Bobby wants everything," and everything went to Bobby from then on . . .'

Bobby Kennedy's elder brother had his own urgent interest. The deputy chief of the CIA's London station, Cleveland Cram, recalled that a 'specific request' had come in from the President himself. He needed to know whether there was any-thing about to be made public in the case, on the grounds of 'forewarned is forearmed'. Cram had no doubt that Washington wanted to find out whether 'one of the Kennedys' was linked to the Profumo girls.

Who inspired the press leaks about Novotny and Suzy Chang? It may have been Robert Kennedy's arch-enemy, J. Edgar Hoover himself. The FBI Director has been called the 'keeper of the keys to the closet where our skeletons are stored'. For nearly four decades, Hoover had been building an astonishing dossier of smear material on some of the most influential men in the United States. These were the 'O and C' – Official and Confidential – files that were kept by Hoover in his own office, and which have never become fully available to researchers. They contained damning ammunition that gave the Director a lasting hold over many men of power – including the Kennedy brothers.

The FBI file on John Kennedy had been opened at the start of World War II, based on reports by Britain's MI5 on the young man's activity while visiting his father, Joe, then the US ambassador to London. Those first reports almost certainly included material on the Kennedy family's association with the Cliveden set. Also during the war, Hoover had personally ordered tape-recorded surveillance of Kennedy as an officer in Naval Intelligence. The recordings included coverage of the hotel bedroom in which Kennedy had sex with Inga Arvad, a Danish woman suspected of being a German agent. The apparently insatiable Kennedy had from then on provided Hoover with a stream of compromising material, culminating most recently – in the early 1960s – in his prolonged affair with starlet Judith Campbell. Now there were Mariella Novotny, Suzy Chang, and the mounting information linking the Kennedys and their friends to the Stephen Ward circle in London.

This was manna from heaven for Hoover, for it apparently

touched not only John but also Robert. Hoover's greatest disdain was for Robert, whom he regarded as an upstart Attorney General, the first ever to treat Hoover as his subordinate and dare to dictate FBI policy. Sexually, Robert had been more restrained than his brother the President. In 1962, though, Hoover had come to the rescue to suppress evidence of both brothers' relationships with Marilyn Monroe. Now, with the apparent links to women in the British scandal, Hoover's hold over the Kennedys was strengthened yet again.

It was very likely Hoover who saw to it that the *Journal-American* got its stories on Novotny and Chang, and that the paper had the confidence to run them. It was a Hearst Corporation newspaper, and throughout the fifties Hoover had seen to it that the Hearst papers were able to fan the flames of the Red Menace. Some Hearst star writers, like Walter Winchell, were personal friends of Hoover's. There were even former FBI men on the newspaper's staff. In 1963, the cosy relationship was still flourishing. Red-baiting continued, as did fierce editorial opposition to the policies of the Kennedy administration.

The *Journal-American* folded four years after the Profumo Affair, and there is now no way to discover how it got its inside information on the alleged Kennedy connection. With the deaths of both reporters involved in the main story, we are left only with coded references in a novel authored by one of them, managing editor James Horan. Entitled *The Right Image* and written on a theme of political fixing in the White House, it includes barely veiled allusions to the Novotny affair, and to an oriental girl called 'Suzy Chu'.

Courtney Evans, the former FBI Assistant Director charged with the delicate task of liaising between Hoover and Robert Kennedy, was legendarily tight-lipped. In retirement, he rarely agreed to speak with writers or the press. On the Profumo Affair, though, he was blunt.

'This was a time,' Evans said, 'when there was a feeling that we had been deceiving ourselves, that we had felt more secure that we should have done, not least because we depended a great deal on the security capability of the British. And then to find that the President was perhaps involved with somebody in the British security scandal. Nobody was grinning . . .'

CHAPTER 29

The Special Relationship Falters

As early as March 1963, President Kennedy's aide Arthur Schlesinger had reported back following a three-day visit to London. He had not been impressed. 'The Conservative Government,' he wrote, 'is in a sad state . . . It sinks steadily in the public opinion polls under the weight of old age, unemployment, Soviet espionage . . . and personal scandal. It reeks of decay; and the press and the opposition, sensing a rout, are moving in for the kill . . . It is hard to overstate the atmosphere of political squalor in London today . . . and the impression that the Government is frivolous and decadent, and that everything is unravelling at the seams.'

To his surprise, when Schlesinger went to see Kennedy to expand on this report, all the President seemed to want to talk about was the Profumo Affair. The views Schlesinger had expressed, however, were by now widely shared in Washington – not least by FBI Director Hoover, with his growing knowledge of the Affair and Kennedy's own possible entanglement. It all dovetailed neatly with his obsession about communist subversion, and the conviction – ever since the defection of traitors Burgess and Maclean – that British security was hopelessly unreliable. In the late 1950s, when Britain was trying to reach an agreement with the United States on sharing nuclear secrets, Hoover's British specialist Charles Bates had told him just the sort of thing he wanted to hear. Bates wrote of a 'British counter-espionage service full of inexperienced "old school-tie" men, who feared probing suspects because of possible political rows . . .'

Now, in early summer 1963, the old-school-tie men at the top were at odds with each other. Lord Chancellor Dilhorne had completed the swift inquiry into the security aspects of the Profumo matter Macmillan had requested, in the hope that it would dispel growing concerns. It had criticised MI5, yet concluded that 'no further enquiry is necessary from the security angle'. That did not satisfy all Cabinet members. William Deedes, Minister without Portfolio, told the Prime Minister in a memorandum that there was 'chilling' evidence of a Soviet plot to enlist 'spies' and sow 'social demoralisation'. Had members of the Cabinet known what was happening in Washington, their concern would have been even greater.

In mid-June, the FBI had received some explosive information from its prized informant within the KGB at the Soviet mission at the United Nations. This was Aleksey Kulak – better remembered today by his code name, 'Fedora'. Shortly after Profumo had resigned, Kulak reported, he had heard a senior KGB colleague say that Soviet naval attaché Ivanov 'had received [through Christine Keeler] . . . a lot of information' from Minister for War Profumo. The colleague, a KGB colonel, said Ivanov 'had established micro-phones in [Stephen Ward's] apartment'.

With President Kennedy's visit to Britain only ten days away, Hoover sent a 'Top Secret' report of this development to his brother the Attorney General, emphasising that the source was usually reliable and that the KGB colonel quoted by the source was a highly experienced veteran. He asked that Robert Kennedy pass the information on to the President. Defense Secretary McNamara, who was also briefed, said he viewed it as 'of extreme importance'.

The FBI did not, however, inform its counterparts in MI5 anything about the development at the time. The British Security Service and the government itself were by then considered so unreliable, so untrustworthy, that the FBI decided it could not risk jeopardising the safety of its agent-in-place. Instead, Director Hoover dispatched two agents to London where their job was, according to the Scotland Yard police officer who liaised with them, 'to interview people about possible security leaks because of the Ivanov connection'.

It may be that the development in Washington was communicated to the Prime Minister . The day the FBI received its information from its agent in the KGB, Macmillan had told the head of MI6, Dick White, he was sure there was 'a conspiracy directed from Moscow to drive me from office'. White told Macmillan that the Soviets 'had no assets to organise a plot involving Profumo', but said he would review the evidence.

The same day, 17 June, a joint MI6-MI5 working party was instructed to 'look into the possibility that the Russian Intelligence Service had a hand in staging the Profumo affair in order to discredit Her Majesty's Government'.

The following day, US Ambassador to London Bruce sent a cable to Washington saying he thought Macmillan had become an 'electoral liability'. He thought, however, that Macmillan would survive until President Kennedy's imminent visit to Britain. By the end of June, however, Macmillan's biographer Richard Lamb has written, the President and his advisers believed that, 'with the Profumo affair, Macmillan's reign was over'.

On Saturday, 29 June 1963, in the same edition that carried the

Novotny-Chang story, the *Journal-American* gave the first news of yet another British security fiasco. In London on the following Monday, the same day the government at last admitted that Kim Philby had defected, the *Guardian* reported on 'a new spy sensation ... a startling new espionage case which is likely to break momentarily and may bring down the Conservatives'. In the midst of harrying Macmillan over the Profumo case, George Wigg – citing American sources – told reporters that there were 'bigger scandals to come'.

Newsweek, then one of the two most powerful American weeklies, went for the story hard, quoting 'an unchallengeable security source in Washington'. According to the magazine, the new case involved 'leaks of a US Skybolt missile critique and other military documents'. Defense Secretary McNamara, the story said, had months earlier shared a Skybolt document with the British Ministry of Defence.

The Skybolt missile programme was highly controversial. Its cancellation, communicated to Macmillan at his Nassau meeting with Kennedy in 1962, had threatened the British leader with political disaster. Without Skybolt, and with no UK-built alternative, Britain's days as a nuclear power seemed numbered. As a sop, Kennedy had given the Prime Minister the Polaris missile, and Profumo had gone to Washington for talks on the technical details. In 1963, when the scandal about Profumo broke, that fact alone caused alarm in the United States. When he learned of the alleged British leak of Skybolt information, it is said Macmillan had telephoned President Kennedy close to tears. If Kennedy were to cancel his forthcoming visit to Britain, he would understand. The visit, of course, went ahead, but confidence was not restored.

The FBI firmly believed that the leaks about Skybolt were emanating from London, and Director Hoover ensured the press reflected that belief. So did the Defense Department, which fed correspondents the line that 'it would be dangerous to allow the sale of Polaris missiles to Britain'.

The *Times*' defence correspondent Alun Gwynne Jones – who was to become Lord Chalfont and a Labour government minister – visited Washington that summer. His numerous contacts included a meeting in the Oval Office with President Kennedy. 'I came upon some alarming repercussions from the Profumo affair,' he wrote later. The case provoked 'a great witchhunt in American intelligence and security circles. American doubts about the effectiveness of British security, never far from the surface, were now widely canvassed, and in several of my conversations with politicians and officials in the United States, our security arrangements in the United Kingdom were described as being "as full of holes as a sieve".'

At home in London, Gwynn Jones' contacts with both MI5 and MI6 led him to the conclusion that they were indeed 'in some disarray . . . hampered by a deteriorating relationship between MI5 and MI6'. The US administration would be 'reluctant to agree to the transfer of sensitive information on nuclear systems to . . . the United Kingdom, while security was seen to be so ineffective'.

The CIA's deputy Station Chief in London, Cleveland Cram, was warned by the Agency's Soviet Division head that year that 'all our secrets pass through here and the security is bad. It's dangerous. It's a mess.' Though he was an Anglophile, Cram could only agree.

The FBI's man in London, another Anglophile, was also by now disillusioned about British security and about MI5 Director General Roger Hollis in particular. 'I'll never forget going to see Hollis one time,' Charles Bates told the authors. 'I said, "Roger, you guys haven't come up with anything since World War II." He said, "Oh, sure we have." I said, "No you haven't. We gave you almost everything, either us or the CIA." ' When Bates asked what Hollis could give the FBI on the Profumo matter, the MI5 chief just said, '"Oh, we looked at that, and there's no security angle . . . We don't have any interest . . ." '

'Now I can see,' Bates said years later, on being shown the releases from his own Bureau's 'Bowtie' file and other research produced for this book, 'that they were deliberately misleading me.'

CHAPTER 30

Damage Control

'The capital and whole nation was mad with hatred and fear,' the historian Thomas Macaulay wrote of a scandal in another century. In the summer of 1963, there was a feeling that Britain's political world had gone mad, a fear that the Profumo Affair would topple the government. 'The "popular" Press,' the Prime Minister wrote in his diary, was nothing but coverage of 'the lives of spies and prostitutes, written no doubt in the office. Day after day the attacks developed, chiefly on me – old, incompetent, worn out.'

At sixty-nine, Macmillan was indeed suddenly weary of it all. His Labour opponent Harold Wilson, however, did not want to be seen to be kicking the incumbent when he was down. Further Opposition attacks on Macmillan, Wilson confided to the First Secretary at the US embassy, 'could easily have the effect of alienating the public and consolidating Conservative ranks in a demonstration of sympathy'. Wilson believed, the First Secretary reported to Washington, that Labour could safely 'allow the post-Profumo plot to boil in a "natural" way. He mentioned several – he said six – ministers who may be mixed up in the Keeler business. Wilson was not certain when (or if) all these floating rumours about high-placed persons could be stilled. But it could take a long time, smudging the Prime Minister's hopes of carrying on . . .'

The Conservative Party Treasurer, Robert Allan, briefed Ambassador Bruce himself on the rumours linking more ministers to the scandal. 'Names mentioned,' Bruce told President Kennedy in note form, 'are Selwyn Lloyd, Sandys, Hare and Marples. Has been told Marples naked masked man who served at banquet. Allan thinks allegations against Selwyn Lloyd ridiculous.'

In fact, the gossip about former Chancellor of the Exchequer Lloyd was not against him personally; Stephen Ward was said to have had a sexual encounter with a member of Lloyd's family. As reported in these pages, moreover, Transport Minister Ernest Marples had not been the Man in the Mask at Mariella Novotny's notorious party. Rumours were flying, though, that it had been him, and some Conservatives claimed Ward was behind the allegation. There is no evidence he made any such claim – not least because, by that time, he was languishing in Brixton Prison awaiting trial.

One man who did tell tales about the Man in the Mask was a Chelsea solicitor who knew Ward, Novotny and her husband, Hod Dibben. Before the scandal, according to Dibben, the lawyer was forever hanging around outside the house in Hyde Park Square, and once threatened Novotny with rape. He claimed falsely that he had himself attended the Mask party. According to *People* journalist Roy East, the man was 'one of the people mainly responsible for putting around false tales'.

On Wednesday, 12 June 1963, the *News of the World*'s chief crime reporter, Peter Earle, was at Christine Keeler's flat. Keeler was now a 'property', for the newspaper had now bought her story. 'She had been out with her black lovers,' Earle recalled, 'and was lying in bed, naked and asleep.' Dragged from her bed at Earle's editor's insistence, to be asked whether she had slept with any ministers other than Profumo, Keeler burst into tears. Profumo, she said, was the only official with whom she had been involved.

The call to Keeler was inspired by Sir Winston Churchill's son Randolph, at the time a political columnist for the *News of the World*, who had received a tip-off that yet more embarrassments would come to light. One Cabinet minister – supposedly Enoch Powell, though he later denied it – reportedly threatened to resign rather than remain a member of a tainted Cabinet.

Another minister, Secretary of State for the Colonies Duncan Sandys, did offer to resign – because he had featured in an unrelated but lurid divorce case. Sandys, German newspapers had reported, had been the 'headless man' having oral sex with the Duchess of Argyll, as depicted in Polaroid photographs produced at the Duchess' recent divorce hearing. The 'headless man' – as the mystery individual was henceforth called – because the photographs that showed the Duchess giving oral sex were close-ups. One could see the Duchess' face, but not the man's.

On 20 June, the Prime Minister's aide Harold Evans arrived at work 'to be greeted with a warning at the 11.30 lobby I should almost certainly have to announce a ministerial resignation. The Minister . . . was not the headless man, but he had been involved with the lady and apparently felt he must expiate the indulgence by resignation . . .' Duncan Sandys decided to ponder his final decision for a few hours.

The following day, when Macmillan announced the appointment of Lord Denning to hold an inquiry into the security aspects of the Profumo case, he asked him to look into the 'headless man' rumours as well. There was no further word of a new resignation; Sandys, who spoken privately with the Prime Minister, had changed his mind overnight. Denning would report that Sandys was not the man in the photograph. A medical examination established that the physical characteristics of Sandys' penis did not match those of the man in the lewd photographs. The Report, however, would discreetly avoid mentioning that – even if he had not been the 'headless man'– Sandys had indeed had a dalliance with the Duchess of Argyll.

In his pursuit of this tacky matter, Denning interviewed four possible candidates other than Sandys: American businessman John Cohane, Peter Coombe, a former Savoy Hotel press officer, Sigismund von Braun, brother of Wernher, the famous German rocket scientist, and the film star Douglas Fairbanks Jr. The handwriting on one of the 'headless man' Polaroids, it turned out, matched Fairbanks' writing. It may be no coincidence that, as reported in an earlier chapter, Fairbanks was the proud possessor of a Polaroid camera.

There is an odd postscript to this sordid story. According to the ghostwriter of Yevgeny Ivanov's 1992 autobiography *The Naked Spy*, a copy of one of the 'headless man' photographs wound up in the archives of the KGB. It was obtained, allegedly, as part of Operation Dom – for blackmail purposes.

The way Denning's Report handled the 'headless man' sideshow exemplified the way it took every opportunity to smear the name of Stephen Ward. While his Report left Sandys looking whiter than white, it gave publicity to the notion that Ward had been in possession of one of the Argyll sex photographs.

While Denning always referred to Profumo as 'Mr', he granted Ward neither 'Dr' – as was his right – nor 'Mr'. He was just plain 'Ward'. Profumo's adultery with the young woman he had seen cavorting with a Soviet diplomat was called an 'indiscretion', balanced against a record that entitled him to 'the confidence of his colleagues'. Ward, however, was characterised as 'utterly immoral', a man of 'vicious sexual activities' whose efforts as a diplomatic go-between were 'misconceived and misdirected'. Ward, of course, would have no way of answering back. By the time the Denning Report had dragged him through the mire, he would have been dead for weeks.

The purpose of the Denning Report, Macmillan was to write, was to serve as 'at least some check in the flood of accusation and rumour'. To Britain's senior Appeal Court judge, this was a patriotic assignment. 'It was my duty,' he would recall, 'to do what I was asked.' There were, he noted in his Report, 'unavoidable limitations'. Since his inquiry was held in secret, his work 'had not the appearance of justice'. He alone was 'detective, inquisitor, advocate and judge'. 'My enquiry,' Denning wrote, 'is not a suitable body to determine guilt or innocence . . . No witness has given evidence on oath. None has been cross-examined . . .'

An advantage, Denning thought, was that – because they were heard in private – witnesses were probably honest with him. He could check individuals' testimony one against the other, and allegations made received no publicity. 'It is, I believe,' Denning wrote at the end of the Report, 'better for the country . . . that this unfortunate episode should be closed'. The Report did just that. It was, in the words of the commentator Ludovic Kennedy, who wrote one of the earliest books on the case, 'a disgrace. Lord Denning produced all sorts of dirt, with no evidence. It was a shambles.'

'Some of the evidence I heard,' Denning would recall, 'was so disgusting – even to my sophisticated mind – that I sent the lady shorthand writers out, and no note of it was taken.'

The 'disgusting' evidence included, Denning wrote, information on Stephen Ward's attendance at sex parties, and on Ward's collection of pornographic photographs. As the Profumo scandal was breaking, his journalist friend and occasional MI6 operative Warwick Charlton told the authors, Ward entrusted a number of photographs to Charlton for safe keeping. He in turn consigned them to the safe at his employers, Odhams Press, part of a group of magazines and newspapers that included the *Daily Mirror*. Later, some time after Ward's arrest, they wound up in the hands of the police.

The photographs Ward handed him, Charlton told the authors, had been taken as long ago as the early 1950s at parties at a house in St John's Wood.* 'They were hardly dirty pictures,' he said, 'but . . . they would have been considered rather daring.' He claimed 'they showed Prince Philip, Vasco Lazzolo, and other people, [Conservative MP] William Rees-Davies, and the photographer Baron. There were all these girls around, stark naked.'

Baron, who had a withered arm, was easily recognisable in the pictures, Charlton said. Oddly, for a similar reason, so was Rees-Davies – he had lost an arm during the war. One of his nicknames was 'the One-Armed Bandit'.

Why would such photographs have come into the possession of Stephen Ward? There is no way now of knowing. A rational speculation, though, is that they may originally have been taken by the photographer Anthony Beauchamp, who had been keeper of the records of the Thursday Club – and Ward's very close friend. Another Ward friend, artist Vasco Lazzolo, had become custodian of the records following Beauchamp's death. Beauchamp is known to have taken nude photographs, Lazzolo to have had a collection of pornographic photographs.

Charlton believed that Ward 'was quite friendly with Prince Philip in the early days'. 'When [Lord] Denning was doing his stuff,' Charlton said, 'he was very worried about it. Stephen protected people he had known. He was very proud of that relationship.'

At the time of the Profumo scandal, whatever the truth about the allegation that there were compromising photographs that featured Prince Philip, word spread far and wide that the Prince

---

* See earlier reference to parties at p.24.

was somehow involved. On 18 June 1963, in New York, an FBI Supervisor noted that there were 'thorny problems involved, inasmuch as there are indications that Prince Philip [and Douglas Fairbanks] may have been involved in the Keeler affair'.

Days later, as Denning started work, the *Daily Mirror* devoted its entire front page to a story replete with innuendo. 'The foulest rumour being circulated about the Profumo scandal,' the article said, 'has involved the Royal Family. The name mentioned in this rumour has been Prince Philip's.' The *Mirror* did not tell readers what the foul rumour was, just assured them it was 'utterly unfounded'.

Was it true that, as Charlton claimed, risqué photographs allegedly featuring the Prince had for a time reposed in the safe of a company in the same group as the *Mirror*? If so, was the article mere coincidence? Though the paper could go no further, this appears to have been a nod and a wink to readers.

Is it possible that the suggestion that the Prince could be compromised was not far-fetched? A detailed report in 2000, the result of a three-month *Daily Mail* investigation on the ground in Russia and elsewhere, described a joint KGB/GRU project of the 1950s and 1960s code-named 'Operation Dom – or in English 'Operation House'. According to the report, which drew on interviews with Soviet intelligence veterans, its purpose had been to collect intimate details on the private lives of British royals, senior politicians and diplomats. The motive was to use compromising information as ammunition for blackmail, or leak it to subvert the Establishment.

What has this to do with the alleged youthful activity of Prince Philip? He had, of course, been associated with the Thursday Club, remembered now for its libertine gatherings in the late 1940s and 1950s. The content of the Thursday Club records –

last known to have been in the hands of Vasco Lazzolo – made their way, according to the 2000 report, to the KGB in Moscow.

The records had been passed to the Soviets, the report said, by the journalist Derek Tangye. Tangye, a sometime editor of the *Daily Express'* William Hickey column, was to claim he had been assigned the task of 'monitoring the mood of people in influential circles' by MI5. However, the Soviet sources said, he and his wife Jean Nicol, the press officer of the Savoy Hotel, turned traitor and passed information to the Soviets. The couple left the high life in London in 1949, but their spying on the rich and famous – including Thursday Club members – is said to have continued into the 1950s.

The Tangyes were the conduit for royal letters, diaries and documents that found their way into KGB files. And the material they shared with the Soviets supposedly included information on Prince Philip. Unsubstantiated or false rumours about the Prince may of course have been spread deliberately – to undermine the monarchy.

Former Soviet assistant naval attaché Ivanov, the Soviet agent at the heart of the Profumo case, made claims – long after his departure from Britain as the case was breaking – that dovetail with the recent information about Operation Dom. In 1992, in his controversial autobiography, he noted that Stephen Ward had 'known the Royal Family for years'. However well Ward did or did not really know the royals, for Ivanov the connection had 'held out the possibility of getting information through provocation and blackmail'.

One of his list of 'top-priority' targets, Ivanov claimed, had been the Queen's sister Princess Margaret. That this could have been so is consistent with references to Princess Margaret in the recent report about Operation Dom. It is also less than surprising, for the Princess' amours were long the talk of the town.

Following an introduction to Margaret by Stephen Ward, according to Ivanov he went on to meet her on multiple occasions. According to Ward, the Russian on one occasion irritated the Princess by first expressing admiration of her 'lovely hair' – then adding that it must surely be dyed.

Ivanov related, too, how he also contrived to meet Prince Philip, by acting as interpreter during a visit to London by a Soviet polar explorer. The Prince, he noted, steadfastly avoided involving himself in conversation about anything sensitive. Ivanov claimed that he did – separately – manage to secure highly sensitive material on Philip himself.

Following the encounter at the function, Ivanov wrote, he and Ward discussed the Prince. The osteopath claimed that he had known Prince Philip early on and that the Prince had at that time lived 'by different rules'. He had then supposedly shown Ivanov an album containing what – the Soviet agent claimed in his autobiography – were 'candid photographs' of the Prince, his cousin the Marquess of Milford Haven 'and the rest of our merry bachelors' company'. There were also two women in the pictures, whom Ward identified as 'Nichole' and 'Maggie' – 'nice girls'.

When left alone at some point, Ivanov claimed, he used his Minox camera to photograph five or six of the pictures. 'Later in the day,' he wrote, 'I sent the photographs and my report to Moscow Centre.'

Did Ivanov really obtain photographs that could have compromised Prince Philip? Did such photos even exist? As recently as this past decade, former KGB officers have approached British reporters claiming to have these photographs and offering to sell them for large sums of money. Negotiations are said to have fallen through when the Russians closed the relevant archive. Whether the claim to have such pictures was true, or just made in the hope of cashing in on an old rumour, remains unknown.

The Denning Report is as interesting for what it omits as much as for what it covers. Though Lord Denning called Prince Philip's former equerry and close friend Michael Parker for interview, his Report does not say why he did so. Lord Denning was told about the American aspects of the Profumo case. He interviewed solicitor Michael Eddowes, and apparently accepted detailed memoranda from him. The documents are not referred to in the Report. He heard testimony about Mariella Novotny's alleged sexual encounters with President Kennedy – and interviewed Novotny herself. 'I do remember that a woman called Mariella came and gave evidence . . .' Denning told the authors in a letter, 'but I'm afraid I cannot add anything of use . . .'

On these matters, and much else, Lord Denning's Report would say nothing. For months before it appeared, however, just the knowledge that he was at work – coupled with Stephen Ward's arrest – served to contain the damage of the Profumo Affair at a vital time. The prosecution of Stephen Ward shifted attention away from the government on to one lone individual.

Ward was kept in prison for a month following his arrest in early June 1963, an inordinately long time in light of the relatively minor – prostitution – offences with which he was charged. The police opposed bail on the grounds that Ward might flee abroad or interfere with witnesses. When bail was finally granted, it was in the sum of £3,000, a huge amount at the time.

Ward had been abandoned by his high and mighty friends. Those who put up the bail money were Pelham Pound, the journalist who was acting as the osteopath's agent; Dominic Elwes, himself a controversial society figure; and, reportedly, Claus von Bülow, oil millionaire Paul Getty's assistant.

Ward's trial began at the Old Bailey on 22 July 1963. It was to be a show trial, an outrageous abuse of the judicial system.

CHAPTER 31

Smokescreen:
The Trial

'All I have left between me and destruction,' Ward wrote before the trial, is a handful of firm friends, my legal advisers, the integrity of a judge, and twelve men on a jury.'

He continued, meanwhile, to try to protect the fair-weather friends who had scurried for cover. He was to cover for them, minimising damaging testimony, drawing the fire on himself, to the bitter end.

Ward hoped, at the start, that Lord Astor would come to his aid. 'I had always believed,' he told Warwick Charlton, 'that Bill wouldn't let me down. I thought he could do something to restore my good name. I thought he might hold a party at Cliveden, collect some notables, and have me down as a sort of gesture of solidarity. Imagine my shock when he at once asked me to let him have a letter vacating the cottage ... I was absolutely flabbergasted. I then began to realise that the waves were coming aboard and soon I would be clinging to the mast. And all the time there was no one at all to turn to ...'

'Expect nothing from the Establishment,' Charlton had warned. Ward had spent nearly twenty years cultivating these 'friends'. Now they dumped him, and Ward belatedly realised their true calibre. 'They are all the same,' he told Charlton. 'They all thought you could buy it with a cheque book.'

Lord Astor, his widow told the authors, stayed silent not only on the advice of his solicitors, but on the 'spiritual direction' of a bishop. 'He could not defend either of them, Ward or Jack Profumo,' said Lady Astor, 'without incriminating both of them . . .'

While, according to his wife, Astor paid Ward's legal expenses, he kept his mouth shut. 'Silence,' the bishop told him, 'is the only possible course.' Astor had recently become a fervent Christian and, Lady Astor said, his 'model' for keeping quiet was Jesus Christ. Like Christ, according to her, Astor did not want to 'start having to involve other people as witnesses . . .'

'By the time the balloon had gone up,' Ward noted, 'no one looked like the same people any more . . . I have lost hope of the basic simplicity of the matter ever emerging . . . The car is out of control. Anything may happen now.'

The setting for the trial was the Old Bailey's Court Number 1, where so many celebrated defendants have entrusted their fate to a jury. Outside the building, the crowds were ten deep. The authoritative account remains that of Ludovic Kennedy, author and respected campaigner for the righting of judicial wrongs. Under a ruling made by Chief Justice Lord Parker, however – and though transcripts of other trials had been made available – Kennedy was refused access to full official transcripts. We did obtain a partial transcript, following repeated application, and will draw on it in this chapter.

'The tiny, tubby judge,' Kennedy wrote, 'came billowing in like a small Dutch *shuyt* under a full spread of canvas, grey and black and scarlet . . . a keen, determined mole, all set for a good day's burrowing . . .' This was sixty-four-year-old Sir Archibald Marshall, nicknamed 'the Hen', a former President of the Oxford Union. 'As a judge,' his *Times* obituary was to note, 'he was an unusual mixture; his upbringing and beliefs perhaps led him to pass or at any rate form, moral judgements which would no doubt be regarded as old-fashioned in this day and age, and yet he never seemed to be out of sympathy with a modern jury. He had the knack of talking to the men and women of a jury as if he were on neighbourly and equal terms with them.'

'Marshall could hardly be expected to make allowances for the renegade son of a canon,' one observer wrote of the judge's attitude to Ward. 'He conducted the trial without overt bias, but his demeanour and the very inflection of his voice implied moral disapproval, emphasised by the scratching of his pen as he laboriously entered questions and answers on a huge pad, like the Recording Angel.'

Judges for trials at the Old Bailey were on occasion selected by the office of the Lord Chancellor – who at the time was none other than Lord Dilhorne, the man who had initially looked into the security side of the Profumo case. It could also be, though, that a word from the Lord Chief Justice determined the selection of a judge. The then Chief Justice, sixty-three-year-old Lord Parker – Rugby School and Cambridge – had his own reason to disapprove of those in Ward's circle.

In summer that year, travel writer Robert Harbinson was having his portrait painted by the artist Gwen le Gallienne, close friend of Ward and well-known lesbian. 'At the time she was doing my portrait,' Harbinson remembered, 'she was also doing the Lord Chief Justice. And she came back from the Strand one day, and told me that Parker had discovered her in bed with his wife.'

Prosecuting barrister at the trial was Mervyn Griffith-Jones – Eton, Cambridge and the Brigade of Guards. 'Square,' wrote Ludovic Kennedy, 'is the word that suits him. He is so ultra-orthodox that some aspects of modern life have escaped him altogether . . . During the *Lady Chatterley's Lover* trial [to decide whether D. H. Lawrence's novel was obscene], as prosecuting counsel, he solemnly asked the jury whether it was a book they would wish their servants to read . . .' At the Ward trial, Griffith-Jones would tell the jury that the accused was a 'thoroughly filthy fellow . . . a wicked, wicked creature'.

Defence counsel was James Burge – Cheltenham and Cambridge. He was not a Queen's Counsel, but a respected criminal barrister. Kennedy thought him 'a jovial, sunshiny, Pickwickian sort of man, who always seemed to be smiling . . .' Some of Burge's practice was devoted to licensing cases. 'Beer and Burgundy,' Kennedy wrote, 'seemed to blend with his beaming face . . . I had been told by one of his colleagues that he was one of the few men at the Bar who could laugh a case out of court.' Burge had a bad back, and Dr Ward gave him treatment for it – on the sofa in his chambers.

It has been said that Burge was a model for the eponymous character in John Mortimer's *Rumpole* series on television, and Mortimer did not deny it. The barrister and his staff soon came to feel, though, that there would be no laughing this case out of court. 'No one liked the trial or the procedure,' one of Burge's former colleagues told the authors. 'It was too political, and it was felt that Ward was a scapegoat,' Burge himself said. 'Ward said to me, "The dice is loaded." And it was. On the other hand, with an English jury, he had a good chance.'

Ludovic Kennedy watched the man with a chance enter the dock. 'There was no mistaking the now familiar figure,' wrote Kennedy, 'the roué of fifty who looked thirty-five, perceptive eyes set in a face rather too full to carry them, boyish hair swept back like the wings of a partridge . . . He was dressed in a sober heather-mixture suit, and one's first and most striking impression was that he was a man of intelligence and dignity.'

'Right at the end,' Ward wrote in his memoir, 'I realised they were out to get me at all costs.' Now, like some heterosexual Oscar Wilde, he listened to the charges against him being read out. He was accused of living on the earnings of prostitution of Christine Keeler between June 1961 and August 1962, on those of Mandy Rice-Davies in late 1962, and on those of two other women between January and June 1963. There were two other charges: of procuring a female under twenty-one to have intercourse, and of attempting to procure another underage woman.

At one stage there had been no fewer than nine charges, including one of keeping a brothel. Two had been that Ward had introduced women to an abortionist – probably his friend Dr Sugden. Those charges were dropped for the time being, with the possibility that they might be revived later. It was all out of proportion. The 1957 Wolfenden Report – ironically Ward had met Sir John Wolfenden at Cliveden – had documented how such cases had in normal circumstances been treated. Of 131 people found guilty of living on immoral earnings in a year, 117 were dealt with in magistrates' courts, and thirteen were conditionally discharged, fined or put on probation. To pursue such an offender in the way Ward had been pursued was unprecedented. Even then, the prosecution failed to find real evidence.

The trial lasted eight days. Two young women identified only as 'Miss X' and 'Miss R' were brought to court to speak of their sex relations with Ward, but the relevant charges – those of procuring a woman under twenty-one – had seemingly been brought only to make the defendant look even more lecherous. But there was worse. 'There is just one possibility that struck me,' Ward had written to a friend, 'that is the danger of false evidence.' It was more than a possibility.

The Metropolitan Police had pursued Ward with a zeal for which these authors can find no parallel – except perhaps in the case of the murder of a fellow officer. The police force's Profumo operation had been headed by Chief Inspector Samuel Herbert and included Detective-Superintendent James Axon. Axon had been responsible for the painstaking trawl of London's underworld, the search for any evidence that might tilt the scales against Stephen Ward.

Extraordinary effort had gone into Ward's prosecution. Inspector Herbert revealed to the court that he personally had interviewed Christine Keeler twenty-four times, and that a senior detective questioned her about the Gordon and Edgecombe cases on fourteen other occasions.

A spy had been infiltrated into Ward's home. Wendy Davies, a twenty-year-old barmaid at the Duke of Marlborough pub, near Ward's flat, knew Ward – he had sketched her – and her boyfriend was a policeman. So it was that Davies had been asked to renew the acquaintance with Ward. 'I went to Stephen's flat practically every night up to his arrest,' she later revealed. 'Each time, I tried to listen in to telephone conversations, and to what Stephen was saying to friends who called. When I got back to my flat I wrote everything down in an exercise book, and rang the police the next day. I gave them lots of information . . .'

Ward knew he was being watched. One day, as he and his journalist friend Pelham Pound walked to his place, he pointed to an upstairs window across the street. 'Do you see it?' he said. 'The telephoto lens?'

'The policeman in charge,' the playwright Michael Pertwee said – like his brother Jon, he was one of Ward's friends – 'had spent most of his recent past operating in Soho against pimps and blackmailers, and his methods were pretty dubious . . .'

Ward had exclaimed when he was arrested, 'Oh, my God, how dreadful! I shall deny it. Nobody will come forward to say it is true.' He had had no idea what savage tricks were to be used against him at the trial.

The prostitute Ronna Riccardo was produced by the prosecution on the third day of the trial. Known as 'Ronna the Lash', Riccardo specialised in flagellation. 'She used to carry her equipment around in a leather bag,' reporter Trevor Kempson recalled. 'She was well known for the use of the whip, and I heard that several of Ward's friends used to like it rough.' John Edgecombe, Keeler's lover, also remembered Riccardo and her equipment. As reported earlier, she had had sex in Ward's flat – perhaps more conventional sex – with the American airman 'Silky' Hawkins.

Initially, in a statement to the police and at the Ward committal proceedings, Riccardo had implicated the osteopath in a series of sex episodes involving money. She spoke of having been invited to a house party on Lord Astor's estate, quoting Ward as telling her it 'would be worth my while'. She said she visited Ward three times at home in London and on one occasion had gone to the bedroom with a man who gave her a 'pony' – £25. 'I went to bed with men at the flat . . . when this did happen . . . I had been invited to go there by Stephen.'

Two days before the Ward trial, Riccardo made a new statement to the police. 'The evidence I gave at the Stephen Ward hearing earlier this month,' she said, 'was largely untrue. I visited Ward at his flat at Bryanston Mews on one occasion. No one received any money. At no time have I received any money on Stephen Ward's premises, or given money to him. The reason the earlier statement was divergent from the truth was my apprehension that my baby daughter and younger sisters might be taken out of my care following certain statements made to me by Chief Inspector Samuel Herbert.'

'Are you suggesting,' Judge Marshall asked when Riccardo appeared at Ward's trial, 'that the police had just put words into your mouth?' 'Yes,' Riccardo replied. '. . . I wanted the police to leave me alone . . .'

'Riccardo,' Ludovic Kennedy wrote, 'was clearly in a state of terror at what the police might do to her for having gone back on her original evidence. After the trial she seldom stayed at one address for more than a few nights for fear the police were looking for her . . .' Riccardo told Kennedy that the police had interviewed her no fewer than nine times before her initial testimony. For days at a time, a police car had sat outside her home.

Traced by the authors during research for this book, Riccardo was even more forthright. 'Stephen didn't have to ponce,' she said. 'He was dead rich, a real gentleman; a shoulder to cry on for me, for a long time. Some of my clients were friends of Stephen's. But it wasn't business, like, more like friends. I was really into costumes then. These blokes would turn up with a costume inside their little briefcases, and I'd dress up as a nanny or a nurse, and smack their bottoms for them.'

Riccardo repeated what she had told Kennedy about pressure from the police, and explained her quandary. 'The police knew I hung around with Stephen,' she said. 'They said they would do me on immoral earnings, but Chief Inspector Herbert, who was running the investigation, was a punter of mine himself. I didn't know he was a policeman for ages. I used to wear a wig, and he always wanted me to take it off and shake my hair around. I was going with another copper, too, who was involved in the enquiry. I couldn't take this pressure by the coppers, and Stephen was a good friend of mine. But Inspector Herbert was a good friend as well, so it was complicated . . .'

So it had been that, at the committal hearing, Riccardo had given false evidence against Ward. At the trial, and after talking with *Daily Express* reporter Tom Mangold – he told her to tell the truth – she withdrew it.

The police denied her claims. Riccardo, for her part, had the letters ACAB tattooed on her wrist. They stood for: 'All coppers are bastards'.

At the time this book was being researched, no transcript of Riccardo's testimony had been released. The Denning Report did not mention her at all.

The court also heard the testimony of a prostitute named Vickie Barrett, who was said to have made multiple visits to Ward's flat and to have had sex with several men for money. Barrett had been arrested for soliciting on 3 July, which was – perhaps by coincidence – the day Ward was committed for trial. The diary she had with her when arrested had allegedly contained Stephen Ward's name and telephone number, and five other names. Vickie Barrett was to testify that Ward had picked her up that year in Oxford Street, when he was cruising the street in his Jaguar. According to her, 'He said he had a man in the flat who wanted to go with a girl, and he said the man would give him the money . . . he said if I visited him two or three times a week he would save the money, and I could live in a flat.' On arrival at the flat, Ward had supposedly given her a contraceptive and told her to go into a room where a man would be waiting. Afterwards, she said, Ward told her the man had paid him, and that he would save the money for her – to help her obtain a flat.

She had met other middle-aged men at the flat, Barrett said, and had beaten several of them with a horsewhip – at a pound a stroke. Ward, again, had allegedly kept the money. Barrett said one of the men had been Ward's artist friend Vasco Lazzolo. Lazzolo admitted having met Barrett, but insisted he had never met her at Ward's flat. It was hardly likely he would have behaved as the witness claimed, he said, at a time he knew Ward was already under investigation.

One of Vickie Barrett's closest friends, Brenda O'Neil, said she had been to bed with Ward for money. Oddly, though, Barrett had never told her of the sex scenes at Ward's flat that had supposedly involved other men. Another woman, Frances Brown, said that – along with Barrett – she had visited both Ward and Lazzolo and had 'helped' in a sex act. She knew nothing, though, of Ward having received any money.

Ward admitted having met Barrett and O'Neil, and having paid them – £2 each – for sex. He vehemently denied entirely, however, the Barrett claim that she had gone with other men at the flat for money, and that he had kept the cash. Barrett's evidence, he said, was 'a tissue of lies from beginning to end'.

After the trial, when Ward to all appearances committed suicide, he was to leave a note addressed personally to Vickie Barrett. 'I don't know,' he wrote, 'what it was or who it was that made you do what you did. But if you have any decency left, you should tell the truth like Ronna Riccardo. You owe this not to me, but to everyone who may be treated like you or like me in the future.'

Immediately after Ward's death, *Daily Telegraph* reporter Barry O'Brien went to see Barrett to show her the dead man's letter. 'She read the note,' he recalled, and began to cry. "It was all lies." she said of her sworn testimony, "But I never thought he would die . . ." She said she had been coerced into giving her evidence by the police. She agreed to go to see Ward's solicitor, then went to another room to get her coat. A few moments later, an older

woman came out, and said Miss Barrett was not going anywhere . . .' Barrett later retracted her retraction.

The best evidence the prosecution could muster against Ward
came from Christine Keeler and Mandy Rice-Davies. They, too,
had been under inexcusable police pressure. Keeler had been
endlessly interrogated. Mandy Rice-Davies had been twice
arrested at London Airport to prevent her from travelling abroad.
On the first occasion, she was remanded in Holloway Prison
for a week – on a driving-licence offence. On the second
occasion, she was charged with having stolen a television set,
which she had not.

'I've never seen anything like the day we brought Christine to
court,' said Keeler's former solicitor Harry Stevens. 'We had
to smuggle her out of the judges' car park to get her away from the
crowds. And still we got the eggs – people were throwing eggs at
the girl. She was not popular. The policemen were getting their
helmets knocked off right, left and centre . . .'

Keeler was in a funk. 'The old matron was plying Christine
with phenobarbitone, the Valium of the day,' Stevens said. 'She
was vomiting in the room there. She was terribly upset about
testifying against Stephen Ward . . . desperately unhappy about it.
She did not want to harm him in any way at all.'

Ludovic Kennedy watched the women as they entered the
courtroom. 'Despite the tarty high-heeled shoes,' he noted,
Keeler 'was tiny, a real little doll of a girl . . . She walked superbly
on long slender legs . . . one could see at once her appeal to the
animal instincts of men . . . It was a terrifying little face, vacant
yet knowing, and it belonged not to a girl of twenty-one but
to an already ageing woman . . .'

Mandy Rice-Davies looked more wholesome. 'Astride her
golden head,' Kennedy wrote, 'sat a little rose-petalled hat, such

as debutantes wear at garden parties . . . Her simple grey sleeveless dress accentuated the impression of modesty – until one looked at it closely. Then one saw that the slit down the front was only held together by a loose knot – when she walked one could see quite a long way up her leg . . .'

The testimony prised out of Keeler established that she had been given a little money by John Profumo. 'On one occasion,' said Keeler, 'he gave me money to give to my mother.' She also admitted having had sex at Ward's flat, on about six occasions, with a Major James Eynon. He had paid her – £15 or £20 a time. Keeler had also had sex – for £50 – with a man referred to in court only as 'Charles'. This, she later confirmed, was the millionaire financier Charles – later Sir Charles – Clore. Clore knew Profumo and Douglas Fairbanks Jr, lived only a few minutes' drive from the Astor mansion at Cliveden and was said to have a prodigious appetite for sex – an encounter with Keeler sounded plausible enough.

Rice-Davies told the court she had had sex 'about five times' with a man referred to at the trial only as 'the Indian doctor'. When someone blurted out his name, however, he was identified as the Ceylonese-born Emil Savundra, the crooked head of Fire, Auto and Marine Insurance. Savundra, Rice-Davies admitted, had paid her for sex – between £15 and £25 in cash. Rice-Davies also spoke of the one occasion she had slept with Lord Astor, an episode the prosecution sought to link with the cheque Astor had once given Ward, and which Ward had used to pay Rice-Davies' and Keeler's rent. There was no such connection, Rice-Davies explained. She had had sex with Astor simply because they both felt like it – two years after the rent episode.

There were two key questions. Had Keeler and Rice-Davies been prostitutes, and – this was the crucial issue – had Ward lived on their immoral earnings? There was no statutory definition of a prostitute. Though the two young women had clearly not been 'professionals', it was also clear they had taken money for sex.

In a pertinent cartoon he drew in the *Daily Express* at the time, the veteran cartoonist Osbert Lancaster portrayed a man asking, 'If I give my wife's lover the winner of the 4.30 [horse-race], would I be living off her immoral earnings?' It was a daft issue, in a trial that should never have taken place, but Ward's fate now hung on such legal hair-splitting.

Laboriously, Keeler and Rice-Davies were taken through the circumstances in which they had met the named men, and the basis on which the money had been paid. The prosecution did not try to make anything of the money given to Keeler by Profumo – his name was kept out of the case as much as possible. As for Major Eynon, Keeler said she passed some of the money she received from him on to Ward – 'because I hadn't paid any rent, and things like that'.

She said she had had sex with Clore 'because I was in a lot of debt at the time . . . and Dr Ward suggested he knew this person who would give me this amount of money to have intercourse. He suggested if I did, that he would give me money.' With Clore's £50, she said, she paid off debts to Ward and to Mandy Rice-Davies.

Savundra, who could afford it, had thrown his money around. 'He came round once or twice, and we did not have sex, and he still gave me money,' Rice-Davies told the court. How much did he give her? 'It depended,' said Rice-Davies, 'because he asked me if I wanted anything. I was taking drama lessons at the time, and he gave me some money to buy a tape-recorder once, which was twenty-five pounds.'

Rice-Davies also mentioned a Mr Ropner, a man she had seen a couple of times. Ward, she said, had suggested she 'borrow'

£250 from him. She had neither had sex with Ropner – because, she said, she did not fancy him – nor had she borrowed money from him. She, like Keeler, admitted having sometimes given Ward money – 'just a couple of pounds, or something like that, but it was not in return for him introducing me to men. You have to pay where you live.' Like Keeler, Rice-Davies had contributed to the rent at Wimpole Mews, and the food bills – 'in all about twenty-five pounds'. Rice-Davies had also slept with the landlord of the flat, John Shepridge, and had once passed on a request by Ward to ask Shepridge to hold off on a rent demand.

How the pair had met their men became a key issue. Profumo and Astor had come on the scene as a result of Ward's socialising. Keeler met James Eynon off her own bat, but Ward, she said, introduced her to Charles Clore – and allegedly suggested that an encounter with Clore would not go unrewarded. It was he, too, who had arranged Rice-Davies' first meeting with Savundra – at a coffee bar in Marylebone – and told her he was 'a very rich man'. Ward also supposedly arranged for Savundra to use Rice-Davies' room at the flat, when she was out, for assignations with yet another woman – the financier allegedly paid Ward £25 to use the room.

Keeler had her own damaging testimony about Savundra. According to her, Ward had suggested she should entertain him once a week – for money. There were, however, no such encounters.

The facts of the matter might have become clear had the men themselves been called as witnesses. Yet Profumo and Astor, who were spoken of in court almost reverentially, were never called. Nor was Savundra, and Clore's surname was never revealed. The only man who had the guts to appear was Major Eynon. He looked, Ludovic Kennedy thought, 'typically English, a cross between Enoch Powell and the man from the Pru, a sort of poor man's

David Niven', in a grey suit and old school tie. Eynon's brief appearance established only that – in her relations with him – Keeler certainly had been a whore. Ward, however, had not been involved at all.

The trial was a national entertainment. In the pubs at lunch-time, the reporters exchanged the latest jokes. Question: 'What newspapers does Christine Keeler take?' Answer: 'One *Mail*, two *Mirrors*, three *Observers*, a *New Statesman* every week, and any number of *Times*.' Flagellation gags flourished. Question: 'What happens when you dial the speaking clock on the telephone?' Answer: 'The voice says, "At the third stroke, it will be three pounds precisely."'

CHAPTER 32

Scapegoat

On the fourth day of the trial, the man with nothing to laugh about moved from the dock to the witness box. Stephen Ward repeated the oath firmly in a voice, Ludovic Kennedy thought, 'of quite extraordinary power, richness and resonance . . . his voice transformed him, gave him magnetism'.

Ward said he had 'a pretty shrewd idea' Keeler was having intercourse at Wimpole Mews, but 'not the remotest idea' she was doing so for money. He had met Major Eynon only once. He had no idea who Keeler meant by a man named 'Charles', and Keeler was lying when she testified that involvement with him would prove profitable. Her statements about Savundra were 'all fabrication' – he said Savundra never did rent a room at the flat, and never paid him any money. Ward scoffed at the notion that he asked Rice-Davies to get money out of Ropner. 'I knew Mr Ropner extremely well,' said Ward. 'If I had wanted money from Mr Ropner I would have asked him myself.'

The only payments to him from Keeler and Rice-Davies, Ward said, had been occasional contributions to the rent, and to the telephone and electricity bills. Rice-Davies' total contribution, over two months at Wimpole Mews, had been 'twenty-four pounds, plus five or six pounds for the telephone'. This was exactly what Keeler and Rice-Davies had said.

'This evidence was not subsequently challenged by the prosecution,' Ludovic Kennedy was to write. 'How *could* they go on asserting that Ward was *living* on Mandy Rice-Davies' *earnings*? It seemed so utterly absurd.' It was absurd – not least when Christine Keeler had said, 'I usually owed him more than I ever made . . .' The show, however, went on. 'There were times,' Kennedy thought, 'when Mr Griffith-Jones . . . became, as it were, the commentator in some mad Victorian melodrama, tracing Good and Evil in letters high enough for any child to see.' Griffith-Jones repeatedly pointed up Ward's promiscuity, which was not what he was on trial for. Nevertheless, doing so probably influenced the jury.

Ward admitted knowing prostitutes Ronna Riccardo and Vickie Barrett and having had sex with them. That, however, was all – he had merely been their client. Vickie Barrett's claim that he got her to have sex with men, then kept the money she earned for himself, was a lie. A defence witness, Sylvia Parker, who had been staying at Ward's flat at the time Barrett claimed she was brought there to have sex with men other than Ward, called Barrett's statements 'untrue, a complete load of rubbish'. Then there are both Barrett's and Riccardo's subsequent admissions that they were pressured into making false allegations.

'This is the bottom of the bucket,' Ward cried at one point. 'A hundred and fifty people have been questioned and these are the people they found. There are other people, a hundred and fifty, who would not say anything detrimental about me. It's easy in most people's lives to find at least half-a-dozen people willing to come forward with some active malice, and they will make these statements against a person, especially a person who had some sort of irregularity in his life as I have. They lay themselves open to this type of misrepresentation.'

If any part of the prosecution evidence was to be taken seriously

– and the jury was required to take it seriously – Christine Keeler's truthfulness or otherwise was a vital issue. There was very relevant information on the point.

Almost two months earlier, in yet another related court case, Lucky Gordon had been tried for assaulting Keeler in the spring, found guilty and jailed. On the morning of 30 July, however, as Ward's trial was ending at the Old Bailey, Gordon's case came up for appeal – and he was freed. One reason for that decision was that there was hard evidence – a tape recording – in which Keeler told a story different to the one she told at the Gordon trial and repeated at Ward's. In court, she had denied that anyone else was present when Lucky Gordon assaulted her, saying that only Gordon was involved. In the tape recording, she admitted that two other men had been there, and that another man had caused her main injuries. This was perjury, for which Keeler would later be tried and found guilty, and serve nine months in prison.

Chief Justice Parker, who presided over the Gordon appeal, telephoned Sir Archibald Marshall, the judge running the Ward trial. According to a clerk who listened in to the call, Parker warned Marshall to take care, because Keeler had lied in another court.

Prosecuting counsel Griffith-Jones did inform the jury of this towards the end of the Ward trial – but in the following way. 'The basis or the grounds of the appeal,' he told the jury of Keeler's evidence in the Gordon case, 'were that her evidence was not true . . . Gordon's appeal has been allowed . . . That does of course not mean to say that the Court of Appeal have found that Miss Keeler is lying. As I understand from the note I have, the Lord Chief Justice said that it might be that Miss Keeler's evidence was completely truthful, but in view of the fact that there were witnesses now available who were not available at the trial, it was felt that the court could not necessarily say that the jury in that case would not have returned the same verdict as they did if those two witnesses had been called. That is all it amounts to. The Court of Criminal Appeal have *not* found whether Miss Keeler was telling the truth . . .'

If legally accurate, this was hardly honest. 'We were all a bit gulled by these words,' Ludovic Kennedy wrote afterwards. 'Later we found out that the evidence was there [on Keeler lying], but that the public were denied hearing it . . . If it had been heard publicly by the Court of Criminal Appeal (and many lawyers think it monstrous that it was not heard), if the Ward jury *had* known that Christine had lied on oath in the witness-box, not only in Gordon's trial but at this trial too, where she had repeated the lies, it is inconceivable that they would have brought in the verdict they did.'

By any standards, Kennedy continued, the case against Ward was feeble. 'It consisted mainly of uncorroborated statements by proved liars: it was a hotchpotch of innuendoes and smears covered by a thin pastry of substance. It was a tale of immoralities, rather than crimes.'

Judge Marshall's summing-up at the trial was lengthy – and disconcerting to those who reported it. In print, in the newspapers, it seemed dispassionate and fair. Yet, said Ludovic Kennedy, 'when I first saw the summary I could hardly believe I had an accurate report of it, so great was the gulf between the words and my memory of them'. A French reporter for *France-Soir* put his finger on it. 'Monsieur Marshall,' he said, 'is a puritan, and Ward, the roué, the libertine, the cynic, appalled him . . . every time M. Justice Marshall explained to the jury the questions they would have to answer, his voice gave it away: M. Marshall did not like Ward, for he had brought a scandal upon England.'

Marshall told the jury they must decide three questions:

1. Were Keeler and Rice-Davies prostitutes?
2. Did Ward know they were?
3. Did he knowingly receive from them or others money for the introduction and facilities for sexual intercourse which he provided?

To decide that a man was guilty of living on prostitution, the judge told the jury, it must be shown that he knowingly assisted a prostitute, and received money for it. Then the judge pointed out that Ward had been abandoned by his friends. 'There may be many reasons,' he said, 'why Ward has been abandoned in his extremity . . . You must not guess at them, but this is clear: if Stephen Ward was telling the truth in the witness-box, there are in this city many witnesses of high estate and low who could have come and testified support of his evidence.' The judge had found a way to turn against Ward the fact that none of his highfalutin friends had had the courage to come and speak up on his behalf.

This struck Ludovic Kennedy as grossly unfair: 'I had no doubts at all,' he wrote, 'of the effect of such a remark on the jury.' The eminent solicitor Sir David Napley, who was on the Council of the Law Society in 1963, wrote after the trial: 'The real source of injustice is the rumour and calumny which abounds when the name is published as the subject of a charge. Stephen Ward faced a wealth of publicity unconnected with any charge or proceedings. Once he was charged, public gossip and rumour was disposed to convict him out of hand. It was confidently disclosed that the evidence would reveal that he had been selling information to the Russians; running a brothel for important persons, procuring abortions. What effect would this currency of falsehood have on potential jurors?'

At half-past four on Tuesday, 30 July, with the summing-up unfinished, the court rose. Ward, who was shattered by the judge's attitude, asked his solicitor Jack Wheatley for a considered opinion as to what the outcome would be. 'Guilty – and a two-year sentence,' replied Wheatley. 'For once,' Pelham Pound remembered, 'Stephen had nothing to say, except a long "Oh . . ."'

The first day of the trial had been marked by the Museum Gallery in Holborn with an exhibition of Stephen Ward's sketches. In the evening, after the court had recessed, Ward himself had shown up, smiling and charming in spite of the stress of the trial. Mandy Rice-Davies was there too – posing for photographers in front of a portrait of herself drawn by Ward.

The collection included Ward's sketches of Prince Philip, Princess Margaret, the Duke and Duchess of Gloucester and the Duke of Kent. 'I knew certain friends would be deeply horrified,' recalled Ward's friend Robert Harbinson, 'so I telephoned Anthony Blunt' – Sir Anthony Blunt, Surveyor of the Queen's Pictures, yet to be unmasked as a traitor. 'I believe,' said Harbinson, 'that Blunt, ever anxious to keep in with Buck House, telephoned Michael Adeane [the Queen's Private Secretary] at the Palace.'

Five days later, an unidentified man arrived at the Museum Gallery, produced a bank draft for £5,000, bought up all the royal portraits and departed. He was acting, it later emerged, as agent for Sir Gordon Brunton, then managing director of the Thompson publishing interests. Ward's royal sketches would remain, for years to come, under lock and key at the offices of the *Illustrated London News*. The remainder of them, saved from destruction by an art collector, were finally made public in 2013.

The osteopath watched a BBC television report on the exhibition of his sketches. 'The commentator,' recalled his friend Frederic Mullally, was 'a young man who would probably have botched a child's colouring book, but who reached millions daily with his special brand of urbane irony. He and his BBC masters chose this day for the most savage public mauling of an artist's work I have ever witnessed. It started with a sneer and built up to defamation. It ended with the Olympian judgement that there was nothing in the exhibition beyond the capabilities of a second-year student at one of London's schools of art. This was the day they axed through Stephen's last lifeline. He hung on, of course, for the miracle of a judge who would sum up against prejudice and hypocrisy.'

On the evening of the final day of the trial, Ward headed off with his girlfriend of the moment, a young singer called Julie Gulliver, to the flat in Chelsea of an advertising executive named Noel Howard-Jones – Ward's place of refuge during the trial. There, at Vale Court in Mallord Street, Ward began writing letters – to be delivered 'only if I am convicted and sent to prison'. There were twelve of them, and Gulliver watched as Ward sealed them and handed them over to Howard-Jones. He seemed restless, 'noticeably upset'.

Daily Express reporter Tom Mangold took a call from Ward that evening, probably between 7 and 8 p.m. Mangold, who had been covering the Profumo Affair for months, was one of the few reporters Ward still trusted. The two men had spent night after night talking into the early hours. That evening, Mangold too was desperately tired and trying to cope with a personal problem, and this call was a damned nuisance. 'He asked me to come round to where he was staying,' recalled Mangold, a *Panorama* reporter and one of the most accomplished British journalists of our time. 'He said it was urgent. I said I would come, but I didn't want to spend another long night talking.'

Mangold drove to Mallord Street. He had been handling the

prostitute Ronna Riccardo, as well as Ward. She had cried on his shoulder and told him, 'I've fitted up Stephen.' 'There were two strands running through the thing, it seemed to me,' Mangold said years later. 'There was some sort of intelligence connection, which I could not understand at the time. The other thing, the thing that was clear, was that Ward was being made a scapegoat for everyone else's sins. So that the public would excuse them. If the myth about Ward could be built up properly, the myth that he was a revolting fellow, a true pimp, then police would feel that other men, like Profumo and Astor, had been corrupted by him. But he wasn't a ponce. He was no more a pimp than hundreds of other men in London. But when the state wants to act against an individual, it can do it.'

Mangold knew Ward was at the end of his tether. 'He felt absolutely betrayed. Until the very last minute he was certain that Lord Astor would turn up and pull him out of the shit. But he was abandoned. That night he asked me to post the letters he had written. I said I knew what they were, suicide notes, and I refused to post them for him.' One letter was addressed to Mangold himself. 'Well,' Ward told the reporter, 'take your letter, but don't open it till I'm dead.'

Then Mangold left Ward, and went home. With hindsight, while sad about what happened that night, he was philosophical. A reporter may be compassionate, but cannot be held responsible for his interviewees. When the phone rang next morning with the news of Ward's apparent suicide, he was not surprised.

Julie Gulliver stayed with Ward until about 11.30 that last night. Then he drove her home, and – as they parted – said 'Goodbye.' 'Usually,' she said, 'he would say something like "Cheerio" or "See you tomorrow."'

The following morning, at 8.30, Ward's host Howard-Jones – still in his bedroom – heard the telephone ringing. It was, he knew, just feet from his guest, who was sleeping in the lounge. Yet the phone rang on and on. Howard-Jones stumbled out to take the call – it was Vasco Lazzolo's wife, calling to wish Ward the best of luck.

'It was only when I hung up,' Howard-Jones would say at the inquest, 'that I turned around and saw him. I thought he was dead. His face was a purple colour. His mouth was open and there was a sort of mark on his face, like dry saliva . . . I slapped his face, and he breathed just once. I tried for a minute or so an amateur type of artificial respiration. He started breathing at long intervals, so I ran for the phone and dialled for the ambulance.'

Ward was carried from the building on a stretcher, covered in a scarlet blanket. The photographs – for the press got there – show his head lolling sideways, eyes closed. On admission to nearby St Stephen's Hospital, twenty minutes after he was found, he was unconscious, not responding to stimuli. An hour later, though, according to one of the medical team, his condition was 'good enough for him to be transferred to a ward'. The doctors thought he might pull through.

At the Old Bailey, the court reconvened. Judge Marshall delayed for a while, then said, 'I want it to be understood that Ward shall be immediately put under surveillance. Bail is withdrawn from now, and the normal steps shall be taken to secure greater security.' Like most of his statements at the trial, the judge's words seemed unrelated to reality. He continued his summing-up – which included the suggestion that Ward, a prominent osteopath with additional income from art, had needed to supplement his income by living on immoral earnings. Hours later, the judge told the jury, 'The ball is in your court.'

The jury deliberated all afternoon, then trooped back with a long note for the judge. Marshall lectured them about prostitution and the problem of proving it. The jury wanted refreshment.

Marshall said they would have to pay for it themselves, 'to avoid any suspicion of favours'.

The jury came back with a verdict shortly after 7.00 p.m. It found Stephen Ward guilty on the first two counts, not guilty on any of the others.

The first two counts had concerned living on the immoral earnings of Christine Keeler and Mandy Rice-Davies. It was an extraordinary verdict. It may have been possible, using abstruse legal technicalities, to argue that Ward was guilty. This, though, was a travesty of natural justice – he was no pimp.

The judge postponed sentence until Ward might recover and be able to appear. Had he survived, he faced a possible seven years in prison. He did not survive.

At the hospital, a sample of Ward's blood told doctors what they already assumed – that he had taken an overdose of barbiturates. A pill bottle had been found at his side. Ward's friend Julie Gulliver knew he had been taking all sorts of pills, including sleeping tablets, during the trial, mostly Nembutal, the fashionable killer of the day. His old friend Dr Sugden – the abortionist – had written a prescription for the Nembutal. Even were Ward to be found not guilty as currently charged, the police had told him they might revive the charges alleging that he had introduced women to an abortionist.

Now Ward clung to life in Ward 3D, at St Stephen's Hospital, with a prison officer sitting nearby. Julie Gulliver, Pelham Pound and Ward's temporary host, Noel Howard-Jones, went to see him. One of his brothers, Raymond, sat at the bedside for a long time. Bunches of flowers were delivered. There was still hope.

Then the patient's condition began to deteriorate. A tracheotomy was performed – and heart massage attempted – but in vain. At 3.45 p.m. on 3 August, after seventy-nine hours in a coma,

Ward died. Outside Ward 3D, a nurse tapped the waiting prison officer on the shoulder.

'The horror, day after day at the court and in the streets,' Ward had written in one of his suicide notes. 'It's a wish not to let them get me. I'd rather get myself – I do hope I haven't let people down too much. I tried to do my stuff.'

The funeral took place a week later, in secret, at Mortlake Crematorium. Only his brother Raymond, his sister Patricia, two cousins, his solicitor and Julie Gulliver were present. A single wreath, with no card, lay on the paved courtyard of the crematorium.

Ward of all people would have been touched and amused to know that his death caused a fuss at Cheltenham Ladies' College, where a shocked headmistress wanted to know which of her charges had left a large wreath beside the town's war memorial. The accompanying note read: 'We three girls of Cheltenham Ladies' College have laid this wreath as a tribute to dear Dr Stephen Ward, who dared to live his life as a human being and not just as a dummy. An outraged society revenged itself upon him.'

Another huge wreath, made of hundreds of white roses, had been delivered to the undertakers who managed the funeral. It was sent by twenty-one writers and artists, including John Osborne, Kenneth Tynan, the singer Annie Ross and Penelope Gilliatt. Their note read: 'To Stephen Ward, a victim of British hypocrisy.'

In 1987, Lord Denning declined to be interviewed for a BBC documentary that raised the possibility that there had perhaps been a miscarriage of justice. 'I refused,' he said in the House of Lords, 'because over twenty-three years ago I heard all the evidence in that case in great detail.' This is not reflected in Lord Denning's Report, which devoted only two paragraphs to the trial for prostitution.

Lord Goodman, former legal adviser to Prime Minister Harold Wilson, was also – by a fine irony – lawyer to John Profumo. Unlike Denning, he did think there had been a miscarriage of justice. Ward's women, he says, 'plainly weren't prostitutes ... The conduct both of the judge and of the prosecution left much to be desired. It was an historic injustice.'

The Rich Wot Gets
The Pleasure ...

John Profumo died in 2006, aged ninety-one. He was predeceased by his wife, Valerie Hobson, in 1998. Much sympathy was expressed for him over the years, largely because of his work for Toynbee Hall, an East London centre for the flotsam of society, alcoholics, drug addicts and dropouts. He began this work, a 'totally voluntary three-day working week', soon after the scandal that bears his name. He had a London home, a place in the country and immense wealth – he remained deputy chairman of the Provident Life Association of London until its sale to a Swiss insurance company in 1982. 'The Profumos,' the *Daily Mail* City editor reported at the time of the takeover, 'should come out with something better than £6 million.'

Once a keen racegoer, Profumo was no longer seen at the tracks. He listed his hobbies as fishing and gardening, and his London club as Boodle's. His wife was active on behalf of Lepra, the organisation that aids victims of leprosy. She dreamed up the Ring Appeal, which prompted wealthy people, including members of the Royal Family, to hand over rings to raise money for Lepra. She wore round her neck a gold medallion that showed Profumo and herself in profile, very close, looking at each other. 'Jack made it for me,' she said.

Astonishingly, or perhaps not, the former War Minister was until 1975 a member of the Board of Visitors of Grendon Prison. That same year, in recognition of his work at Toynbee Hall, he was made a Commander of the British Empire. The CBE is awarded for public service. The Queen made a point of talking to Profumo when she opened a new home for social workers established by the Attlee Foundation, of which Profumo was a trustee.

Profumo did not talk about the events of 1963. 'Jack Profumo was so greatly hurt,' said his wife. 'My husband certainly got to know about spiritual things when he retired from public life.'

Of the Affair that bears his name, Profumo told a reporter in 1977: 'I have my own personal papers relating to those events. For many years now they have been locked in a bank vault, and that is where they will stay.' In 2006, however, his journalist son David authored a family memoir, *Bringing the House Down*, which relied on his father's papers, and on conversations with his father.

Yevgeny Ivanov, who died in January 1994 – reportedly as a result of his heavy drinking – was not reliably sighted for years after leaving England in 1963. 'I was told,' Ward's Czech friend Ilya Suschenek said at the height of the Affair, 'that Ivanov is dead. It is very sad.' Press reports later said variously that he was under house arrest in the Soviet Union, working in the Navy Ministry or in a mental hospital. Later again, he was reported to be suspended from the Communist Party, pending an inquiry into his role in the Profumo case. He was also reported in Egypt, on special assignment.

It was all hogwash. On his return to Moscow, his activities were exploited by the KGB. He would recall, however, that the GRU – in which he had served – was, following the exposure of

Penkovsky's spying for Britain and the US, 'in for a dark time'. Though he was made captain, 1st rank, there were to be no rewards. His affair with Christine Keeler ultimately displeased his masters, who felt it had wrecked Moscow Centre's operation against Profumo.

As reported in these pages, Ivanov's autobiography, *The Naked Spy*, ghostwritten by Russian journalist Gennady Sokolov, was published in 1992. The following year, after three decades, he and Christine Keeler met in Moscow for dinner. He later wrote to her, apologising for the way he had used her to try to obtain military secrets.

Harold Macmillan held on to office only until the autumn of 1963, when he resigned on the grounds of ill health. Privately, he felt that he had been hounded from government by members of his own party. He lived on until 1987.

The Prime Minister had been apprehensive, in the summer of 1963, as to what the Denning Report would reveal, and what the consequences might be for him. He did not wish, he wrote in his diary, to 'go down in history as a Prime Minister who had been destroyed by filth which had seeped up from the sewers of London.' He contemplated resigning on at least two and possibly three occasions.

One moment of great anxiety was when he received from Lord Denning a letter suggesting there were problems over allegations against two more of his ministers. As reported in these pages, there was Transport Minister Ernest Marples who – Denning said – 'had an association with a prostitute' and whose conduct was 'of such a nature as to constitute a security risk'. A junior minister at the Ministry of Science, Denzil Freeth, had 'participated in homosexual conduct'.

Three more of Macmillan's ministers offered to resign on

publication of the Denning Report, which said they and colleagues had failed in their duty when they had simply accepted – at their meeting with Profumo in the early hours – that he had not had sex with Christine Keeler. The Prime Minister, however, asked them to stay on.

The Report itself, meanwhile, proved to be something of a damp squib when it was published in September 1963. Public interest had moved on – there was now the Great Train Robbery to keep the newspapers busy. Nevertheless, the Affair had left the Conservative government and the personal standing of the Prime Minister damaged beyond repair.

Lord Astor died in 1966. At the height of the scandal, he had the face to show up at Ascot looking – as the William Hickey column reported – 'urbane and relaxed'. His Lordship toasted the winning jockey of the Gold Cup, Lester Piggott, in champagne, then drove to Cliveden for the party he gave every year during Ascot Week. Astor's widow painted a less rosy picture of her husband's life following the Affair. At her manor house in Surrey, surrounded by books on religion, she told the authors that the pressure of the Profumo case drove her husband to an early death. So far as she was concerned, she said, Stephen Ward had always been anathema to her.

Colin Coote, the editor of the *Daily Telegraph*, who introduced Ward to Ivanov, was knighted the following year. He died in 1979.

Keith Wagstaffe, the MI5 officer who handled Ward in 1961, retired to the south of England. He was prepared to be interviewed for this book, but was denied permission to do so by MI5. 'I'm sorry about this,' he wrote. 'But I am sure you will understand that in the circumstances I cannot agree to see you . . .' 'Yes, Ward might still be alive today,' said a former senior MI5 officer, when asked if his organisation could have helped the osteopath by owning up to how they had used him. 'We didn't expect the final outcome, and we were very cut up when we learned he was dead.'

Lord Denning died in 1999, weeks after his 100th birthday. He lived to the end in a splendid house in Hampshire, with a trout stream where Isaac Newton himself once fished. He left the Court of Appeal in 1982. Denning had urged in the 1960s that his dossier on the Profumo case be destroyed, and in 1977 claimed that the papers had indeed been jettisoned. The then Prime Minister James Callaghan, however, stated that the papers had in fact been placed in the Cabinet Office, where they remained closed until 1994.

Relevant Cabinet papers have been released to the National Archives at Kew, but many of the documents remain censored in full. Denning did allow Harold Macmillan's biographer, Richard Lamb, limited access to his private papers on the case. In an exchange about Denning's papers in the House of Lords in 2013, Lord Wallace stated that he had been told by officials that 'there are still some sensational personal items ... which would be embarrassing if released'.

In 2013, one of Denning's aides, Assistant Home Office Secretary Thomas Critchley, allowed the author and journalist Tom Mangold access to a journal he had kept during the inquiry. Critchley had described Stephen Ward as 'osteopath, artist, demon, socialite, pervert'. Yet he also thought him 'highly intelligent, anxious to please and be liked, extrovert, gay even now, with a streak of cruelty in his look and manner ... however, there was much about him that was appealing'.' In 1964 Critchley had told Ludovic Kennedy, 'I daresay we were a bit unfair to Ward.'

A Royal Commission in Tribunals of Enquiry reported in 1966

that 'Lord Denning's report was generally accepted by the public. But this was only because of Lord Denning's rare qualities and high reputation.'

Mervyn Griffith-Jones, who had been prosecuting counsel in the Ward trial, died in 1979. He wept, it is said, when told of Ward's death.

James Burge, the defence counsel, died in 1990. 'When Ward committed suicide,' Sir David Napley has written, 'Jimmy Burge was very affected. He never seemed to be the same man again . . . It was not long after this that he left the Bar and took up residence abroad.' Ironically, Burge is a holder of the Profumo Prize, the name given to a Bar scholarship set up ninety years ago by John Profumo's father.

John Lewis, the former Labour MP who did so much to bring about Ward's ruin, was delighted at the news of Ward's death. 'He was celebrating,' said Warwick Charlton. 'He made no bones about it.' He died of a heart attack in 1969, following the collapse of his business, leaving £63,000 in his will.

Ward always blamed Lewis for his ruin, according to *Daily Telegraph* journalist R. Barry O'Brien, who knew the osteopath. 'He said he was the author of all his misfortunes . . . He regarded Lewis as an evil man who had pursued him unjustly with malevolence . . .'

George Wigg, the Tory government's persecutor in Parliament during the scandal, became Postmaster-General in the Wilson government of 1964. He was made a life peer three years later, and became Chairman of the Horserace Betting Levy Board. In 1976, by then long out of the limelight, Wigg was charged with kerb-crawling near his London home. He had merely been trying to buy a newspaper, he said, and was found not guilty. Wigg died in 1983. His papers, which were given to the London School of Economics, are now at last open. Many security-related files, however, remain closed to researchers.

Christine Keeler is now seventy-one. Her life after the Affair was for a long time a trail of dole queues and broken marriages. She lived for a time at World's End in London, in one of the appalling council blocks there deemed suitable for the British working classes. Her flat had good views but little furniture. She has had two husbands, one a labourer, one a company director. She has two sons, who are estranged from her.

In 1984, the National Portrait Gallery paid £1,000 for a portrait of Keeler by Stephen Ward. In March 1987 she was arrested and fined for drunkenness and causing damage near her home.

When Stephen Ward died all those years ago, she has said, she had 'the worst attack of asthma . . . And I hated people, I went to buy a paper and I heard some people say, "He's dead, the old ponce." I was so furious that I wanted to kill them. I drove my car at them, but at the last minute I hooted and they jumped out of the way.' Ward, Keeler said, 'really was a gentleman.'

Asked whom, of the all the men she has known, she loved best, she replied, 'Oh, I loved Stephen. Always, I'm very loyal.' Keeler believed Ward was working for the Soviets, not MI5. As for Ivanov, she remembered him as 'a bit of a bore really, very serious, and Red . . .'

Profumo she thought 'a bit overpowering, not really exciting'. She did not think he had the right to live in peace after the scandal. 'He knew exactly what he was doing, even if I didn't,' she has said. 'I've never felt any remorse about what happened to him. I've had just as much trouble rebuilding my life.'

She has produced a number of accounts of her life. The latest, *Secrets and Lies*, published in 2012, was an updated version of her 2002 book, *The Truth at Last*.

'I regret it terribly,' she has said of her past. 'It's been a tough life, but it's something that could have happened to anybody, any good-looking girl.'

Her tragedy, perhaps, is that she can never be anybody *but* 'Christine Keeler'.

Mandy Rice-Davies is sixty-eight and – unlike Keeler – is the quintessential survivor. She lives with her third husband in Virginia Water, Surrey. Early in 2013, she was spotted dining with composer and impresario Lord Lloyd-Webber, discussing his forthcoming musical based on the life of Stephen Ward. After the Profumo Affair, she worked on the nightclub circuit, then went to Israel, where she married her first husband and opened a successful nightclub and restaurant business. She helped found Israel's first glossy magazine, then returned to England to appear in plays on television and in the West End. In 1986 she had a part in the film *Absolute Beginners*. Like Keeler, she has seen her autobiography published, and also novels.

She is extremely intelligent, and in control of her life. She saw herself, rightly, as just 'a bright, bubbly sidekick' to the events of 1963. The memory of Yevgeny Ivanov telling her, 'What you've got is more powerful than the atom bomb' made her giggle. She thought of herself as having been at best 'passably pretty'.

Rice-Davies told the authors she had little sympathy for rich politicians who fall because of their involvement with a woman. She did not understand why people sympathised, for example, with former Conservative Party Chairman Cecil Parkinson, who was brought down in the 1980s because of his affair, as a married man, with his secretary. 'Why,' Rice-Davies asked, 'is the secretary not important? Why is his career so important? Why is the woman always told to go away in a corner and shut up? . . . She's a victim. Like Christine and myself. Victims of hypocrisy and egotism.'

Rice-Davies said she thought the sort of people who suppressed the truth about the Profumo Affair still have a hold on power in Britain. 'That group still exists in the shadows,' she says. 'The people who pressed the buttons remain a shadowy group who inhabit the labyrinths of Whitehall. The sheer ego of it drives me crazy to this day.'

Mariella Novotny, the woman who claimed she was bedded by John Kennedy, and who wanted to be London's most celebrated hostess, died in 1983. She was forty-two, still living with her husband, Hod Dibben, who had been her co-host at the Feast of the Peacocks in 1961. Novotny took too many sleeping pills, got up in the night to fetch a bowl of jelly from the fridge, then toppled face down into the jelly. Death was due to inhalation of vomit and a drug overdose. Novotny's psychiatrist, Dr Joan Gomez, told the inquest that she had been suffering from a 'hysterical personality disorder'. Dr Gomez thought it unlikely that she was – as she claimed – involved in an operation designed to trap corrupt policemen. The psychiatrist was wrong. Novotny was a police informant, involved in the celebrated investigation of corrupt policeman, Operation Countryman. Research shows that, while Novotny embroidered the facts in later years, there was an element of truth to most of what she said.

Hod Dibben, Novotny's husband, died at the age of 85, shortly after the first edition of this book was published.

Suzy Chang, the other woman linked in the press to both the Profumo Affair and John Kennedy, was living quietly under a new name, in a grand house on the eastern seaboard of the United States, when last interviewed by the authors in 2006. For all the passing of the years, her beauty was still evident.

Julie Gulliver, the young woman who stood by Stephen Ward at the end, was pregnant when he died – she said by him. They had slept together just once. In October 1963, three months after Ward's death, she took an overdose of sleeping pills and lost the baby. She drifted through the so-called Swinging Sixties in a haze of drugs, then got married in 1972. The following year, after another drug overdose, she was found naked and dead on the floor of her home. She was given a pauper's funeral in the London Borough of Southwark.

While Ward was dying, Gulliver had told the press, 'I'll make sure it is not in vain. He is not going to die to let a whole lot of people get off scot-free. There is a whole crowd of them, right now, praying for Stephen to die so their names won't be mentioned. Stephen used to call them his friends. But in this crisis he found out who his friends really are.' Gulliver made a tape recording of her knowledge of the Affair, and was questioned by Lord Denning. Her name, however, did not appear in the Denning Report.

Yvonne Brooks, yet another girlfriend of Ward's, attempted suicide when she heard that Ward was dead. 'A very sweet girl,' Ward had called her. 'She knows more important men than I do. We've had a lot of fun together down at my cottage at Cliveden.' At the height of the Affair, Brooks went to Spain to stay with Lord Willoughby de Eresby, a cousin of Lord Astor and a godson of Sir Alec Douglas-Home, the Foreign Secretary at the time of the Affair. Brooks survived the 1963 suicide attempt, which was her second. After Lord Willoughby disappeared on a boat trip in the Mediterranean, she moved to Rome, where she lived on the borderline between prostitution and the high life. In 1964, while staying at London's Hilton Hotel, she called the switchboard operator and asked not to be disturbed. She was later found dead, having downed numerous sleeping pills and most of a bottle of gin.

Ronna Riccardo, the prostitute whom the police pressured into giving false testimony against Stephen Ward, is said still to be alive. She bore three children, by different fathers. She became dramatically overweight, and – by her own admission – remained 'on the game', on a part-time basis. She said, and FBI documents confirm, that she went to the United States in the wake of the Profumo Affair to marry her American airman lover 'Silky' Hawkins. 'I was desperate to leave England,' she said, 'because I was still under a lot of pressure from the police.' Riccardo did not stay in the States for long. She left in early 1964, says the 'Bowtie' dossier, on advice that 'her departure would be best for all concerned'.

'In Washington,' Riccardo said, 'I was dragged into the offices of the CIA, and they said they knew all about me, from the cops in England.'

In the early days of MI5's honeytrap operation, she said, she too was taken down to Cliveden by Stephen Ward. 'Astor gave us the free run of the place,' she told the authors. The purpose, she believed, was to involve her in plans to compromise Soviet attaché Ivanov. She claimed, 'Christine never went to bed with him. She used to lie about posing, and looking lovely, but she never went to bed with him. But he was really innocent – he'd never seen anything like it. That was the way they wanted to get someone like him involved. They wanted to blackmail Ivanov. My role in the set-up was to look after Ivanov – a minder, I suppose. Stephen got involved before he knew what was happening.

When he realised what was happening, he was too far in to get out . . .'

Vickie Barrett, who testified against Ward, retracted her evidence and then retracted her retraction, proved impossible to trace.

Frances Brown, the prostitute, did not live long after testifying that she had been involved in a sex act with Ward and the artist Vasco Lazzolo. In November 1964, Brown's decomposing corpse was found on wasteland in Kensington, apparently strangled. On her forearm was the tattoo 'Helen', over a design of red flowers and green leaves, and the legend 'Mum and Dad'. A dustbin lid had been placed over her face. She was reportedly the seventh victim in the series of killings between 1959 and 1964 known as the 'Jack the Stripper' murders, in which eight prostitutes died.

The woman believed to have been the third victim in the Stripper murders, Hannah Tailford, had reportedly been one of the women supplied for orgies organised by Prince Philip's cousin the Marquess of Milford Haven. Tailford allegedly featured in 8mm pornographic films. Her memories of life as a prostitute included the experience of being purchased by a young man in a Rolls-Royce near the Embankment for £25, a pricey sum in 1960. She was driven to a luxurious apartment and told to wait nude in a darkened bedroom for the client. When he arrived, she felt a strange furry outline, then the light went on and the room filled with laughing people. The man was dressed as a gorilla, and Hannah Tailford was left to find her way out of the house in tears.

In February 1964, her corpse was found on the mud beside the Thames at Hammersmith, naked except for a pair of stockings.

Police investigating the Stripper murders questioned Christine Keeler. Commander John du Rose, who headed the inquiry, said,

'Every person connected with the Stephen Ward scandal was traced and questioned by the police, but all enquiries proved fruitless.'

The Metropolitan Police file on the case, which had become available by 2006, is a catalogue of broken lives, mental illness, abortions, unwanted pregnancies, venereal disease, drug addiction, downmarket prostitution, pimping and violence towards women.

So ends this shabby history of corruption and death – and the survival of the richest.

A Final Mystery – The Last Hours of Stephen Ward

The Establishment roared its disapproval when this book was first published. Seven public figures, all former holders of high office in politics, business and the law, three of them old Etonians and all but two products of Oxford and Cambridge, joined in a letter to *The Times*.

Lords Hailsham, Carrington, Goodman, Weinstock, Prior and Jenkins and the Earl of Drogheda held forth as follows:

> Sir,
>   The undersigned have noted the current publicity . . . and feel it is a good time to place on record their sense of admiration for the dignity and courage displayed by Mr and Mrs Profumo.
> This letter also records our feeling that it is now appropriate to consign the episode to history.

Here was the British Establishment calling for three cheers for 'poor Jack', the Minister whose folly had triggered the scandal in the first place. The oddest voice in the chorus was that of Profumo's own legal adviser, Lord Goodman. It was only weeks since he had characterised the conduct of the judge at the Ward trial as having 'rivalled Judge Jeffreys' and called the trial 'an historic injustice'.

Stephen Ward should be rescued from history, not consigned to it.

Information that came in following the first publication of this book made the end of the Profumo case – and of Ward's life – look even murkier. It may suggest that British intelligence perpetrated further skulduggery – and even that Ward's death was not a simply case of suicide.

It certainly looked straightforward at the time. The inquest jury was shown a glass vial that had contained sleeping pills, which had been found near Dr Ward's body empty but for 'three or four' tablets. The autopsy pathologist, Dr Donald Teare, told the inquest that death had followed softening of the brain as a result of barbiturate poisoning. He said the softening was 'due to the deprivation of oxygen for three or four minutes'.

The autopsy indicated that Ward's system had contained the barbiturate equivalent of fourteen to twenty 1.5 grain sleeping tablets. Dr Teare said 'twenty grains would be dangerous and thirty very dangerous'. The medical evidence aside, there were the notes Ward left behind, twelve in all, the last – though unsigned – clearly a suicide note.* There were also the attempted suicides – if they had not been just cries for help – in the distant past. And there was the testimony of the people who were believed to have been the last to see Ward – including his host that night, and a respected reporter with whom the osteopath had discussed killing himself.

---

* See second photo section.

The inquest verdict was that Ward's death was caused by barbiturate poisoning, self-administered, that he had committed suicide. The coroner's jury would, however, have been thrown into confusion had it heard the information that follows.

First there is the account of a late-night meeting between Ward and Bryan Wharton, a well-known Fleet Street photographer who long worked on the *Sunday Times*. In 1963, he covered the Profumo case for the *Daily Express*.

Late on the night of Ward's apparent suicide, Wharton told the authors, his picture desk instructed him to go to meet Ward, who had telephoned the paper – apparently following his earlier meeting with *Express* reporter Tom Mangold. The rendezvous was at Ward's own flat in Bryanston Mews, not at the Mallord Steet address where Ward was currently staying and where Mangold had seen him that evening.

Wharton said he hurried to the address, and arrived about 11.30 p.m. Ward was there, accompanied by another man 'dressed in a topcoat with a velvet collar'. Wharton thought the second man was Noel Howard-Jones, Ward's host at Mallord Street. Howard-Jones declined to give the authors a comment for quotation on Ward's last hours.

'It was clear,' said Wharton, 'that Ward was under a tremendous amount of pressure. He felt that he had been let down. I photographed him at the table. He was writing a letter to Henry Brooke, the Home Secretary. It contained a lot of names, though I don't recall whose they were. I didn't read it all – it was about three pages long. I took various shots, various angles, so that it could be seen that it was Ward who was writing. I took great care to get it right.

'Ward was extremely upset,' Wharton said, 'and was insistent that I should meet him the next morning. He wanted me to go with him to the Home Office to deliver the letter. He kept on about me being there at 7.30 a.m., so as to be at the Home Office before going to Court.'

Wharton left Ward some time after midnight, believing he had a scoop on his hands, and headed for the offices of the *Express*. 'I processed the films,' he said, 'and hung them up. I was going to wrap up the story the next day.' He did not get home until the early hours of the morning, and arrived somewhat late to accompany Ward to the Home Office – only to learn that Ward had been taken to hospital in a coma.

At the *Express*, according to Wharton, he found that his scoop pictures had vanished. They were never found. He came to believe that British intelligence had had a hand in their disappearance. 'The *Express* in those days,' he asserted, 'was close to MI5, and "5" had people in the office. The paper also had close contact with a number of policemen.'

Mangold, the reporter who had been with Ward at Mallord Street earlier in the evening, told the authors he learned nothing of Wharton's experience at the *Express* office the following day. One might doubt there was anything to Wharton's account – were it not that the known time frame does have a gap during which Ward's movements are unknown, a period that fits Wharton's recollection.

When Ward dropped his girlfriend Julie Gulliver at her Bayswater home at about 11.30 p.m., he drove straight off again – destination unclear. 'He had told me,' Noel Howard-Jones said at the inquest, 'he would go for a drive after he had run Miss Gulliver home.' Where Ward's 'drive' took him remains unknown, but Howard-Jones testified that it was not until 'about one o'clock' that he heard someone – he assumed it was Ward – enter the flat.

There is other evidence that, the alleged letter to the Home Secretary aside, Ward was frantically trying to reach people in authority. Sometime that last evening he got through to Tom

Critchley, a Home Office bureaucrat working with Lord Denning on the official investigation. Critchley declined to comment to the authors on that conversation.

There is no reference to the Critchley call in the Denning Report, and it was not mentioned at the Ward inquest. Nor were journalists Mangold or Wharton heard at the inquest, though their evidence and Critchley's would have been very pertinent to any assessment of Ward's state of mind during his final hours.

Did something occur that night to push Ward over the edge, to contribute towards his death? And was *Express* photographer Wharton the only other person Ward saw during his final frantic hours?

The entertainer Michael Bentine, who was close to Ward for many years, told the authors that – for all the evidence pointing to a simple case of suicide – he did not believe Ward died by his own hand. Bentine, a former Air Force intelligence officer who said he kept up his contacts after the war, quoted a police source. 'A Special Branch friend of mine,' he said, 'told me Ward was "assisted" in his dying. I think he was murdered.' Bentine declined to be drawn further.

Following publication of the first edition of this book, the authors received information suggesting that Ward was indeed helped on his way to death, or murdered. Because – then – it appeared to fly in the face of the facts, we did not initially publish the material. Here it is now, for readers to evaluate in the context of all the other information.

Earlier in these pages, the authors reported their interviews with Lee Tracey, a former MI6 operative who told how – under journalistic cover – he handled Ward as a potential MI6 asset. The operative's information on other matters that over time proved reliable to colleagues in national journalism and at the BBC.

'It was decided that Ward had to die,' Tracey told the authors. 'The man who was with Ward, when he took those tablets, worked for MI5. This agent told me what happened . . . He admitted that Ward was killed on the instructions of his department. He convinced Ward that he ought to have a good night's sleep and take some sleeping pills. The agent said he let Ward doze off and then woke him again and told him to take his tablets. Another half an hour later or so, he woke Ward again, and told him he'd forgotten to take his sleeping pills. So it went on until Ward had overdosed.

'It might sound far-fetched,' Tracey said, 'but it's the easiest thing in the world to do. Once the victim is drowsy he will agree to almost anything . . .' Just fantasy? Doctors specialising in suicide prevention say many apparent suicides are really victims of confusion, people who return again and again to the pill bottle, not realising they have taken more than the safe dosage. Ward at the end of his trial, though a qualified doctor, may have been a prime candidate for such confusion. Behind the dark glasses there were red-rimmed eyes, the result of too little sleep and too many pills.

'He was strung out,' said his friend Pelham Pound. 'During the trial he was taking all sorts of pills, bombers or uppers mostly.' Is it possible that – rather than meaning to go through with his talk about suicide – Ward simply miscalculated? Or could it really be that he was persuaded into the overdose by some dark emissary of an intelligence organisation?

Former MI6 operative Tracey named the man who – he claimed – deliberately caused Ward's death. 'Stanley Rytter is the one who killed Ward,' he said, 'I know because he told me. I don't quite know how he managed it. I wasn't there. But Rytter was with Ward the night he died, and Rytter told me he was paid to kill Ward. He was paid by our mob.'

Rytter? Our mob?

Stanley Rytter, born in Poland in 1927, joined the small flood of his contemporaries who settled in England after the war. This was the man who, as reported earlier, had apparently at one stage taken over Warwick Charlton's assignment of handling Ward for MI6. Like fellow operatives Charlton and Tracey, he made his overt living as a journalist – largely as a press photographer. He specialised in 'glamour shots', the kind of slightly risqué pictures that were in those days the stock-in-trade of some Sunday newspapers.

Rytter, who – Tracey said – worked for Polish intelligence before coming to Britain, had been an associate of another Polish émigré, property racketeer Peter Rachman. He managed Rachman's 150 Club in the Earls Court Road, lost money gambling there and was bailed out by Rachman.

Ward, as reported earlier, had also known Rachman. According to Serge Paplinski, another of Rachman's Polish associates, Ward and the racketeer were for a time in the mid-1950s partners in the Paintbox, a London coffee bar. Like its successor, the Brush and Palette, it featured a small dais on which a nude girl used to pose – as a service for artistic customers who might wish to draw her. It was there that Ward first met Noel Howard-Jones, then an impoverished law student moonlighting as a wine waiter, one day to be Ward's host on his last night alive.

British intelligence was interested in Rachman's shadowy world, in his émigré friends. The book *Spycatcher*, by MI5's Peter Wright, provided details on how MI5's D Branch, charged with counter-espionage, ran Russian, Czech and Polish exiles as agents. They were easy to recruit, and – in the case of those already run by the KGB – had potential as double agents.

MI6's Tracey said it was Rachman who first pointed Ward in the direction of the Security Service, MI5. A Polish businessman, Angus Labunski, who knew Rytter well, said he received funds from mysterious sources. In the course of research, among Polish exiles and in Poland itself, it emerged that Rytter was remembered for his occasional involvement with British intelligence. He was apparently an operative for hire, who answered to whichever organisation contracted him. On occasion MI6, although – one Pole said – his principal link was to MI5.

'Rytter,' Tracey said, 'had been trying to sell his services to us [MI6]. But he was more likely to succeed in selling his services to MI5. He was a useful person to infiltrate the Russian and Polish émigrés here . . .'

The name 'Rytter' had cropped up at Ward's trial, in an ominous context that has never been explained. It came up in questioning, very briefly, and was forgotten until we obtained transcripts for the first time. Prosecuting counsel Griffith-Jones asked Ward about an affidavit by the prostitute Ronna Riccardo, in which she admitted having given false evidence against the osteopath. Rytter's name appeared in her affidavit.

Ward had referred during his trial to a letter he had written, a letter that mentioned Rytter, in which he claimed 'false things were being piled up against me . . . intentional false evidence'. The letter, Ward said, also named a man called Marshall, who had allegedly been asked by Rytter to 'find a girl willing to swear an affidavit that I had employed her'. A few sentences later, Ward said Rytter had later explained the 'story' to his satisfaction. This odd exchange hung there in the trial transcript, incomplete and mysterious.

MI6's Tracey said he first learned of Rytter's involvement in Ward's death from the man himself, years afterwards. Rytter turned up at his home, 'extremely nervous, apprehensive and sweating', and gave him a sealed package. 'He had written the whole story in Polish, and sealed it with sealing wax, and gave it to me to hold for him.'

In 1980, according to Tracey, Rytter came to reclaim the package. He died, following a stroke, in 1984 – in the same hospital as had Stephen Ward. His daughter Yvonne told the authors she threw away all his papers without reading them. She did recall, though, that her father took her to wait outside St Stephen's Hospital when Ward was dying. 'Someone came to us and said, "That's it. He's dead," she recalled, 'then we drove away . . .'

Yvonne Rytter suggested the authors consult Bill Lang, the film producer who had given Ward refuge at his Hertfordshire home just before his arrest. Lang, she said, had been close to her father. Asked about Rytter, Lang requested time to think it over. Then he responded: 'I don't want to get involved. I have absolutely no statement to make. I'm going to leave things as they are. Stanley [Rytter] would have wanted that. I don't want to be rude, but I'm saying nothing at all.'

Rytter's fellow Pole Serge Paplinski was more forthcoming. He said, 'Stanley was there with Ward on the last night . . . he always said that Ward was poisoned.' Paplinski also thought Rytter was linked to British intelligence.

There the Rytter trail ends, as does the allegation that Ward was 'assisted' in his dying. Except for an even more dramatic allegation, by a key player in the Profumo case, Ward's friend Paul Mann. Mann, the dead man's bridge partner, a visitor to Cliveden and a negotiator with Ward's lawyer during legal efforts to prevent the scandal from breaking, went on to become a businessman in the Midlands. During the Profumo scandal, Mann told the authors, he was repeatedly approached by members of the security services trying to keep tabs on what was going on.

Shortly after Ward's death, Mann told the authors, he was told that 'Ward was injected with an air bubble, by hypodermic, with the intention of causing a fatal embolism. The needle broke, and the assassins left in a hurry. It was enough, though, to send the drugged Ward on his way. It was a botched affair.'

Mann claimed he learned this from the individual who committed the crime, who said he did it in the company of another person. Mann would not divulge the alleged killer's name to us, but said – this was in 1988, when further official action seemed not impossible – he would do so to a properly constituted official inquiry.

What would the motive have been? According to Lee Tracey, Ward remained a threat to the Macmillan government, the British Royal Family and to British intelligence. Specifically, there were sex photographs that could damage both the government and the Royal Family.

As revealed in these pages, Ward had entrusted compromising photographs – including one or some supposedly featuring Prince Philip – to his friend Warwick Charlton, of Odhams Press, who also took on assignments for MI6. The photographs were eventually seized by the police – never to be seen again – although according to Ivanov copies of some reached the KGB in Moscow.

Did Ward have more evidence to reveal, more secrets to tell? The flat at Bryanston Mews, where Ward allegedly met *Express* photographer Wharton before the fatal overdose, was where he had first stashed the photographs given to Charlton – and some jewels linked to Peter Rachman, which were found hidden in the ceiling. Did Ward have something else secreted there, something he could have produced in court following a guilty verdict?

MI5 certainly did have an intense interest in Ward's actions and statements. His phone calls were bugged, and there were probably microphones in his various flats. Did someone in British intelligence, on learning what Ward had said in his conversations, decide that he should be silenced?

Lee Tracey of MI6 said Ward had 'started to make veiled threats, asking for money . . . and generally making himself a nuisance to the security services. The Establishment's view has always been to take a tough line against such people – squash them! Ward thought that because of what he knew, and the pictures in his possession, he was indispensable. He was wrong.'

Fifty years on, it would be naïve to expect any further, open, government inquiry into this case. Whether Ward was murdered or not, though, the information in this chapter – had it been known at the time – would have demanded an airing in the coroner's court. There is no statute of limitations on murder.

Stephen Ward not only lost his life. As the consequence of an unjust trial he also lost what Shakespeare's Othello called the 'immortal part' of himself, his reputation. As with Othello, 'what remains is bestial', and that suited the Establishment just fine.

Acknowledgments

Before listing those who did help during the writing of this book, we prefer to note the names of those principal players who were not helpful: John Profumo, Lord Denning, Lord Wilson of Rievaulx, and Lord Home of the Hirsel. Profumo did not answer our letter.

Generous with their time, however, were the Hon. David Astor and the 4th Earl of Dudley. We thank Mandy Rice-Davies, who cheerfully disinterred her youth; Mariella Novotny's husband Hod Dibben; and Christine Keeler's sometime lover Johnny Edgecombe. Ronna Ricardo, the prostitute who had the guts to retract her false testimony in 1963, bravely spoke with us – for the first time since then. Stephen Ward's friends Warwick Charlton, Jon Pertwee and Dr Ellis Stungo gave very generously of their time. So did Robert Harbinson, better known as the travel writer Robin Bryans.

Of those who reported the scandal in 1963, we appreciated the help of Peter Earle, then chief crime reporter of the *News of the World*, Trevor Kempson of the *News of the World*, Roy East, then chief crime reporter of *The People*, Tom Mangold, then with the *Daily Express*, later to go on to become a star reporter for *Panorama*, Brian McConnell of the *Daily Mirror*, Barry O'Brien of the *Daily Telegraph*, Alastair and Sheila Revie, then freelance journalists, and Tom Tullett, who then headed the *Daily Mirror* crime bureau. We are grateful to the late Ludovic Kennedy for permission to quote from his book *The Trial of Stephen Ward*.

Interviewees and correspondents included: former Police

Commissioner Sir Ranulph Bacon; Michael Bentine; Paul Boggis-Rolfe; Derek Brook; John Broxholme; Mrs David Bruce; James Burge; Mrs Derek Cooper; Thomas Corbally (through his lawyer); Glen Costin; John Cummings (of the CID Officers' Association); Dr Eric Dingwall; Alfred Donati; John Doxat; Michael Eddowes; Walter Elder; Courtney Evans; David Floyd; Nina Gadd; Logan Gourlay; John Grigg; Lord Harrington; Brian Innes; Mandy Kearney; Lord Kennet; Angus Labunski; David Lewis; Paul Mann; former CIA Director John McCone; Dr William McClurg; Bobby McKew; Michael Mordaunt-Smith; Frederic Mullally; Sir Godfrey Nicholson; Clive Nicol; former Detective Inspector Thomas O'Shea; Serge Paplinski; Michael Pertwee; Chapman Pincher; Pelham and Philip Pound; the Right Hon. Enoch Powell; Jocelyn Proby; 'Victoria Regine' (the pseudonym of a source on London sexual activity); Max Robertson; Archibald Roosevelt (former CIA Station Chief, US embassy); Gerhards Seedorff of the Black Star Picture Agency; Harry Stevens; Donald Stewart (former FBI supervisor); prostitute 'Sue'; Sir Edmund Tompkins; Harry Alan Towers; Andrew Tully; Mike Wallington; and Nigel West.

We thank those members of the intelligence services, British and American, who helped but cannot be named here.

Of the institutions consulted, we thank especially the Huddersfield Public Library. Also the British Library, the Canadian High Commission information service, the British Newspaper Library at Colindale, the *Daily Telegraph* Information Service, the actors' union Equity, Kensington and Chelsea Library, Eddie Pedda, the *TV Times* Picture Department, *Queen* magazine, the staffs of St Catherine's House and Somerset House, *Spotlight* magazine, *Stage*, Torquay Central Library, and the Virginia Historical Society. In the United States, the FBI's Freedom of Information staff were very helpful.

Of those who made major contributions to the project we

thank especially Claire Powell, who left a job on the *Wolverhampton Express & Star* to work with us, and Gay Watson, who had worked with Summers at the BBC in the sixties. Powell found herself trawling some of London's sleaziest backwaters in pursuit of the prostitutes and pimps of 1963 – and found some of them still busy more than twenty years later. She proved to be not only a true gumshoe but also a fine reporter – she is now in a senior position at the BBC. Watson made many things elementary – even when her house burned down.

We are indebted to Anthony Frewin, a personal assistant in the film industry, and to Dick Brewis, an academic, who in the 1970s began their own citizens' inquiry into the Profumo Affair. Frewin has swapped information with us over a thirty-year period. Fred Vermorel has also been a mine of information. In recent years, filmmaker Harvey Lilley has been steadily supportive and helped with research. In Russia, journalist Gennady Sokolov, who continues to research the Soviet aspects of the case, has been a valued contact. In the United States, we thank Lori Winchester of WCJ Inc., which provides investigative and protection services worldwide. Robert Fink, a Washington investigative journalist with long experience of research in the labyrinth of US government agencies, conducted vital interviews.

Crucial to the project, too, were Palace Pictures, producers of the television series *Scandal*. At Palace, Joe Boyd opened up difficult research roads.

The editor of the first hardback edition, Victoria Petrie-Hay of Weidenfeld & Nicolson, brought skill and energy to the project. We thank, too, Rose Scott, Yvonne Holland and Tomás Graves, who discovered obscure pictures. At Coronet, Peter Strauss and Anna Benn helped us to become enthusiastic all over again at paperback time.

For having confidence in the revival of the book in 2013, we thank Jane Friedman and Pete Beatty of Open Road Media in New York and Headline publisher Simon Thorogood in London. Jonathan Lloyd, chairman of Curtis Brown Ltd, agented with his usual skill and wise advice.

Stephen Dorril thanks above all his wife Stephanie, not least for her help and infinite patience as a small house overflowed with research materials. His mother was a mine of information on ancient scandals, and Marilyn Webb typed. The work of that speedy and accurate typist Ritchie Finney was invaluable when – this year – we needed an electronic version.

Anthony Summers thanks his friends Fanny Dubes, the late Paul Sutton, Kathy Castle and Cecily O'Toole, who – the first time around – helped more than they knew. Above all, though, he thanks his wife and indispensable colleague Robbyn Swan, who proofread this new edition and made perceptive suggestions. Last but by no means least he thanks his long-suffering children Colm, Fionn and Lara, who put up with their father revising the book during their annual summer holiday.

A.S.
S.D.
August 2013

Photo Credits

The photographs are reproduced by permission of the following: Mirrorpix: 1 (*above*), 3 (*above*), 8 (*above*); Topfoto: 1 (*below*); Getty Images: 3 (*below*), 4, 8 (*below*); Camera Press London: 1 (*below right*), 3 (*below right*); Antony McCallum, WyrdLight Photography: 2 (*above*); Illustrated London News Ltd/Mary Evans: 5; FBI: 6; Courtesy of Lee Tracey: 7 (*top*).

Sources

The following source notes are intended for the general reader and not so much for the scholar. While every fact has been meticulously sourced, these notes are not a catalogue of each small point but more a guide to let readers know what our major sources were and who was interviewed or contacted in person. At their request, some sources in intelligence have not been named. We have not specified citations from newspaper coverage.

Interviewees

Bridget Astor
Lady Bronwen Astor
David Astor
Charles Bates
Michael Bentine
Paul Boggis-Rolfe
Clive Bossom
James Burge
Connie Capes
Suzy Chang
Warwick Charlton
Thomas Corbally (through lawyer)
Glen Costin
Robin Dalton
Horace Hod Dibben
Dr Eric Dingwall
Alfred Donati

John Doxat
Lord Dudley
Peter Earle
Roy East
Michael Eddowes
John Edgecombe
Walter Elder
Courtney Evans
David Floyd
Nina Gadd
D. Goulding
Logan Gourlay
John Grigg
Robert Harbinson
William Hitchcock IV
Trevor Kempson
Angus Labunski
Vasco Lazzolo
David Lewis
Nicholas Luard
John Lyle
Tom Mangold
Paul Mann
Jeanne Martin
Dr W. M. McClurg
John McCone
Brian McConnell
Bobby McKew
Arnold Miller
Michael Mordaunt-Smith
Frederic Mullally
R. Barry O'Brien
Thomas O'Shea
Serge Paplinski

Jon Pertwee
Michael Pertwee
Barbara Pistalo
Pelham Pound
Philip Pound
Jocelyn Proby
Alastair and Sheila Revie
Ronna Riccardo
Mandy Rice-Davies
Max Robertson
Archibald Roosevelt
Yvonne Rytter
William Shepherd
Gennady Sokolov
Harry Stevens
Donald Stewart
Dr Ellis Stungo
Bill Sykes
Sir Edward Tomkins
Felix Topolski
Harry Alan Towers
Lee Tracey
Andrew Tully
Alfred Wells
Bryan Wharton
Roger Whipp
Matt White

Correspondents

William Burdett
Thomas Critchley
Douglas Fairbanks Jr
Brian Freemantle

Tommy Friend
Drs Harvey and E. N. Coomes
Noel Howard-Jones
Bill Lang
Keith Wagstaffe

Principal Documentary Sources

The Denning Report, Cmmd 2152, HMSO, September 1963

'Notes for an Autobiography,' by Dr Stephen Ward [compiled from mid-May 1963, some of it on tape, some typewritten in prison]

Stephen Ward's Officer's Record of Service, supplied by Ministry of Defence

Stephen Ward trial transcripts, as released February 1987 to authors by Lord Chancellor's Office

Unpublished handwritten manuscript by Mariella Novotny [supplied to authors by Hod Dibben]

Stephen Ward Inquest, report by Anthony Frewin

Vasco Lazzolo, outline for planned autobiography

FBI files, series 31–88538

FBI ('Bowtie' file) 65–68218. In addition to the main file released in 1986, the authors obtained further material in 2010.

John Lewis file, supplied by Labour Party Headquarters

Unpublished Robin Drury interview

Hansard (daily record of the House of Commons)

Ambassador David Bruce journals, Virginia Historical Society, by permission of Mrs Bruce

Suzy Chang, Immigration & Naturalization documents, INS A 1372612

'The KGB's Spy at the Palace,' by Jason Lewis and Kim Willsher, *Mail on Sunday*, 20/2/2000 and see 24/7/2010

Burke's Peerage and Debrett's

The Times obituaries, 1945–2013

Bibliography

Allason, Rupert (Nigel West), *The Branch: A History of the Metropolitan Police Special Branch, 1883–1983* (Secker & Warburg, 1983)

Andrew, Christopher, *The Defence of the Realm: The Authorized History of MI5* (Allen Lane, 2010)

Astor, Michael, *Tribal Feeling* (John Murray, 1963)

Baker, Bobby, *Wheeling and Dealing: Confessions of a Capitol Hill Operator* (W. W. Norton, 1978)

Baron, *Baron* (Frederick Muller, 1956)

Barron, John, *The Secret Work of Soviet Agents* (Corgi, 1975)

Barron, John, *KGB Today: The Hidden Hand* (Coronet, 1985)

Bartok, Eva, *Worth Waiting For* (Putnam, 1959)

Bayliss, John, *Anglo-American Defence Relations 1939–84* (Macmillan, 1984)

Bentine, Michael, *The Long Banana Skin* (Wolfe, 1975)

Bentine, Michael, *The Door Marked Summer* (Granada, 1981)

Birmingham, Stephen, *Jacqueline Bouvier Kennedy Onassis* (Fontana, 1979)

Booker, Christopher, *The Neophiliacs: A Study of the Revolution in English Life in the Fifties and Sixties* (Collins, 1969)

Boothroyd, Basil, *Philip: An Informal Biography* (Longman, 1971)

Bower, Tom, *The Perfect English Spy: Sir Dick White and the Secret War 1935–90* (Mandarin, 1996)

Bradlee, Ben, *Conversations with Kennedy* (Quartet, 1976)

Cate, Curtis, *The Ides of August: The Berlin Crisis of 1961* (Weidenfeld & Nicolson, 1978)

Catterall, Peter (ed.), *The Macmillan Diaries, Vol. 11: Prime Minister and After, 1957–1966* (Macmillan, 2011)

Cecil, Lord David, *The Young Melbourne* (World Books, 1955)

Chalfont, Alun, *The Shadow of My Hand* (Weidenfeld & Nicolson, 2000)

Charlton, Warwick, *Stephen Ward Speaks* (special paperback, *Today*, Odhams Press, 1963)

Churchill, Sarah, *Keep on Dancing* (Weidenfeld & Nicolson, 1981)

Clutterbuck, David, with Devine, Marion, *Clore, The Man and His Millions* (Weidenfeld & Nicolson, 1987)

Collis, Maurice, *Nancy Astor: An Informal Biography* (Faber & Faber, 1960)

Collis, Maurice, *The Journey: Reminiscences 1944–68* (Faber & Faber, 1970)

Connell, Jon, and Sutherland, Douglas, *Fraud: The Amazing Career of Dr Savundra* (Hodder & Stoughton, 1978)

Coote, Colin, *Editorial: The Memoirs of Colin Coote* (Eyre & Spottiswoode, 1965)

Coote, Colin, *The Other Club* (Sidgwick & Jackson, 1971)

Cowles, Virginia, *The Astors* (Weidenfeld & Nicolson, 1979)

Craig, Mary, *Longford: A Biographical Portrait* (Hodder & Stoughton, 1978)

Crawford, Iain, *The Profumo Affair* (White Lodge Books, 1963)

Croft-Brooke, Rupert, *The Dogs of Peace* (W. H. Allen, 1973)

Davenport-Hines, Rupert, *An English Affair: Sex, Class and Power in the Age of Profumo* (HarperPress, 2013)

Davis, John H. *The Kennedy Clan* (NEL, 1985)

De Feu, Paul, *Let's Hear It for the Long-Legged Woman* (Angus & Robertson, 1975)

Dempster, Nigel, *HRH The Princess Margaret: A Life Unfinished* (Quartet, 1981)

Denning, Lord, *The Due Process of Law* (Butterworths, 1980)

Detzer, David, *The Brink: The Cuban Missile Crisis of 1962* (J. M. Dent, 1980)

Dickie, John, *The Uncommon Commoner: A Study of Sir Alex Douglas-Home* (Pall Mall, 1984)

Dors, Diana, *Behind Closed Doors* (Star, 1979)

Dunleavy, Stephen and Brennan, Peter, *Those Wild, Wild Kennedy Boys* (Pinnacle, 1981)

Du Rose, John, *Murder is My Business* (W. H. Allen, 1971)

Egremont, Lord, *Wyndham and Children First* (Macmillan, 1968)

Eddowes, Michael, *November 22nd: How They Killed Kennedy* (Neville Spearman, 1976)

Eddowes, Michael, *The Oswald File* (Clarkson N. Potter, 1977)

Evans, Harold, *Downing Street Diary: The Macmillan Years 1957–63* (Hodder & Stoughton)

Freemantle, Brian, *The Fix* (Corgi, 1986)

Frischauer, Willi, *Margaret: Princess without a Cause* (Michael Joseph, 1977)

Fryer, Peter, *Private Case, Public Scandal* (Secker & Warburg, 1966)

Gelb, Norman, *The Berlin Wall* (Michael Joseph, 1986)

Glenton, Robert, and King, Stella, *Once Upon a Time: The Story of Antony Armstrong-Jones* (Anthony Blond, 1960)

Gordon, Charles, *The Two Tycoons* (Hamish Hamilton, 1986)

Gosling, John, and Warner, Douglas, *The Shame of the City: An Enquiry into the Vice of London* (W. H. Allen, 1960)

Gould, Tony, *Inside Outside: The Life and Times of Colin MacInnes* (Penguin, 1986)

Graham, Philip, and Fisher, Heather, *Consort: The Life and Times of Prince Philip* (W. H. Allen, 1980)

Grantley, Lord, *Silver Spoon* (Hutchinson, 1954)

Green, Shirley, *Rachman* (Hamlyn Paperback, 1981)

Grigg, John, *Nancy Astor: Portrait of a Pioneer* (Sidgwick & Jackson, 1980)

Grimes, Sandra & Vertefeuille, Jeanne, *Circle of Treason* (Naval Institute Press, 2012)

Hamblett, Charles, and Deverson, Jane, *Generation X* (Tandem, 1964)

Hancock, Robert (Douglas Howell), *Ruth Ellis: The Last Woman to be Hanged* (Weidenfeld & Nicolson, 1985)

Harrison, Rosina, *Rose: My Life in Service* (Cassell, 1975)

Hersch, Burton, *The Mellon Family: A Fortune in History* (William Morrow, 1978)

Hopkins, Harry, *The New Look: A Social History of the Forties and Fifties in Britain* (Readers Union, Secker & Warburg, 1964)

Horan, James, *The Right Image* (Crown Publishers, 1967)

Howard, Anthony, and West, Richard, *The Making of the Prime Minister* (Jonathan Cape, 1965)

Humphry, Derek, and Tindall, David, *False Messiah: The Story of Michael X* (Hart Davies, McGibbon, 1977)

Hutchinson, George, *The Last Edwardian at No. 10: An Impression of Harold Macmillan* (Quartet, 1980)

Irving, Clive, Hall, Ron, and Wallington, Jeremy, *Scandal '63: A Study of the Profumo Affair* (Heinemann, 1963)

Israel, Lee, *Killgallen* (Dell Publishing, 1980)

Ivanov, Yevgeny, *The Naked Spy* (Blake, 1992)

Jackson, Stanley, *The Old Bailey* (W. H. Allen, 1978)

Jakubait, Muriel, *Ruth Ellis: My Sister's Secret Life* (Constable & Robinson, 2005)

Judd, Dennis, *Prince Philip: A Biography* (Michael Joseph, 1980)

Kaufman, William, *The McNamara Strategy* (Harper & Row, 1964)

Kavaler, Lucy, *The Astors: A Family Chronicle* (George G. Harrap, 1966)

Kearney, Patrick J., *The Private Case* (Jay Landesman, 1981)

Keeler, Christine, and Meadley, George, *Sex Scandals* (Xanadu, 1985)

Keeler, Christine, with Fawkes, Sandy, *Nothing But . . .* (New English Library, 1983)

Keeler, Christine, *Secrets and Lies* (John Blake, 2012)

Kelleher, Catherine, *Germany and the Politics of Nuclear Weapons* (Columbia University Press, 1975)

Kennedy, Ludovic, *The Trial of Stephen Ward* (Gollancz, 1964)

Knightley, Phillip & Kennedy, Caroline, *An Affair of State: The Profumo Case & the Framing of Stephen Ward* (Jonathan Cape, 1987)

Knightley, Phillip, *The Second Oldest Profession: The Spy as Bureaucrat, Patriot, Fantasist and Whore* (André Deutsch, 1986)

Lamb, Richard, *The Macmillan Years, 1957–1963: The Emerging Truth* (John Murray, 1985)

Lambert, Derek, *Just Like the Blitz* (Hamish Hamilton, 1987)

Lane, Peter, *Prince Philip* (Robert Hale, 1980)

Langhorne, Elizabeth, *Nancy Astor and Her Friends* (Arthur Barker, 1974)

Leaman, G., *The Horn Book* (University Books, 1964)

Lee, Carol Ann, *A Fine Day for a Hanging: The Real Ruth Ellis Story* (Mainstream, 2012)

Levin, Bernard, *The Pendulum Years: Britain and the Sixties* (Jonathan Cape, 1970)

Lewis, David, *Sexpionage: The Exploitation of Sex by Soviet Intelligence* (H. Hanau, 1976)

Lucas, Norman, *Britain's Gangland* (Pan, 1969)

McConnell, Brian, *Found Naked and Dead* (New English Library, 1974)

Macmillan, Harold, *Pointing the Way* (Macmillan, 1972)

Macmillan, Harold, *At the End of the Day* (Macmillan, 1973)

Malone, Peter, *The British Nuclear Deterrent* (Croom Helm, 1984)

Mander, John, *Berlin, Hostage for the West* (Penguin, 1962)

Margaret, Duchess of Argyll, *Forget Not* (W. H. Allen, 1975)

Martin, Ralph G., *A Hero for Our Time: An Intimate Story of the Kennedy Years* (Macmillan, 1983)

Masters, Anthony, *Nancy Astor: A Life* (Weidenfeld & Nicholson, 1981)

Minney, R. J., *The Biography of the Hon. Anthony Asquith, Aristocrat, Aesthete, Prime Minister's Son and Brilliant Film Maker* (Leslie Frewin, 1973)

Morgan, Janet (ed.), *The Backbench Diaries of Richard Crossman* (Hamish Hamilton and Jonathan Cape, 1981)

Morrison, Majbritt, *Jungle West 11* (Tandem, 1964)

Mure, David, *The Last Temptation* (Buchan & Enright, 1984)

Napley, David, *Not Without Prejudice* (Harrap, 1982)

Nicol, Jean, *Meet Me at the Savoy* (Museum Press, 1952)

Nunnerley, David, *President Kennedy and Britain* (Bodley Head, 1972)

O'Donnell, Kenneth, and Powers, David F. with McCarthy, Joe, *Johnny, We Hardly Knew Ye: Memoirs of John F. Kennedy* (Little, Brown, 1972)

Parmet, Herbert S., *JFK: The Presidency of John F. Kennedy* (Penguin, 1984)

Penrose, Barry, and Freeman, Simon, *Conspiracy of Silence: The Secret Life of Anthony Blunt* (Grafton Books, 1986)

Pertwee, Michael, *Name Dropping* (Leslie Frewin, 1974)

Pincher, Chapman, *Treachery: Betrayals, Blunders & Cover-ups: Decades of Espionage Against American and Great Britain* (Random House, 2009)

Playfair, Giles, *Six Studies in Hypocrisy* (Secker & Warburg, 1969)

Power, James, *Against Oblivion* (Fontana, 1981)

Powers, Robert, *The Man Who Kept the Secrets: Richard Helms and the CIA* (Weidenfeld & Nicolson, 1979)

Profumo, David, *Bringing the House Down: A Family Memoir* (John Murray, 2006)

Rice-Davies, Mandy, with Flack, Shirley, *Mandy* (Sphere, 1980)

Rice-Davies, Mandy, *The Mandy Report* (Confidential Publications, 1964)

Roth, Andrew, *Sir Harold Wilson: Yorkshire Walter Mitty* (Macdonald & Janes, 1977)

Salinger, Pierre, *With Kennedy* (Garden City, 1972)

Sampson, Anthony, *Anatomy of Britain* (Hodder & Stoughton, 1963)

Schlesinger, Arthur, *A Thousand Days: John F. Kennedy in the White House* (Mayflower Dell, 1967)

Seabrook, David, *Jack of Jumps* (Granta, 2006)

Sinclair, David, *The Astors and Their Times* (J. M. Dent, 1983)

Slater, Frank, *Getting a Likeness* (Seeley Service, 1952)

Smith, Jean Edward, *The Defence of Berlin* (Oxford University Press, 1963)

Sorenson, Theodore C., *Kennedy* (Harper & Row, 1965)

Sullivan, William C., *The Bureau: My Thirty Years in Hoover's FBI* (Norton, 1979)

Summers, Anthony, *Goddess: The Secret Lives of Marilyn Monroe* (Open Road, 2012)

Sykes, Christopher, *Nancy: The Life of Lady Astor* (Granada, 1979)

Tangye, Derek, *When the Wind Blows* (Michael Joseph, 1980)

Thompson, Douglas, *The Hustlers: Gambling, Greed & the Perfect Con* (Pan, 2007)

Thorpe, D. R., *Supermac: The Life of Harold Macmillan* (Chatto & Windus, 2010)

Thurlow, David, *Profumo: The Hate Factor* (Robert Hale, 1992)

Tully, Andrew, *White Tie and Dagger* (William Morrow, 1967)

Ungar, Sandford J., *FBI* (Atlantic Monthly Press, 1976)

Van den Bergh, Tony, and Marks, Laurence, *Ruth Ellis: A Case of Diminished Responsibility* (Macdonald & Janes, 1977)

West, Nigel, *A Matter of Trust: MI5 1945–72* (Weidenfeld & Nicholson, 1982)

West, Rebecca, *The Meaning of Treason* (Penguin, 1965)

Wigg, Lord, *George Wigg* (Michael Joseph, 1972)

Williams, Charles, *Harold Macmillan* (Phoenix, 2009)

Wills, Gary, *The Kennedys: A Shattered Illusion* (Orbis Publishing, 1983)

Winn, Godfrey, *The Positive Hour* (Michael Joseph, 1970)

Wright, William, *The Von Bülow Affair* (Arlington Books, 1983)

Wyatt, Woodrow, *Confessions of an Optimist* (Collins, 1985)

Wynne, Greville, *The Man from Odessa* (Granada, 1983)

Wynne, Greville, *Wynne and Penkovsky (The Man from Moscow)* (Corgi, 1985)

Young, Kenneth, *Sir Alec Douglas-Home* (J. M. Dent, 1970)

Young, Wayland, *The Profumo Affair: Aspects of Conservatism* (Penguin, 1963)

Ziegler, Philip, *Mountbatten* (Collins, 1985)

Index